Calcium Signalling in the Nervous System

Calcium Signalling in the Nervous System

P.G. KOSTYUK AND A.N. VERKHRATSKY

Bogomoletz Institute of Physiology, Academy of Sciences of the Ukraine, Kiev, Ukraine

JOHN WILEY & SONS

Chichester · New York · Brisbane · Toronto · Singapore

Copyright © 1995 by John Wiley & Sons Ltd,
Baffins Lane, Chichester,
West Sussex PO19 1UD, England

Telephone: National   01243 779777
             International   (+44) 1243 779777

Other Wiley Editorial Offices

John Wiley & Sons, Inc., 605 Third Avenue,
New York, NY 10158-0012, USA

Jacaranda Wiley Ltd, 33 Park Road, Milton,
Queensland 4064, Australia

John Wiley & Sons (Canada) Ltd, 22 Worcester Road,
Rexdale, Ontario M9W 1L1, Canada

John Wiley & Sons (SEA) Pte Ltd, 37 Jalan Pemimpin #05-04,
Block B, Union Industrial Building, Singapore 2057

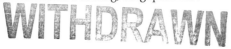

British Library Cataloguing in Publication Data

A catalogue record for this book is available from the British Library

ISBN 0 471 95941 3

Typeset in 10/12 Palatino by Vision Typesetting, Manchester, UK
Printed and bound in Great Britain by Bookcraft Ltd, Bath, Avon

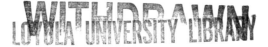

Contents

Preface

For many years the Bogomoletz Institute of Physiology of the Ukrainian Academy of Sciences in Kiev has been known as a distinguished research centre in cellular physiology. This research line was started by the late professor Daniel Woronzov, a famous pupil of Wedensky, who created the Department of General Physiology at the Institute and attracted many talented young scientists; in a few decades the Department became dominant in the scientific activity of the Institute. Investigations have been extended to all aspects of cellular and molecular physiology, and the Institute has become internationally recognized.

Despite the economic difficulties which science is facing in the newborn states after the disintegration of the USSR, the Bogomoletz Institute still continues most active research in its traditional fields. This became possible due to a large extent to international collaboration and valuable support from the world scientific community. Here we would like to extend our appreciation for the help provided by the Physiological Society of the UK, the German Physiological Society, the US Neuroscience Association, the US Physiological Society, the Sandoz Gerontological Foundation, the International Soros Foundation, the European INTAS Foundation, the Wellcome Trust Foundation and Bayer AG (Leverkusen). We are grateful personally to the scientists involved in the organization of this international support for our Institute; in particular to Prof. W. Almers (Germany), Prof. A.C. Dolphin (UK), Prof. D. Eisner (UK), Prof. B. Hille (USA), Prof. G. Isenberg (Germany), Dr M. Kano (Japan), Prof. H. Kettenmann (Germany), Dr F. Kirchhoff (Germany), Prof. M. Klee (Germany), Prof. A. Konnerth (Germany), Prof. M.T. Miras-Portugal (Spain), Prof. E. Neher (Germany), Prof. M. Nowycky (USA), Prof. O. Petersen (UK), Prof. B. Sakmann (Germany), Dr F. Seuter (Germany), Prof. A.D. Smith (UK), Prof. L. Tauc (France), Prof. J. Traber (Germany) and Prof. S. Wray (UK).

We are also grateful to all members of the scientific team of the Bogomoletz Institute of Physiology who participated greatly in our experiments, which became the basis for the present book. We are grateful to Prof. O. Krishtal, Prof. N. Veselovsky, Dr P. Belan, Dr O. Garaschuk, Dr O. Gerasimenko, Dr S. Fedulova, Dr A. Fomina, Dr S. Kirischuk, Dr E. Lukyuanetz, Dr O. Lyuabnova, Dr A. Martynyuk, Dr N. Pronchuk, Dr A. Shmigol, Dr Ya. Shuba; Dr A. Tarasenko, Dr A. Tepikin, Dr Yu. Usachev and Dr N. Voitenko. We also greatly appreciate the excellent technical assistance provided by Mrs L. Grigorovitch, Mrs E. Kovaleva; Mrs L. Vikhreva and Mr R. Nagorny.

Kiev, 1995

Introduction

The idea that calcium plays a special role in the maintenance of the basic functional properties of living matter was expressed almost a century ago. As had been noticed in the pioneering observations of Ringer (1873) and Loeb (1906), a definite relation between monovalent (sodium) and divalent (calcium) elements in the external medium is necessary for the execution of active cellular reactions. If this ratio is too high (at the expense of calcium), contraction becomes impossible; on the other hand, they are depressed also if calcium is excessive.

The way to an understanding of the mechanisms of this crucial role of Ca^{2+} ions has been long and complicated. Obviously, the simplest way of thinking was to assume that they exert their effects from outside—for instance by preferential binding to the cell surface. This action really takes place, and its intimate features are still a matter for detailed analysis. However, several pioneering observations made clear that penetration of Ca^{2+} ions into the cell by specific pathways may be of crucial importance for cellular activity. Among them we have to quote the findings by Fatt and Katz (1953) that the action potential in crayfish muscle can be evoked in a sodium-free solution and depends on influx of calcium (as well as other divalent cations) into the fibre; the observation of Hagiwara's group (Hagiwara and Naka, 1964; Hagiwara and Nakajima, 1966) that this process is substantially enhanced when calcium buffers are introduced inside the fibre, elevating the transmembrane gradient for Ca^{2+} ions; the findings by Coraboeuf and Otsuka (1956) that in cardiac muscle the long-lasting plateau of the action potential depends on extracellular Ca^{2+} and is necessary for triggering contraction, and similar findings for smooth muscle by Hollman (1958); finally the classic experiments by Katz and Miledi (1967a, 1967b) demonstrating that synaptic transmission is crucially dependent on influx of Ca^{2+} into the presynaptic terminal.

An important step in the clarification of the mechanisms of calcium influx was made by the development of a technique for reliable separation of calcium transmembrane currents (I_{Ca}) from other types of membrane permeabilities. This has been achieved by the perfusion (or dialysis) technique based on the finding that soluble ingredients in the cytosol can be removed from the cell if a constant microhole is made in the membrane, and replaced by other substances (Kostyuk et al., 1975). The immediate advantage of the application of this technique was the washout of potassium ions from the cellular interior, with the subsequent possibility of measuring inward transmembrane currents in a pure form. A parallel elimination of sodium from outside revealed the net Ca^{2+} currents. This technique has been successfully applied to a huge variety of cells and soon enabled a detailed description of the properties of calcium current pathways. An important advantage of this was that large intracellular molecules remained in the cytosol and continued to exert their action, which could be important for maintenance of normal channel activity.

The next important step was the development of the patch-clamp technique (Hamill *et al.*, 1981), which combined intracellular perfusion with low-noise current measurements and for the first time opened the way to recording the activity of single ion-conducting membrane channels, including Ca^{2+} channels. A parallel investigation of ionic currents at the macro' and micro' levels became the dominant technique in modern cellular physiology.

This technical success, however, posed the next question: what happens to Ca^{2+} ions when they enter the cell? Obviously, their fate might be completely different from that in aqueous extracellular medium. Thus a search for a way to estimate directly the status of ions in the cytosol became inevitable. Initial attempts to measure free Ca^{2+} concentration in the living cytoplasm were made in the late 1920s, using the calcium-sensitive dye alizarin (Pollack, 1928). The first effective step in this respect was the use of the calcium-binding protein aequorin, which emits light after binding Ca^{2+} ions (Shimomura *et al.*, 1962). Later came the light-absorbing dye arsenazo III. Finally, the most effective fluorescent indicators, constructed on the basis of Ca^{2+} chelators, were proposed (Grynkiewicz *et al.*, 1985). The important point was that these substances could be specially modified in a way to penetrate freely the cellular membrane, and they become impermeable following de-esterification by intracellular enzymes. Glass calcium-selective microelectrodes filled with highly specific ion exchangers have also been manufactured (Corey *et al.*, 1980). All these techniques clearly indicated that after entering the cell Ca^{2+} ions are subjected to a powerful influence from intracellular processes. These obviously include a very effective buffering, as the resting level of intracellular calcium has been shown to be almost four orders lower than in the extracellular medium. Furthermore, capacious intracellular compartments greedy for Ca^{2+} ions and equipped with effective mechanisms for Ca^{2+} uptake and storage were detected. Finally, Ca^{2+} ions immediately meet mechanisms trying to expel them back to the extracellular medium (Ca^{2+} pumps and ion exchangers). Competition between all these mechanisms changes the characteristics of the injected bulk of Ca^{2+} ions and creates a new quality which might be called the 'calcium signal', and which in fact is the main messenger for coupling the events on the cell surface with the intracellular machinery. In parallel, a whole family of other intracellular messenger systems has been detected during recent years, like cyclic nucleotides and phosphoinositides (Greengard, 1978; Berridge, 1993), produced by a complex cascade of enzymatic reactions. Some components of these cascades have been shown to exert their own messenger effects (such as GTP-binding proteins). Surprisingly, practically all of these systems have been shown to involve intracellular calcium in their function. In fact, they form a completely integrated polyfunctional machinery capable of coordinating all aspects of cell life.

It is impossible to give an overview of all aspects of this system; hundreds of specialized reviews dealing with the intimate mechanisms of intracellular calcium signalling have been published in recent decades. However, most of them were devoted to calcium signalling in muscle and secretory cells. The function of these systems in neural elements, although being the subject of thousands of experimental works, has not been generalized yet to the same extent. In the present book we shall try to give an up-to-date account of the most fundamental aspects of calcium signal generation in the nervous system, including pathways for Ca^{2+} influx, buffering in the cytosol, involvement of intracellular calcium stores and Ca^{2+} extrusion. At the same time, the most important aspects of the interaction of Ca^{2+} ions with other messenger systems, the functional meaning of Ca^{2+} ions, as well as pharmacological tools for their dissection and modulation, will also be overviewed.

1 Ca²⁺ Influx Through the Plasmalemma

VOLTAGE-GATED Ca^{2+} CHANNELS

FUNCTIONAL DIVERSITY

Calcium-selective voltage-operated ion channels form a main pathway for transmembrane calcium currents (I_{Ca}). A comprehensive analysis of the function of these channels became possible after the elaboration of special techniques allowing the recording of I_{Ca} separately from other types of transmembrane currents (I_{Na}, I_K). The intracellular perfusion (or dialysis) approach (Kostyuk et al., 1975; Kostyuk and Krishtal, 1977a) was especially helpful in this respect. Quite soon it became obvious that calcium channels, contrary to previously analysed sodium channels, are not homogeneous in their properties and actually form a whole family of different channels.

The presence of two main subtypes of Ca^{2+} channels was first detected in our laboratory when analysing the current–voltage characteristics of I_{Ca} in dorsal root ganglion (DRG) neurones: this current could be clearly separated into low-voltage and high-voltage activated (LVA and HVA) components (Veselovsky and Fedulova, 1983; see Fig. 1.1). Contrary to already known HVA currents, the LVA current could be activated at very negative membrane potentials (between -60 and -40 mV) and rapidly inactivated in a potential-dependent way. Separation of Ca^{2+} channels into these two main groups according to their potential dependence has been confirmed in several subsequent papers (Carbone and Lux, 1984; Fedulova et al., 1985; Nowycky et al., 1985). The existence of both groups of channels has been demonstrated in a large variety of excitable cells, including retinal ganglion cells (Karschin and Lipton, 1989), pituitary melanotrophic cells (Keja et al., 1991) and many others, including cells from invertebrates.

Concerning their functional properties, LVA channels seemed to form a quite homogeneous group. However, recently in some neurones a component in the corresponding I_{Ca} has been observed with different kinetics: somewhat slower activation and extremely slow inactivation with an almost potential-independent rate constant (thalamic reticular neurones—Huguenard and Prince, 1992; DRG neurones—Kobrinsky et al., 1994). Very slowly-inactivating LVA I_{Ca} were observed also in *Xenopus* oocytes injected with mRNA from the thalamic complex (see below).

The situation with HVA channels is much more complex. Nowycky et al. (1985) separated the corresponding component of I_{Ca} into an inactivating and a steady component and denoted them as N and L currents. These symbols together with symbol T for the LVA current are now widely used in the literature. The three types of calcium channels have been distinguished in mouse and rat DRG (Kostyuk et al.,

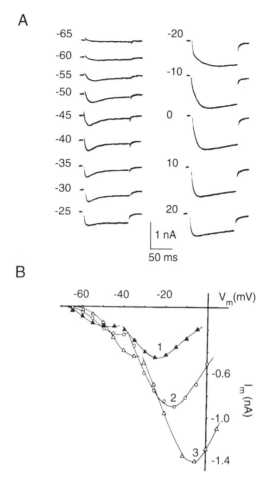

Figure 1.1. Separation of low- and high-voltage activated Ca^{2+} currents in rat dorsal root ganglion neurone recorded at a holding potential of -90 mV (from Veselovsky and Fedulova, 1983, reproduced by permission of Plenum Press, New York). (A) Examples of current recordings. (B) Current–voltage characteristics at $[Ca^{2+}]_o$ 2 mM (1), 5.4 mM (2), 14.8 mM (3). Intracellular perfusion with 150 mM Tris-PO_4

1988a) and dorsal horn (Ryu and Randic, 1990) sensory neurones, rat or guinea-pig granule (Blaxter *et al.*, 1989) and pyramidal (Fisher *et al.*, 1990; Mogul and Fox, 1991; Takahashi *et al.*, 1991) hippocampal neurones, clonal endocrine cells (Biagi and Enyeart, 1991) etc. The situation seemed to be more or less clear and convenient for functional analysis. However, when other methods for differentiation of Ca^{2+} channels became popular, they rapidly prompted the conclusion that the present classification is too simple and that Ca^{2+} channels are much more diverse. The recognition of this fact coincided with a rapid increase in the list of cellular functions triggered or modulated by the influx of Ca^{2+} through calcium channels. Therefore the question concerning the diversity of Ca^{2+} channels and their functional implications is still under consideration.

BASIC FUNCTIONAL PROPERTIES

Permeation

The conductance of Ca^{2+} channels is one of their most fundamental properties, and its measurement seems to correspond well to their separation into three basic types. The statistics of such separation are highly significant in DRG neurones; in 60 mM Ba^{2+} (as a charge carrier) their mean unitary conductance is 7.2 pS for LVA, and 11.4 and 18.4 pS for HVA channels (Kostyuk et al., 1988a; see Fig. 1.2). In isotonic Ba^{2+} solutions hippocampal neurones yielded corresponding values of 8, 14 and 25 pS (Fisher et al., 1990);the value for LVA channels in retinoblastoma cells was about 7 pS (Barnes and Haynes, 1992). In pancreatic β cells, channels with a unitary conductance of 6.4 and 21.8 pS (Sala and Matteson, 1990) and in rat pituitary melanotrophic cells of 8.1 and 24.7 pS (Keja and Kits, 1994) were found. Three mean values of unitary conductances for Ca^{2+} channels were demonstrated in chromaffin cells (Artalejo et al., 1991a) and even in brain membranes of *Drosophila* (Pelzer et al., 1989). Recently a channel with very low unitary conductance (5 pS) has been shown in chromaffin cells and designated a 'G-channel' (Cena et al., 1991), but it may belong to receptor-operated channels. Channels with such low conductance (about 5.6 pS) were recorded in inside-out patches from cerebellar Purkinje neurones; it has been shown that they can be activated from the cytosolic side by inositol trisphosphate (Kuno et al., 1994).

A possible source of error should be kept in mind during such measurements: the property of some channels to pass into a subconducting state, showing only a fraction of the total conductance. This property is prominent for inactivating HVA channels in DRG neurones, in which about 10% of the total number of channel openings showed a conductance attaining an intermediate level of 5.7 pS (Shuba and Savchenko, 1987). An example of such activity is shown in Fig. 1.3. Transitions from the state of partial conductance to either a completely non-conducting state or to a state of maximal conductance were possible. In clonal pituitary cells transitions to at least five subconductance levels were observed (Kunze and Ritchie, 1990). Thus, in some cases additional criteria should be used to verify the principal type of channel conductance.

Despite these differences in unitary conductance, all Ca^{2+} channels seem to share a common molecular mechanism allowing them to select effectively divalent cations. It is now widely accepted that this mechanism is based on the binding of penetrating ions in the channel. Model simulation of the energy profile may predict two separate binding sites (Kostyuk et al., 1982; Rosenberg and Chen, 1991) or a single site (Lux et al., 1990; Armstrong and Neyton, 1991) in the channel; the energy 'well' here should be about 5 E/RT units. The suggestion about two closely located binding sites has been used to explain the high rate of penetration of Ca^{2+} ions through the channel: it has been proposed that mutual repulsion of two bound ions is important here (Kuo and Hess, 1993a). Do these sites (or site) differ in different types of Ca^{2+} channels? It is well known that HVA channels pass Ba^{2+} better than Ca^{2+} (Kostyuk et al., 1982 and others); the situation is opposite in LVA channels (Fedulova et al., 1985; Carbone and Lux, 1987; Fox et al., 1987; Akaike et al., 1989; Takahashi et al., 1991). This difference may indicate that binding sites in HVA and LVA channels are actually different in structure; however, one cannot exclude that different effects of Ba^{2+} and Ca^{2+} on the gating mechanism of the channels could also be involved (see below).

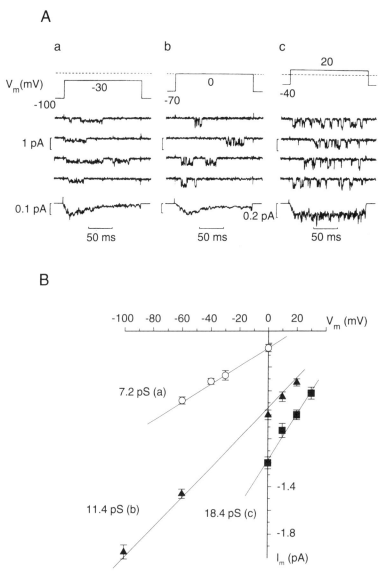

Figure 1.2. Activity of single Ca^{2+} channels in mouse dorsal root ganglion neurones (from Kostyuk *et al.*, 1988a with permission from Springer-Verlag). (A) Three types of single-channel currents recorded by whole-cell patch technique at holding and testing potentials indicated in the pulse protocol; lower traces show the averages of corresponding current records: (a) LVA, (b) HVA inactivating and (c) HVA non-inactivating channels. (B) Current–voltage relations for the same types of channels; mean unitary conductance is indicated near each curve

The binding sites in Ca^{2+} channels are responsible for the well-known blocking effect of Co^{2+}, Ni^{2+}, Cd^{2+}, La^{3+} and some other cations on I_{Ca}. This block is obviously due to more effective binding of these ions, preventing their own permeation through the channel. Analysis of single channel activity indicates that the blocking ion may

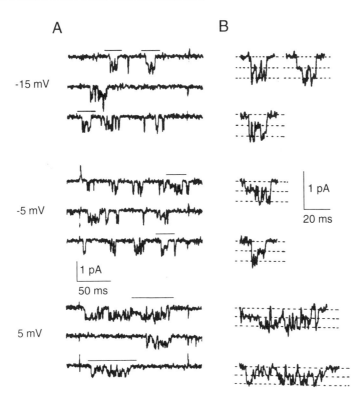

Figure 1.3. Two subconductance states of a single Ca^{2+} channel (from Shuba and Savchenko, 1987). Bursts of channel openings in (B) are taken from parts of records in (A) marked by continuous lines. Test potentials are indicated near each group of records

enter and leave the pore so that the channel starts to fluctuate between fully open and shut states, entry rates being insensitive to membrane potential and the exit rates increasing with membrane hyperpolarization (Lansman, 1990). Smaller ions enter the channel more slowly (dehydrate more slowly?) and bind more tightly. Protonation of the site ($pK_H = 5.8$) may also depress the permeation of HVA Ca^{2+} channels (Kostyuk *et al.*, 1982; Kuo and Hess, 1993b); similar effects have been shown recently on LVA channels (Tytgat *et al.*, 1990). Again, some differences in the blocking effect of alien cations may distinguish different types of channels: LVA channels in DRG neurones are more sensitive to Cd^{2+} (Nowycky *et al.*, 1985), while LVA channels in hypothalamic neurones to La^{3+} (Akaike *et al.*, 1989) as compared with HVA channels. Ni^{2+} and all trivalent metal cations are also effective blockers of LVA channels (Mlinar and Enyeart, 1993). An interesting feature is the inhibition of HVA Ca^{2+} channels from inside by Mg^{2+} ions in concentrations above 0.5 mM, which has been shown on cultured rat cerebellar granule neurones (Pearson and Dolphin, 1993); this has been confirmed also on phaeochromocytoma cells and explained on the basis of already mentioned mutual repulsion of ions inside the channel: between Mg^{2+} ions such repulsion is much weaker compared with Ca^{2+} ions (Kuo and Hess, 1993c).

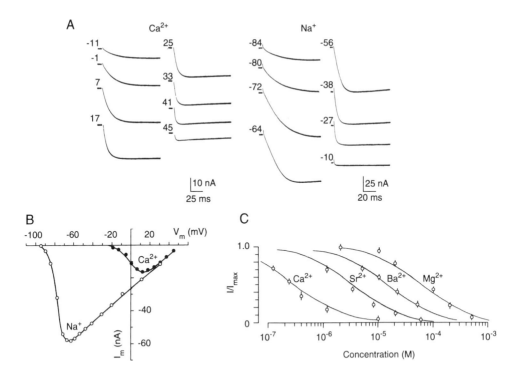

Figure 1.4. Transformation of HVA Ca^{2+} channels into the Na^+-conducting mode in snail neurones (from Kostyuk *et al.*, 1983 with permission from Springer-Verlag). (A) Recordings of currents obtained in Na^+-free solution containing 30 mM $CaCl_2$ and Ca^{2+}-free EDTA-containing solution with 30 mM NaCl. (B) Corresponding current–voltage characteristics. (C) Dose–effect dependences for the blocking effect of different divalent cations on the induced Na^+ current through Ca^{2+} channels

The most striking feature of this mechanism is the immediate loss of selectivity upon removal of divalent cations from the extracellular medium (Kostyuk and Krishtal, 1977b). The described transformation occurs in all types of Ca^{2+} channels studied *in situ* as well as in those transplanted into lipid bilayers (Rosenberg and Chen, 1991), and the affinity of the selectivity-supporting action of external cations is extremely high. K_D values for Ca^{2+}, Sr^{2+}, Ba^{2+} and Mg^{2+} were 0.2, 3.5, 14 and 60 μM, respectively (Kostyuk *et al.*, 1983; see Fig. 1.4). This may indicate that another high-affinity binding site is present in the channel molecule which is normally occupied by a divalent cation. When the latter is taken away, a conformational change occurs which modifies completely the energy profile of the channel and transforms it into a sodium-permeable mode (Kostyuk and Mironov, 1986; for a more extensive model see Mironov, 1992). The presence of substantial conformational changes in the channel molecule is obvious from other changes in channel function, for instance in its pharmacological sensitivity (Carbone and Lux, 1988; Davies and Lux, 1989). Although we suggested in the beginning that this site is located near the external mouth of the channel, it now looks more probable that it is inside the channel (Lux *et al.*, 1990; Kuo and Hess, 1993a) but easily accessible for external ions. A large-diameter external mouth of the Ca^{2+} channel has been suggested, so that diffusion does not limit currents even at low concentrations of divalent cations in the external medium (Kuo and Hess, 1992). It has been shown earlier that lowering of extracellular pH may also trigger a sodium inward current (Krishtal and Pidoplichko, 1981). This current was suggested to pass through Ca^{2+} channels transformed into a sodium-conducting mode by protonation of their high-affinity binding sites (Konnerth et al., 1987; Davies et al., 1988). However, detailed measurements of the blocking effect of divalent cations on the proton-induced I_{Na} gave values different from those characteristic of the transformation of genuine Ca^{2+} channels (Akaike et al., 1990).

Gating

Potential-dependent gating is the next basic property of all calcium channels, which seems to be quite similar in nature to gating in previously studied sodium channels. It operates by displacement of some charged components in the channel molecule, opening or closing the way for permeation. This displacement ('gating current') can be visualized by recording of the asymmetric intramembrane charge displacement triggered by membrane potential shifts normally activating Ca^{2+} channels (Kostyuk et al., 1977, 1981). Their separation from similar events happening in Na^+ channels can be achieved by intracellular introduction of fluoride, which selectively blocks the function of Ca^{2+} channels. The kinetic characteristics and potential dependence of these currents fit well to the activation kinetics of I_{Ca} (see examples in Fig. 1.5); however, the amount of displaced asymmetric charges seems to be much higher than expected from the amount of opened channels (see also Bean and Rios, 1989). This may indicate that the displacement of gating charges is a necessary but not sufficient step in channel opening; channels may remain in a 'pre-opened' state.

The simplest kinetic model which can reconcile these and some other features of Ca^{2+} channel gating can be as follows:

$$R \underset{\beta}{\overset{2\alpha}{\Leftrightarrow}} C \underset{2\beta}{\overset{\alpha}{\Leftrightarrow}} A \underset{b}{\overset{a}{\Leftrightarrow}} O$$

where C and A represent two 'pre-open' states with potential-dependent transition rates α and β between them, and O the final open state reached by fast transitions a and b with less potential dependence (Kostyuk et al., 1988b). The assumption of two 'pre-open' states comes from the fact that activation kinetics of I_{Ca} in most cases can be best described by taking a square power for the m variable, indicating that two gating particles should be displaced simultaneously in order to make the channel ready for opening (Kostyuk et al., 1979; Byerly and Hagiwara, 1982; Kay and Wong, 1987 and others). Two different closed and one open states were suggested also for LVA Ca^{2+} channels (Chen and Hess, 1990).

A mathematical formalism has been elaborated in our laboratory for calculation of all constants of this model using different characteristics of single channel activity (Shuba and Teslenko, 1987); the results were compared for the three types of Ca^{2+} channels (Kostyuk et al., 1988b). The analysis has shown that gating in all types of Ca^{2+} channels can be adequately described by this model. At the same time, there are some differences between them. The mean open time of HVA channels (determined by

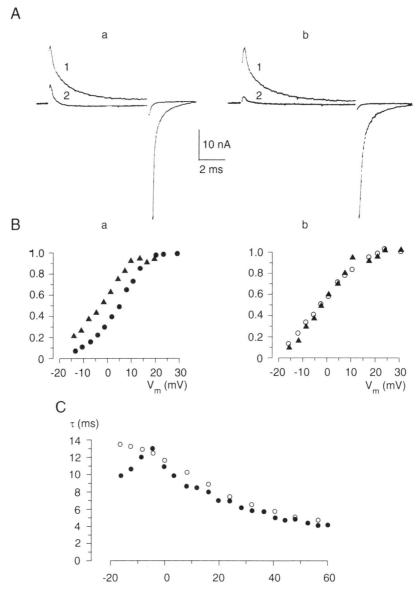

Figure 1.5. 'Gating currents' of HVA Ca^{2+} channels in snail neurones (from Kostyuk *et al.*, 1981; reproduced by permission of The Physiological Society) (A) Asymmetric charge displacements before (1) and after (2) introduction of fluoride into the cell; holding potential −90 mV (a) and −40 mV (b). Difference between 1 and 2 represents the 'gating current' of Ca^{2+} channels. (B) Voltage dependence of asymmetric charge displacement (triangle) and Ca^{2+} conductance (open circle) normalized; in (b) the square root of conductance is presented. (C) voltage dependence of the rate constants of Ca^{2+} currents activation (open circle) and on- asymmetric charge displacement (solid circle)

transition processes a, b) is found to be completely potential-independent, whereas for LVA channels it decreased with increasing depolarization (see below). It is now difficult to speculate about the nature and functional meaning of this finding; more extensive measurements should be done on different kinds of cells to show whether this is a constant property of the main Ca^{2+} channel types. According to Droogmans and Nilius (1989) and Kawano and DeHaan (1990), in guinea-pig and chick cardiac LVA channels the mean open time demonstrates no potential dependence.

A specific feature of gating in HVA Ca^{2+} channels which was demonstrated in PC12 phaeochromocytoma cells and should be added to the model is the possibility of their transition into two different (short- and long-lived) open states (Kostyuk *et al.*, 1988b). A special long-opening state is also characteristic for this type of channel in cardiomyocytes (Pietrobon and Hess, 1990).

Unfortunately, the determination of possible differences between the channels in their intermediate closed states cannot be strict enough. In contrast to our findings, there are data about the possibility of describing the activation kinetics of HVA (N-type?) Ca^{2+} channels in bullfrog sympathetic neurones with a single gating particle mechanism (Jones and Marks, 1989). However, LVA currents in rat thalamocortical relay neurones could be better described by m^3 formalism, indicating a more complicated gating mechanism (Coulter *et al.*, 1989; Wang *et al.*, 1991).

Interaction between permeation and gating

Are permeation and gating really independent mechanisms in Ca^{2+} channels? Analysis of single channel currents provided some answers to this question. Replacement of some divalent cations by others evoked definite changes in transition rates between different states of the channel. They included changes in the slope of the dependence of a and b rate constants on membrane potential as well as in the relation $a(V)/b(V)$. This may indicate that different divalent cations bound to the intrachannel binding site change the potential relief of the channel, thus affecting in a different way the intramembrane movement of charged gating particles (Kostyuk *et al.*, 1988b). However, the data available are not sufficient to allow a conclusion if such changes can explain the observed variations in permeation of Ca^{2+} channels.

Very specific changes were observed in the last kinetic stage of channel transitions after its transformation into an Na-selective mode. The mean open time of the channel became drastically reduced and current-dependent (decreasing with an increase in sodium current, as shown in Fig. 1.6). At the same time, no changes were observed in the mean closed time. We suggested that these changes demonstrate the most effective interaction between permeation and gating in the Ca^{2+} channel. Na^+ ions passing with a high rate through the channel may cause deformations of its steric region and displace charged molecular groups of a selectivity filter at a distance proportional to the ion radius. This will lead to formation of dipoles along the ion trajectory which will exist during the time of dipole relaxation ($\sim 10^{-7}$ s) comparable to the rate of ion transit through the channel. As a result, the dielectric constant of the steric region of the channel may largely increase (up to 20–30) and correspondingly change the transition rate. After transition of the channel from open into the nearest closed state, the steric region of the selectivity filter becomes narrow and the ion flux through it is no longer

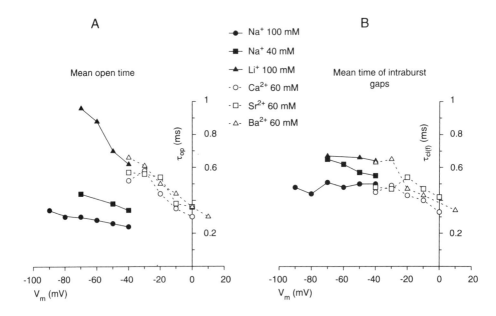

Figure 1.6. Potential dependence of rate constants of single LVA Ca^{2+} channels in mouse dorsal root ganglion neurone before and after their modification into sodium-conducting mode (from Kostyuk *et al.*, 1988a with permission from Springer-Verlag). (A) Mean open time. (B) Mean time of intraburst gaps. Charge carriers are indicated near the curves

possible. That is why the values of mean closed times are practically independent of both the species and the concentration of the permeant ion (Shuba *et al.*, 1991a).

Inactivation

The mechanism of time-dependent inactivation seems to be a reliable criterion for separation of LVA and HVA I_{Ca}: the low-voltage component is rapidly inactivating in a potential-dependent way, whereas the high-voltage one inactivates slowly depending on the current (Veselovsky and Fedulova, 1983; Fedulova *et al.*, 1985). This difference has been observed in many investigations (Matteson and Armstrong, 1984; Kalman *et al.*, 1988; Williams *et al.*, 1991; Takahashi *et al.*, 1991), although in skeletal and cardiac muscle fibres HVA Ca^{2+} channels seem to inactivate also in a potential-dependent way at least partly (Sanchez and Stefani, 1983; Cavalie *et al.*, 1983; Kass and Sanguinetti, 1984; Lee *et al.*, 1985). In frog DRG neurones Akaike and his colleagues (1988) also detected a small voltage-dependent component in the inactivation of HVA currents. One may expect that the existence of such a dual mechanism corresponds to the participation of different channel types in the generation of HVA I_{Ca}; however, this suggestion failed to be proved in recent experiments on rat intermediate pituitary cells (Williams *et al.*, 1991). In guinea-pig cardiomyocytes Ca^{2+} and voltage seem to inactivate the same HVA Ca^{2+} channels through independent mechanisms: one acts via dephosphorylation or modulation of protein kinase A, another by action on the gating machinery (Hadley and Lederer, 1991). The situation may be even more complicated due to recent observations on cerebellar granule cells that a single 22 pS channel can produce both decaying and non-decaying whole-cell currents, dihydropyridine (DHP) Ca^{2+} channel agonists markedly increasing the second mode of activity (Slesinger and Lansman, 1991). On cultured embryonic hippocampal neurones marked bursts of channel reopenings were observed following depolarizing pulses from −40 to +20 mV, which could be potentiated by DHP Ca^{2+} channel agonists and represent probably an unusually long-lived mode of channel gating not susceptible to inactivation; however, the intervention of a different type of channel cannot be excluded (Kavalali and Plummer, 1994).

The intimate mechanism of Ca-dependent inactivation in neuronal cells is still a matter for clarification. It has been shown that HVA Ca^{2+} channels purified from rabbit brain and incorporated into lipid bilayer reproduce selectivity, open time duration and pharmacology, but show sustained activity without inactivation or 'run-down' (De Waard et al., 1994b). If Ca^{2+} level is elevated inside, the main change in channel functioning is a shift in channel gating to low open probability (more than 100 times reduction of entry rate to open state); this happens even when calmodulin and channel phosphorylation are excluded and obviously represents a direct binding of Ca^{2+} ions to the channel (Imredi and Yue, 1994). Experiments with photorelease of Ca^{2+} ions from caged substances in Aplysia neurones have shown that ion concentration near the channel necessary for its inactivation must be quite high (with K_D in the range of dozens of micromoles), and the inactivation site must be about 25 nm from the channel internal mouth (Fryer and Zucker, 1993). Probably, something like a 'shell' (a microscopic space) is formed below the functioning Ca^{2+} channel providing the necessary conditions for its inactivation (Sherman et al., 1990). The Ca^{2+} binding site is located obviously at the main α_1 subunit (see below), as it is present even when this subunit is expressed alone without the additional ones. Of course, all these data do not exclude at all the participation of more complex enzymatic mechanisms related to channel phosphorylation–dephosphoryation, as in many investigations changes in the rate of inactivation have been demonstrated during interference with the activity of Ca^{2+}-dependent phosphatases or protein kinases (Yakel, 1992; Werz et al., 1993). Participation of cytoskeletal structures also cannot be excluded, as it has been shown in some cases that inactivation of L-type channels can be modulated by such factors as colchicine and taxol (Galli and DeFelice, 1994).

Subunit composition

The basic understanding of the structural composition of the voltage-operated Ca^{2+} channel has been obtained mainly from studies of channels purified from skeletal muscle; principal features are the same for channels in other tissues (see Catterall et al., 1988; Glossmann and Striessnig, 1988; Hofmann et al., 1990 and others). All Ca^{2+} channels are composed from five subunits, from which the largest one is α_1 (212–273 kDa). It contains the ion-conducting pore and binding sites for most Ca^{2+} channel antagonists. This subunit contains four membrane-spanning repeats, each of which includes six transmembrane helices. The next in size are the α_2/δ dimer (125 kDa), the intracellularly located β subunit (57 kDa) and transmembrane γ subunit (25 kDa). Schematic presentation of their co-localization is given in Fig. 1.7.

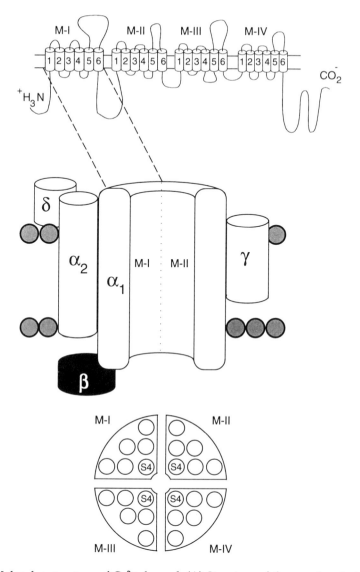

Figure 1.7. Molecular structure of Ca^{2+} channel. (A) Structure of the α_1 subunit showing six transmembrane helices assembled in four membrane-spanning repeats. (B) Spatial arrangement of different channel subunits. (C) Channel formation in the α_1 subunit

Despite this general identity, subsequent isolation of subunits from different tissues and cloning of corresponding cDNAs have shown substantial variation in their primary structure; a comparison of these variations with the functional properties of Ca^{2+} channels expressed in artificial systems is a hot point of many modern studies (see below).

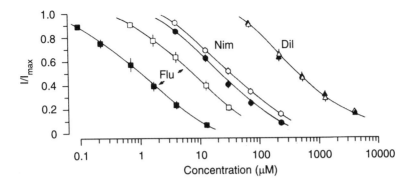

Figure 1.8. Pharmacological sensitivity of LVA and HVA Ca²⁺ channels in rat hypothalamus neurones (from Akaike *et al.*, 1989; reproduced by permission of The Physiological Society). Solid symbols, LVA currents; open symbols, HVA currents. Flunarizine (Flu), nimodipine (Nim), and diltiazem (Dil) were tested. Currents were evoked by voltage steps from -100 mV to -30 mV and from -60 mV to 0 mV, respectively

PHARMACOLOGICAL SEPARATION

The analysis of basic properties of Ca²⁺ channels gives us some ground for the identification of different channel types. LVA and HVA Ca²⁺ channels can be well separated in this respect; the distinction between channels within the HVA group is more vague. The same problem can be approached in a different way: by using pharmacological probes.

In the beginning, pharmacological data seem to fit quite well to the biophysical ones in separation of LVA and HVA channels. HVA channels are more or less sensitive to organic agonists and antagonists, especially DHPs, whereas LVA are not (Fedulova *et al.*, 1985; Nowycky *et al.*, 1985 and others). However, a more extensive screening of Ca²⁺ channels in different objects has shown clearly that such a parallelism is not quite strict: pharmacological properties reflect to some extent also the type of cells in which Ca²⁺ channels are expressed. So, LVA channels in neurones from certain brain structures (hypothalamus, cerebellum) were found to be even more sensitive to DHPs than HVA ones (Akaike *et al.*, 1989; Kaneda *et al.*, 1990). An example is shown in Fig. 1.8. Some DHPs (nicardipine, nimodipine) block LVA channels also in DRG neurones (Richard *et al.*, 1991; Formenti *et al.*, 1992), the effect here being different in different types of cells (Formenti *et al.*, 1993). An increase in sensitivity of these channels to DHPs could be induced in neuroblastoma cells simply by changing the solvent (Wu *et al.*, 1992). Organic antagonists known as antiepileptic drugs were found to exert specific inhibitory action on LVA channels in brain neurones (flunarizine—Akaike *et al.*, 1989; ethosuximide—Coulter *et al.*, 1990; Kostyuk *et al.*, 1992a). One micromole of flunarizine selectively blocked LVA channels in neuroblastoma cells (Wang *et al.*, 1990) and hippocampal neurones (Takahashi and Akaike, 1991), although in hippocampal neurones it also blocked inactivating HVA channels (Tytgat *et al.*, 1991); however, such a popular antiepileptic drug as valproic acid did not exert specific action on these channels (Zona and Avoli, 1990). LVA channels in neonatal rat DRG neurones were also reversibly inhibited by the volatile anaesthetic halothane (EC₅₀ about 100 μM); for HVA channels higher concentrations were needed (Takenoshita and Steinbach, 1991). A novel LVA channel blocker (tetrandrine) has been recently isolated from a Chinese herb (Liu, Q.Y. *et al.*, 1991).

Much more complicated are the results of pharmacological screening of HVA Ca^{2+} channels. An important first step here was the use of a natural Ca^{2+} channel antagonist, ω-conotoxin, isolated from the tropical fish-hunting mollusc *Conus geographicus* (ω-conotoxin, fraction GVIA). In many cases the persistent L-type channels (unitary conductance of about 31 pS) are found to be preferentially blocked by DHPs, whereas the completely inactivating N-type channels (unitary conductance about 16 pS) are preferentially blocked by ω-conotoxin (posterior pituitary nerve terminals—Lemos and Nowycky, 1989; chromaffin cells—Bossu *et al.*, 1991a, 1991b; giant terminals in the ciliary ganglion—Stanley and Atrakchi, 1990; Stanley and Goping, 1991; frog and rat sympathetic neurones—Boland *et al.*, 1994). The latter were even denoted as 'ω-channels' (Bean, 1991) or N-PT channels (Stanley, 1991). The specificity of binding of ω-conotoxin and DHPs was substantiated by immunoprecipitation studies on brain homogenates: both substances revealed different receptors (Hayakawa *et al.*, 1990). Experiments on purified N-type channels from rat brain reconstructed in lipid bilayers revealed high sensitivity of the corresponding receptor sites (K_D about 0.06 nM), which are not located within the channel pore and are allosterically linked to the Ca^{2+} binding site of the channel (Witcher *et al.*, 1993). However, data are accumulating about a much lower specificity of ω-conotoxin and DHP action on Ca^{2+} channels in other types of cells. No clear separation of the action of both drugs was found in hippocampal neurones (Jones *et al.*, 1989; Toselli and Taglietti, 1990). In pituitary peptidergic terminals ω-conotoxin also blocked L-type channels (Wang *et al.*, 1992); the same has been found in cockroach neurones (Wicher and Penzlin, 1994). In frog sympathetic neurones DHPs affected N-type channels (Jones and Jacobs, 1990), and in chromaffin cells ω-conotoxin blocked Ca^{2+} channels that did not seem to be N-type (Artalejo *et al.*, 1991b).

There have been several attempts to find other natural toxins specific for these channels. Thus a toxin isolated from the spider *Tarantula*, ω-grammatoxin, did not affect L-type Ca^{2+} channels in DRG neurones, but completely occluded inhibition of channels sensitive to ω-conotoxin (Lampe *et al.*, 1993; Piser *et al.*, 1994). Obviously, the action of this toxin should be studied in more detail. Conversely, a toxin from the black mamba snake, calseptine, specifically blocked only DHP-sensitive L-type Ca^{2+} channels (de Weille *et al.*, 1991).

Later, Ca^{2+} channels were identified which are insensitive both to DHP and to ω-conotoxin. In cerebellar Purkinje neurones typical HVA channels were found to be insensitive to both agents (Llinas *et al.*, 1989; Usowicz *et al.*, 1992), and the authors preferred to give them a special name (P channels); a toxin from the spider *Agelenopsis aperta* as well as its purified fraction ω-Aga-IVA was found to be a specific blocker for these channels. This finding has been confirmed by many groups (Bindokas *et al.*, 1993, on dendrites of cultures cerebellar neurones, and others). Synthetic ω-Aga-IVA toxin was as effective as the naturally purified one (Mintz and Bean, 1993a), and recently an even more effective natural fraction, ω-Aga-TK, has been extracted (Teramoto *et al.*, 1993). Conversely, fraction ω-Aga-IIIA blocked only N- and L-type channels, with about equal potency (Mintz *et al.*, 1991). According to Hillman *et al.*

(1991), P channels are present in neurones from the entorhinal and pyriform cortex and some brain stem structures but seldom in neocortical ones, although in the latter case HVA Ca^{2+} channels mostly do not belong to L- or N-type, as they are only weakly affected by DHPs or ω-conotoxin (Hoehn *et al.*, 1993). However, Brown *et al.* (1994) when applying ω-Aga-IVA in saturating concentrations (100 nM) succeeded in blocking about 30% of HVA I$_{Ca}$ in acutely isolated rat neocortical neurones; synthetic FTX toxin blocked up to 84% of this current (Brown *et al.*, 1994). In rat thalamic neurones synaptic transmission also involves mainly presynaptic Ca^{2+} channels which are insensitive both to DHPs and ω-conotoxin (Pfrieger *et al.*, 1992); the same is true for neurones from rat frontal cortex (Ye and Akaike, 1993); however, in this case the effectiveness of ω-Aga-toxin has not been tested. Probably, in all brain neurones a fraction of Ca^{2+} channels exists which is insensitive to ω-conotoxin and DHPs, and cerebellar Purkinje neurones are an extreme case in this respect in the sense that here most HVA channels are not blocked by DHPs or ω-conotoxin (Regan *et al.*, 1991). It is interesting that granule cells in the same structure show HVA channels sensitive to both ω-Aga- and ω-conotoxin (Scott *et al.*, 1990a); on the other hand, in many cases a component of Ca^{2+} current remains which cannot be blocked by both types of antagonists, indicating that HVA Ca^{2+} channels cannot be easily fitted into one of the three groups (L, N or P). A DHP and toxin-resistant component of I$_{Ca}$ has been found also in rat insulinoma and human β cells (Pollo *et al.*, 1993). Recent screening of Ca^{2+} current components in rat globus pallidus neurones has shown 21% to be sensitive to DHPs (L-type), 25% sensitive to ω-conotoxin (N-type), 22% sensitive to ω-Aga-IVA toxin (P-type) and the rest resistant to all these toxins (Surmeier *et al.*, 1994). Recently the conclusion about the existence of a novel type of HVA Ca^{2+} channel has been substantiated by the finding that the new synthetic ω-conopeptides SNX-111 and SNX-230 (which correspond to natural *Conus magnus* toxins MVIIA and MVIIC) bind to specific binding sites in rat brain synaptosomes different from binding sites for the already mentioned toxins. Ca^{2+} channels and Ca^{2+} influx have been inhibited very effectively by ω-conotoxin MVIIC also in chick synaptosomes (Grantham *et al.*, 1994; Lundy *et al.*, 1994). They may represent this novel HVA Ca^{2+} channel resistant to blockers of L-, N- and P-type channels (Kristipati *et al.*, 1994).

Because of the quite specific distribution of different types of Ca^{2+} channels in different cellular structures, an effective means for their selective investigation is to extract mRNA from the corresponding structures, which can be then used for cloning of parent cDNA (see below) as well as for direct expression of channels in *Xenopus* oocytes. A peculiar feature in the latter case is substantial amplification of expression (may be because of intervention of additional β subunits which do not increase transcription or translation but apparently affect 'maturation' of functional channels—Nishimura *et al.*, 1993). The expression of channels predominant in the corresponding structure becomes especially amplified, and their activity can be analysed even better than in parent neurones (Gezasimenko *et al.*, 1995).

Brain structures effectively used for this procedure in our laboratory were rat cerebellum and neocortex. The difference in pharmacological sensitivity of induced HVA I$_{Ca}$ was quite remarkable despite identical kinetic and potential-dependent characteristics: those expressed from cerebellum were completely insensitive to ω-conotoxin and could be blocked by *Agelenopsis aperta* venom, whereas those from

A   B

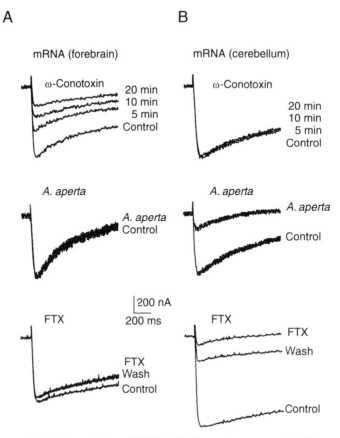

Figure 1.9. Pharmacological sensitivity of HVA Ca^{2+} channels expressed in *Xenopus* oocytes by injection of mRNA from rat forebrain and cerebellum (from Gerasimenko *et al.*, 1995; reproduced by permission of Naukova Dumka Publishers, Kiev). Time after application of 1 mM ω-conotoxin is indicated near the records. Ba^{2+} currents through Ca^{2+} channels were evoked by voltage steps from −60 mV to 0 mV

forebrain were insensitive to the latter and quite sensitive to ω-conotoxin (Gerasimenko *et al.*, 1995; see Fig. 1.9). However, ω-conotoxin failed to block completely I_{Ca} generated in oocytes injected with neocortical mRNA, and the spider toxin those in oocytes injected with cerebellar mRNA. Thus, in addition to predominant N- and P-type channels, HVA Ca^{2+} channels from these brain structures resistant to known organic calcium antagonists were also expressed. Recently LVA Ca^{2+} channels were also expressed in this way, using thalamohypothalamic complex as mRNA donor (Dzhura *et al.*, 1994). The characteristics of induced I_{Ca} were typical for such currents in neurones from the corresponding brain structures, except for a much slower time course of inactivation. The expressed currents were blocked by pharmacological antagonists specific for LVA channels (amyloride, flunarizine), but remained resistant to ω-conotoxin and ω-Aga-toxin (Fig. 1.10).

Finally, it should be pointed out that the application of the pharmacological tools described above for functional classification of HVA Ca^{2+} channels in invertebrate

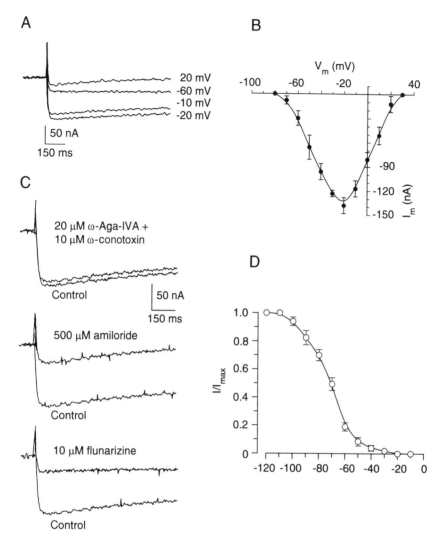

Figure 1.10. Current–voltage characteristics and pharmacological sensitivity of LVA Ca²⁺ channels expressed in *Xenopus* oocytes injected with mRNA from thalamohypothalamic complex of adult rats (from Dzhura *et al.*, 1994 with permission of Rapid Communications of Oxford, Ltd.). (A) Examples of current recordings. (B) Current–voltage characteristics. (C) Pharmacology. (D) steady-state inactivation curve

nerve structures (hydrozoan neurones, squid giant synapses, leech Retzius cells etc.) can be made only very approximately, as has been pointed out by several authors (Bookman and Liu, 1990; Charlton and Augustine, 1990; Przysienzniak and Spencer, 1992).

Obviously, this extreme dependence of pharmacological effects on the type of cells in which Ca²⁺ channels are expressed indicates that their differences are determined mostly by some variations in the structure of the peripheral part of the channel-forming molecule not involving its main functional elements. Recent studies with covalent binding of irradiated DHP to the purified α_1 complex of the Ca^{2+} channel from skeletal muscle and further digestion and sequencing of the peptides have shown that they bind predominantly to the cytosolic tail of the last (IVth) transmembrane-spanning region of the protein (between amino acids 1390 and 1437). It is close to the putative Ca^{2+}-binding domain of the channel responsible for Ca^{2+}-dependent inactivation (see above), and this may explain the requirement of Ca^{2+} ions for such binding. However, contradictory results have been published by other groups. Thus Kass et al., (1991) have shown that ionized DHPs act on the Ca^{2+} channel only exracellularly and the corresponding binding site must be close to the extracellular surface. Obviously, several parts on the channel-forming protein must interact to form the complete 'receptor' (cf. Spedding and Kenny, 1992).

At the same time, the variability in pharmacological sensitivity may be of high applied significance, allowing specific alterations to the functioning of different Ca^{2+} channels in selected cells and tissues.

STRUCTURAL SEPARATION

As has been already mentioned, the structure of the α_1 subunit is most important for the differentiation of different types of Ca^{2+} channels. Complete cDNA clones of this subunit were first made using DHP receptors of rabbit skeletal muscle (Tanabe et al., 1987). It has 55% primary sequence similarity to the α subunit of Na^+ channels with amino and C terminals located inside and long cytosolic loops connecting individual repeats (Tanabe T. et al., 1993). This subunit could not be expressed in oocytes, even with coexpression of auxiliary subunits. More effective was the expression in mouse L cells; however, the kinetics of induced currents was extremely slow (Perez-Reyes et al., 1989). Normalization of the latter was achieved by coexpression of the corresponding β subunit (Lacerda et al., 1991). The α_1 subunit was found to be the key target for regulation by protein kinase A (PK-A) and protein phosphatase 1C (Zhao et al., 1994).

This success started a flood of cloning and expression experiments with different types of Ca^{2+} channels from different tissues. The nomenclature proposed by different authors became quite confusing; recent agreement between several laboratories about simplifying seems to be very useful (Birnbaumer et al., 1994). According to it, the α_1 subunits should be named by numbers or capital roman letters (CaCh1 or α_{1S} for the one described above).

Two more cDNAs for the α_1 subunit generating L-type DHP-sensitive I_{Ca} were cloned: α_{1C} (CaCh2) from cardiac tissue (showing two alternative splice variants 2a and 2b) and α_{1D} (CaCh3) from endocrine cells (Mikami et al., 1989; Hui et al., 1991; Williams et al., 1992a). The α_{1C} showed 66% similarity to skeletal muscle subunit, and α_{1D} is very similar in structure to α_{1C} (about 70% similarity). Both can also be obtained from brain tissue and expressed in oocytes. Northern blot analysis of various brain structures revealed substantial differences in the distribution of these subunits. They were found in soma and proximal dendrites, but α_{1C} subunits were more significant in distal ones, often forming clusters (Hell et al., 1993). A surprising result was the finding of Williams et al. (1992a) that α_{1D} expressed from human brain could be partially blocked by high concentrations of ω-conotoxin GVIA. However, it cannot be excluded that the toxin was blocking an endogenous Ca^{2+} channel overexpressed after injection of foreign RNA.

Brain-specific α_1 subunit cDNAs were cloned by Mori et al. (1991) and Starr et al. (1991). They show only 30–40% similarity with that of α_{1S} and are highly expressed in cerebellum (but also in hippocampus, olfactory bulb and spinal cord). Designated as α_{1A} or CaCh4 (initial index BI), they induced currents insensitive to DHPs and ω-conotoxin but blocked by crude venom from *Angelenopsis aperta* and specially by its fraction ω-Aga-IVA which is, as mentioned already, specific for P-type Ca^{2+} channels (Mintz et al., 1992). However, the oocyte-induced currents appeared almost 100 times less sensitive to this blocker, and at the same time 10 times more sensitive to a special fraction of ω-conotoxin (MVIIC) from *Conus magnus* (Sather et al., 1993). This led to a suggestion that this subunit is responsible for a special type of Ca^{2+} channel (Q-type). Specific binding of synthetic ω-conopeptides similar to that of MVIIC to rat brain synaptosomal preparations has already been mentioned; recently the presence of a ω-conotoxin MVIIC-sensitive binding site in rat brain has been shown by autoradiography (Filloux et al., 1994), and specific effects of a synthetic form of this toxin on epileptiform discharges in rat cortical wedges were observed (Robichaud et al., 1994). On the other hand, the strange properties of the induced currents could be also a result of improper post-translatory modifications of the expression process by the oocyte.

Another brain-specific α_1 subunit has been purified using ω-conotoxin GVIA; it has been identified as α_{1B} or CaCh5 (original BIII) (Williams et al., 1992a; Dubel et al., 1992., Fujita et al., 1993; Coppola et al., 1994). This subunit contains 2289–2339 amino acids (molecular mass 257–261 kDa) and the structure appears to be very similar to that of α_{1A} (82% similarity) but very different from muscle-derived subunits. Several variations of this subunit were detected in different brain tissues. Currents induced by this subunit in oocytes showed specific sensitivity to N-type Ca^{2+} channel blockers but quite different (slow) kinetics. Changes in expression of other subunits could be the reason for such differences; most effective expression was observed when α_{2b} and β_1 subunits were coexpressed with α_{1B} (Brust et al., 1993).

A third brain-specific α_1 subunit was obtained from rabbit brain and identified as α_{1E} (CaCh6, initially BII) (Niidome et al., 1992; Niidome and Mori, 1993). The corresponding mRNA is expressed in different brain tissues (cerebral cortex, hippocampus, corpus striatum, thalamus etc.) but not in muscles, and the subunit exists in two isoforms (2259 and 2178 amino acids, correspondingly 254 and 246 kDa). However, the correspondence of this structure to any type of Ca^{2+} channel is still a mystery. Expression in oocytes by Soong et al. (1993) induced a current with current–voltage characteristics different from the well-known HVA I_{Ca}. It could be activated at voltages about 15 mV more negative and was insensitive to DHPs, ω-conotoxin and synthetic spider venom and could be partially blocked by Ni^{2+} or Cd^{2+}. The authors suggested that the induced current represents the activity of expressed LVA channels. However, it differed substantially from typical T-type currents which normally activate at much more negative potentials; some specific blockers for LVA channels which now exist were not tested in these experiments. Therefore it is quite possible that this subunit also belongs to the HVA group and is responsible for the pharmacologically resistant component of Ca^{2+} current observed in many experiments. The corresponding channels may be called 'R' (resistant) channels. In fact, recently a new set of Ca^{2+} currents has been described in cultured cerebellar granule cells with current–voltage characteristics very similar to those induced by expression of the α_{1E} subunit. The activation threshold varied for different components of this current (designated by the authors as G1, G2 and G3) between -40 and -10 mV, and complete steady-state inactivation was observed at -40 mV. They were insensitive to DHPs and slightly sensitive to ω-conotoxin GVIA (Forti et al., 1994). Probably, members of the same group are also channels isolated from cerebellar granule cells of marine ray and indicated as doe-1 (Zhang et al., 1993). They were also insensitive to DHPs and ω-Aga-toxin, but could be partially blocked by high concentrations of ω-conotoxin and very effectively by Ni^{2+}. Calcium channels of this type were recorded in bullfrog sympathetic neurones; they differed substantially from T-type channels in unitary conductance and potential dependence of inactivation (Elmslie et al., 1994). The most extensive study of the structure and functional expression of Ca^{2+} channels based on the α_{1E} subunit has been published recently by Williams et al. (1994). They found four variants of the corresponding cDNAs in mouse and human brain which induced in HEK293 cells and Xenopus oocytes the expression of HVA Ca^{2+} channels insensitive to drugs and toxins previously used. The corresponding currents revealed very rapid inactivation (τ about 20 ms), and their size was enhanced about 40-fold by coexpression with human α_2 and β subunits.

As LVA Ca^{2+} channels with typical current–voltage characteristics have been expressed in oocytes by injecting total mRNA from certain structures (Dzhura et al., 1994), one may suggest that a special α_1 subunit forming the corresponding channel may still exist and has yet to be identified.

A new promising approach towards correlation between structural and functional characteristics of different α_1 subunits is based on extraction and amplification of individual mRNAs from neurones showing different spectra of Ca^{2+} channels. Such measurements on adult rat neostriatal neurones have shown a good correlation between the presence of α_{1A} and α_{1B} mRNAs and the expression of ω-Aga-toxin IVA and ω-conotoxin GVIA-sensitive Ca^{2+} currents. However, despite the presence of a substantial nifedipine-sensitive component (about 30%), only low or undetectable levels of α_{1C} mRNA were revealed. No significant levels of LVA Ca^{2+} currents were observed in these neurones and obviously no mRNA was present which could be responsible for their expression (Bargas et al., 1994). In experiments on different cell lines (GH$_3$, PC-12, NIE-115, AtT-20) a correlation was found between an increase in the levels of α_{1A}, α_{1B} and $\alpha_{1C/D}$ mRNAs and the expression of P-, N- and L-type Ca^{2+} channels respectively (Lievano et al., 1994).

A summary of structurally identified α_1 subunits and the corresponding Ca^{2+} currents is presented in Table 1.1.

The β subunits are now also structurally differentiated into four subgroups which are identified as CaB1–CaB4 and all are located intracellularly. The skeletal muscle subunit (CaB1) consists of 524 amino acids (Ruth et al., 1989); the two cardiac ones (CaB2 and CaB3) show 71% and 66,6% homology to CaB1 (Hullin et al., 1992). CaB2 is expressed in peripheral tissues, whereas CaB3 is also expressed in brain. The CaB4 subunit is a predominant brain structure (Castellano et al., 1993). During expression in oocytes the coexpression of β_4 increases substantially the amplitude of Ca^{2+} currents with a small effect on kinetics. Conversely, the cardiac/brain β_2 dramatically slowed

Table 1.1. Molecular diversity of calcium channels (modified from Hofman et al., 1994b; Birnbaumer et al., 1994)

Calcium channel	α subunit	Conventional name	Sites of expression	Pharmacological sensitivity
CaCh1	α_{1S}	HVA L type	Skeletal muscle	DHPs, diltiazem, verapamil
CaCh2 family				
CaCh2a	α_{1C-a}		Heart	DHPs
CaCh2b	α_{1C-b}		Smooth muscle, lung	
CaCh2c (CaCh2-III)	α_{1C-c}		Brain	
CaCh3	α_{1D}	HVA L type	Brain, pancreas, GH3, PC12	DHPs; ω-conotoxin GVIA; ω-Aga-TX (IVA); FTX
CaCh4	α_{1A}	HVA P type; HVA Q type (?)	Cerebellum, kidney	ω-Conotoxin MVIIC; ω-Aga-TX IVA
CccCh5	α_{1B}	HVA N type	Brain, peripheral neurones	ω-Conotoxin GVIA; ω-conotoxin MVIIC
CaCh6	α_{1E}	HVA R type	Brain, heart	Ni^{2+}
CaCh?	?	LVA T type	Brain, peripheral neurones, heart	Ni^{2+}, amiloride

down current inactivation, obviously owing to stimulation of reopening of channels (Lacerda *et al.*, 1994). It has been shown that a conservative 30 amino acid domain located at the amino-terminus of the subunit is important for the described changes in channel functioning; it binds to a conserved motif in the I–II cytoplasmic linker of the α_1 subunit (De Waard *et al.*, 1994a).

PHYSIOLOGICAL MODULATION OF DIFFERENT TYPES OF Ca²⁺ CHANNELS

A natural way to distinguish different types of voltage-operated Ca²⁺ channels could be a possible modulation of their activity by physiologically active substances (transmitters, hormones and metabolites). The presence of such modulation is a unique property of Ca²⁺ channels, differentiating them from many other types of ion channels; the classical example is the potentiation of Ca²⁺ channel activity in cardiomyocytes by β-adrenoreceptor agonists mediated through cAMP-dependent protein phosphorylation (Reuter, 1974).

   Again, the division of Ca²⁺ channels into LVA and HVA types seems to fit well with their susceptibility to metabolic modulation. HVA channels are very sensitive to interruption of their connections with cytoplasmic processes; if the cell is perfused with saline solutions, these channels rapidly pass into a 'silent' state (channel 'run-down'). Conversely, LVA channels continue to function even in isolated membrane patches (Fedulova *et al.*, 1985). This difference may indicate that HVA Ca²⁺ channels have to be continuously phosphorylated in order to remain in an active state. This has been clearly demonstrated in cardiac cells (Ono and Fozzard, 1992); in neuronal cells also dephosphorylation by phosphatases 'downregulates' HVA channels, and phosphatase inhibition may 'run-up' these channels (Hescheler *et al.*, 1988; Mironov and Lux, 1991). A systematic study of possible tonic regulation of HVA Ca²⁺ channel activity was made in our laboratory on identified snail neurones (Kostyuk and Lukyanetz, 1993), and some results are presented in Fig. 1.11. Upregulation of I_{Ca} could be induced by lowering [Ca²⁺]ᵢ, injection of calmodulin (CM) antagonists (TFP), inhibition of phosphodiesterase by isobutylmethylxanthine (IBMX) and inhibition of Ca-CM-dependent phosphatase (calcineurin) by okadaic acid. It is important to notice that additional upregulation of I_{Ca} remained possible by application of a natural Ca²⁺ channel modulator in these neurones: 5-hydroxytryptamine (5-HT, serotonin). 5-HT obviously exerted its action through the same channel-phosphorylating system based on Ca²⁺-CM-dependent enzymes, as its effect could be blocked by elevation of [Ca²⁺]ᵢ or supported by inhibition of the activities of phosphodiesterase and phosphatase. In

---

Figure 1.11. Up- and downmodulation of HVA Ca²⁺ channels in identified snail neurones by factors affecting channel phosphorylation (from Kostyuk and Lukyanetz, 1993 with permission from Springer-Verlag). (A) 'Run-down' of Ca²⁺ currents measured in control conditions and on the background of application of 10 μM 5-HT during cell perfusion with standard intracellular solution ([Ca²⁺]ᵢ about 0.05 μM). (B) I_{Ca} 'run-up' after intracellular administration of 10 mM EGTA ([Ca²⁺]ᵢ lowered approximately to 0.01 mM). (C) Acceleration of 'run-down' by elevation of [Ca²⁺]ᵢ to 10 mM by intracellular introduction of the corresponding Ca²⁺ buffer. (D–F) Prevention of 'run-down' during high [Ca²⁺]ᵢ after inhibition of calmodulin by TFP (D), phosphodiesterase by IBMX (E) and phosphatase by okadaic acid (F). Examples of current records taken at different intervals after the beginning of the experiment are also shown

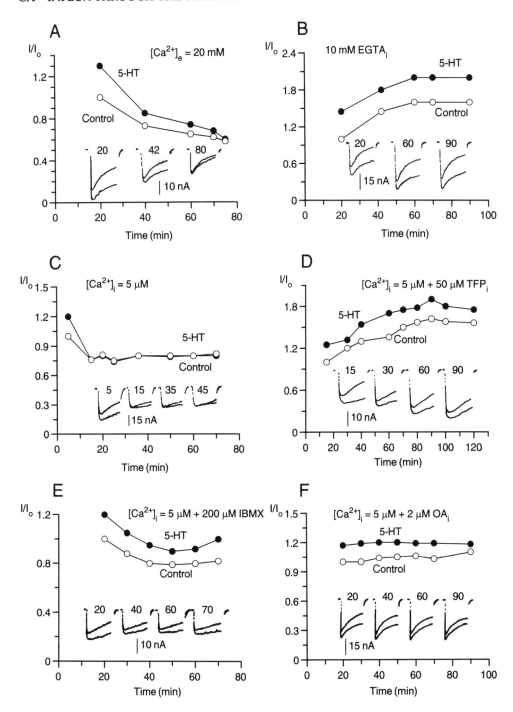

fact both enzymes form here a negative feedback system for tonic downregulation of Ca^{2+} channels activated by elevation of $[Ca^{2+}]_i$; the intervention of both enzymes may occur in subsequent order, as the K_D's of their activation by Ca^{2+} differ substantially (0.04 μM and 0.69 μM respectively).

Experiments on identified snail neurones have shown that different secondary messenger systems may be involved in Ca^{2+} channel modulation in different cells. There are neurones in which HVA Ca^{2+} channels are upregulated by a cAMP-dependent mechanism triggered by activation of 5-HT receptors in the neuronal membrane (Kostyuk et al., 1992b). In other snail neurones upregulation is exerted through activation of protein kinase C (PK-C), and the natural agonist can be a parathyroid hormone-like peptide (Kostyuk et al., 1990, 1992c). Parathyroid hormone is an endogenous upregulator of calcium channels also in cardiomyocytes (Rampe et al., 1991) and identified Helisoma snail neurones (Wang et al., 1994), however, in neuroblastoma cells and smooth muscle fibre synthetic parathyroid hormone inhibited the activity of L-type Ca^{2+} channels (Pang et al., 1990). In some neurones both mechanisms could be found; they were additive and had a different time course. Mediation of the response to 5-HT through activation of cGMP-dependent protein kinase has also been demonstrated in certain neurones (Paupardin-Tritsch et al., 1986). Finally, upmodulation of HVA Ca^{2+} channels triggered by activation of muscarinic receptors and mediated through a still unknown secondary messenger system may also occur (Gerschenfeld et al., 1991).

The molecular mechanisms of the effect of phosphorylation on channel function are still unknown; this process remains after transplantation of the HVA channel in phospholipid bilayer and is manifested mainly by prolongation of the mean open time (Mundina-Weilenmann et al., 1991). In skeletal muscle it is connected structurally to the C terminal of the α_1 subunit, as the cleavage of its main part removes the major site for cAMP-dependent phosphorylation (De Jongh et al., 1994).

Much more complicated are the results obtained in vertebrate neuronal cells. Here the possibility of direct interaction between GTP-binding proteins (G proteins) involved in the adenylate cyclase complex and Ca^{2+} channels has been postulated (see review by Ewald et al., 1988). Therefore the activity of Ca^{2+} channels can be modulated here both through a short intramembrane and a longer cytosolic pathway, which has been shown for cardiomyocytes (Shuba et al., 1990, 1991), DRG neurones (Dolphin, 1990) and other structures. Both effects can be opposite in nature (Gross et al., 1990a). Rapid β-adrenergic potentiation of cardiac Ca^{2+} channels by a fast G_s protein pathway has been demonstrated on cardiomyocytes (Yatani and Brown, 1989) and their inhibition by activation of cGMP-dependent PK (Mery et al., 1991). However, for cardiac Ca^{2+} channels the possibility of direct regulation by G proteins is still questioned (cf. Hartzell and Fischmeister, 1992).

The possible effects of G proteins on neuronal Ca^{2+} channels were studied mostly by testing the influence of application of pertussis-toxin (PTX) or intracellular introduction of GTP analogues (GTPγS or GDPβS) which either promote or inhibit their action. The results indicated the possible existence of a tonic inhibitory action of G proteins on neuronal Ca^{2+} channels which can be removed by loss of intracellular GTP and subsequent inactivation of the corresponding G protein (Pollo et al., 1991; Netzer et al., 1994). After initial inhibition by GTPγS a delayed augmentation of Ca^{2+} channel

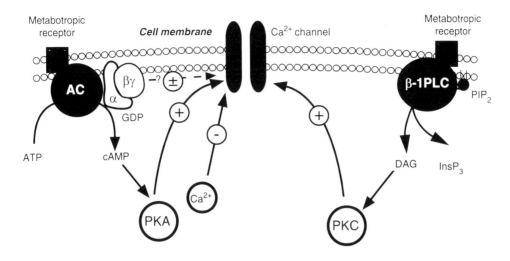

Figure 1.12. Schematic presentation of intracellular mechanisms modulating the functioning of Ca^{2+} channels. AC, adenylate cyclase; GDP, G protein; PKA, protein kinase A; PKC, protein kinase C; DAG, diacylglycerol

currents has been observed in chick sensory neurones, which represent not relief from inhibition but a distinct upregulatory process prevented by PK-C inhibitor (Zong and Lux, 1994); its mechanism is unclear and may involve intracellular phosphorylating systems (see below). More complicated mechanisms of the action of G proteins have been also suggested: promotion of the effects of different receptor agonists on Ca^{2+} channels (Scott and Dolphin, 1987) and involvement in the interaction between DHPs and channels (Schettini *et al.*, 1991). The possible mechanisms of physiological modulation of the functioning of Ca^{2+} channels are presented schematically in Fig. 1.12.

The effects of direct interference with intracellular protein-phosphorylating systems have been studied in several types of neuronal cells. In rat nodose neurones the catalytic subunit of cAMP-dependent PK-A increased both N- and L-type Ca^{2+} currents without effect on T-type; the effect appeared in 7–9 min after rupture of the membrane and could be blocked by protein kinase inhibitor (Gross *et al.*, 1990b). A similar upregulatory effect was observed in P-type channels expressed in *Xenopus* oocytes after injection of cAMP (Fournier *et al.*, 1993). Conversely, activation of PK-C reduced L-type Ca^{2+} channel activity in GH₃ pituitary cells; the PK-C blocker staurosporine blunted this effect (Haymes *et al.*, 1992). In phaeochromocytoma (PC-12) cells activation of PK-C downregulated only DHP-sensitive (L-type) currents, the effect being prevented by staurosporine (Bouron and Reber, 1994). Data have been obtained by Swartz (1993) about a possible complicated mechanism of PK-C action: disruption of the G protein-mediated effects on Ca^{2+} channels leading to reduced G protein-dependent inhibition of Ca^{2+} channels by different receptor agonists (see below).

Extremely variable up- and downmodulatory effects were shown on different neuronal structures under the action of various receptor agonists. In fact, all known neurotransmitters and hormones modulate the activity of voltage-gated Ca^{2+} channels, mainly inhibiting it.

Acetylcholine

Activation of nicotinic receptors in bovine chromaffin cell decreased HVA I_{Ca}, the effect being not influenced by GTP; muscarinic agonists were not active here (Klepper *et al.*, 1990). Conversely, in rat sympathetic neurones N- and L-type Ca^{2+} currents could be inhibited by muscarinic receptor activation (Mathie *et al.*, 1992). Carbachol and muscarin decreased HVA currents also in rat hippocampal neurones (Fisher and Johnson, 1990).

Dopamine

Inhibition of HVA Ca^{2+} currents through activation of D_2 receptors has been shown in many types of cells. It occurs with P-type currents in Purkinje neurones and N-type ones in sympathetic neurones (Sah and Bean, 1994), with N-type currents (but not L- or T-type) in pituitary pars intermedia melanotrophic cells (Williams *et al.*, 1990; Keja *et al.*, 1992; Valentijn *et al.*, 1993) and with HVA currents in differentiated neuroblastoma cells (Seabrook *et al.*, 1994b). In malignant pituitary cells (HGH$_4$C$_1$) HVA Ca^{2+} currents were inhibited by activation of both D_2 and D_4 dopamine receptors (Seabrook *et al.*, 1994a). Peculiar results were obtained on retinal horizontal cells: here dopamine increased L-type and reduced T-type currents; the effect could be mimicked by D_1 receptor agonists and membrane-permeable cAMP derivatives (Pfeiffer-Linn and Lasater, 1993).

γ-Aminobutyric acid

GABA$_B$ receptor agonists inhibit different components of HVA Ca^{2+} currents in peripheral and central neurones. This has been shown for the N-type in DRG neurones (Tatebayashi and Ogata, 1992; Menon-Johansson *et al.*, 1993, Gruner and Silva, 1994), P-type in central neurones (Mintz and Bean, 1993b) and an unidentified type in spinal cord (Sah, 1990) and hippocampal neurones (Toselli and Taglietti, 1993; Pfrieger *et al.*, 1994). In all cases the effect was sensitive to PTX and mediated obviously through the G protein mechanism, probably G$_0$. A depression of both LVA and HVA channels has been reported in lamprey neurones (Matsushima *et al.*, 1993).

Noradrenaline

Noradrenaline reduced HVA I_{Ca} in frog sympathetic (Lipscombe *et al.*, 1989) and rat parasympathetic (Akasu *et al.*, 1990b) neurones, rat spinal cord neurones (Sah, 1990), olfactory bulb neurones (Trombley, 1992), human neuroblastoma cells (Pollo *et al.*, 1992) as well as in insulin-secreting cell lines (Schmidt *et al.*, 1991). The participation of a G protein-coupled mechanism has been also shown in some cases, as the effect could be blocked by PTX and mimicked by injection of GTPγS (Pollo *et al.*, 1992). Potentiating effects from adrenoreceptors have been also observed in hippocampal neurones: isoproterenol increased the activity of N- and L-type, but not T-type channels; this effect might be mediated through the intracellular phosphorylating systems (Fisher and Johnston, 1990).

Serotonin

5-HT inhibited HVA Ca²⁺ currents in rat spinal cord neurones (Sah, 1990) and both the ω-conotoxin-sensitive and -insensitive HVA currents in rat dorsal raphe neurones, predominantly its transitory component (Kelly and Penington, 1989; Penington *et al.*, 1991).

Glutamate

According to Chernevskaya *et al.* (1991), in rat hippocampal neurones N-methyl-d-aspartate (NMDA) agonists inhibited only the ω-conotoxin-sensitive component of I_{Ca}. Metabotrophic glutamate receptor agonists (*trans*-ACPD) in hippocampal neurones affected both N and L components of the current (Sahara and Westbrook, 1993); the effects could be mimicked by quisqualate, but not by kainate or NMDA, and involved the G protein mechanism (Swartz and Bean, 1992). In striatal neurones activation of metabotropic receptors inhibited both Ca²⁺ currents and GABA-mediated synaptic potentials (Stefani *et al.*, 1994a). In cultured mice retinal ganglion neurones only ω-conotoxin but not DHP prevented the inhibitory effect of *trans*-ACPD (Rothe *et al.*, 1994). The inhibition of HVA currents by NMDA and non-NMDA receptor agonists in brain neurones has been shown to depend on the presence of Ca²⁺ in the extracellular solution and could be blocked by intracellular perfusion by rapid calcium chelator BAPTA; calmodulin antagonists also prevented the inhibitory effects. Therefore it has been suggested that Ca²⁺ influx into the neurone participates in this mechanism, probably by activating Ca²⁺ calmodulin-dependent phosphatases (Zeilhofer *et al.*, 1993). PK-C also modulates glutamate receptor inhibition of Ca²⁺ channels in hippocampal pyramidal neurones, reducing G protein-dependent inhibition and enhancing currents through N-type channels (Swartz *et al.*, 1993).

Adenosine

Adenosine and its derivatives are also effective inhibitors of HVA Ca²⁺ channels, acting through A_1 receptors. This has been shown on hippocampal pyramidal neurones (Scholz and Miller, 1991a), spinal dorsal horn neurones (Sah, 1990; Salter *et al.*, 1993) and motoneurones (Mynlieff and Beam, 1994), sympathetic neurones (Zhu and Ikeda, 1993) and ciliary ganglion nerve terminals (Yawo and Chuhma, 1993). The effect has been expressed mainly on N-type channels, and is based on PTX-sensitive mechanisms.

Somatostatin and bradykinin

Somatostatin depressed HVA I_{Ca} in rat spinal cord (Sah, 1990) and neocortical (Wand *et al.*, 1990) neurones, chick ciliary ganglion neurones (Dryer *et al.*, 1991; Meriney *et al.*, 1994) and both LVA and HVA currents in somatotrophs from rat pituitary gland (Chen *et al.*, 1990). In chick ciliary neurones this effect was dependent on an intracellular pathway involving cGMP-PK (Meriney *et al.*, 1994). Bradykinin depressed I_{Ca} in neuroblastoma hybrid cells, probably via a PTX-sensitive mechanism (Wilk-Blaszczak *et al.*, 1994).

Neuropeptide Y

This peptide, widely distributed in the nervous system, inhibited Ca^{2+} currents in rat sensory neurones, the effect being PTX-sensitive (Walker et al., 1988; Wiley et al., 1993). The inhibitory action affected only the transient component of HVA channels; T- and L-type currents were not affected. NRY-2 receptor subtype was involved; activation of NPY-1 receptors seemed to exert an opposite, enhancing effect (Wiley et al., 1993).

Luteinizing hormone-releasing hormone

LHRH inhibited the N-type Ca^{2+} channels in sympathetic neurones (Boland and Bean, 1993; Kuo and Bean, 1993). The effect was quite specific for this type of channel and could be mimicked by internal GTPγS.

Thyrotrophin-releasing hormone

TRH inhibited HVA Ca^{2+} channels in GH_3 cell line; it has been suggested that this effect is mediated by triggering inositol trisphosphate-dependent Ca^{2+} release and stimulation of Ca^{2+}-dependent channel inactivation, as it could be blocked by introduction of Ca^{2+} buffers (Kramer et al., 1991).

Parathyroid hormone

Synthetic parathyroid hormone (1–34 amino acid segment) inhibited L-type Ca^{2+} channels in neuroblastoma cells, the effect being thus quite different from in the above mentioned invertebrate neurones (Pang et al., 1990).

Vasopressin

Contrary to most of the above-mentioned factors, vasopressin potentiated L-type Ca^{2+} channels in an insulin-secreting cell line (Thorn and Petersen, 1991); however, no definite effect has been observed on spinal cord neurones (Sah, 1990).

Steroid hormones

The effects of steroid hormones are exerted obviously by different mechanisms, as they develop much more slowly as compared with most above-mentioned factors which involve changes in synthesis of channel-forming proteins or their processing and incorporation into the acting site. Glucocorticoids (hydrocortisone and dex-amethasone) induced in GH_3 cells a strong (up to five-fold) and long-lasting potentiation of predominantly HVA Ca^{2+} channels, which could be removed by blocking protein synthesis with actinomycin. LVA channels were also potentiated, but to a lesser extent (Fomina et al., 1993). Conversely, oestrogens in the same cells potentiated mainly LVA channels; in this case the effect could be blocked by cycloheximide (Ritchie, 1993). At the same time, rapid inhibitory effects were also observed in some experiments: in acutely isolated hippocampal neurones neurosteroid pregnenolone blocked Ca^{2+} currents (Spence et al., 1991).

Arachidonic acid

This polyunsaturated fatty acid liberated from membrane phospholipids by activation of phospholipase C or other lipases is known to exert several actions, especially in some pathological states. Among them is also modulation of Ca^{2+} channel activity. In GH3 cells at low concentrations (1 μM) it increased HVA I_{Ca}, but at higher ones (10–50 μM) it inhibited them probably by direct action on Ca^{2+} channels (Vacher et al., 1989; Korn and Horn, 1991; see also Meves, 1994 for review).

Most of the described effects were observed on HVA channels. However, data are accumulating about possible selective *upregulation* of LVA Ca^{2+} channels. Carbachol, muscarin and 5-HT quickly increased LVA I_{Ca} in hippocampal neurones (Fisher and Johnston, 1990; Fraser and MacVicar, 1991); 5-HT had a similar effect in spinal motoneurones (Berger and Takahashi, 1990). ACTH depressed LVA current in cultured glomerulosa cells, increasing the HVA current (Durroux et al., 1991). Thy-1 (a major cell surface glycoprotein formed in mammalian brain) was found to play a definite role in modulation of LVA currents: anti-Thy-1,2 monoclonal antibody increased their amplitude in cultured mice DRG neurones (Saleh et al., 1988). According to Scott et al. (1990b), in cultured DRG neurones LVA Ca^{2+} channels can be both up- and downregulated by photoactivation of intracellular guanosine 5--O-(3-thio)triphosphate depending on concentration. In other experiments on rat sensory neurones it was found that LVA I_{Ca} can be diminished by activation of PK-C without affecting HVA currents (Schroeder et al., 1990). However, no data are available about possible natural agonists triggering these effects. Recently it has been shown that simply adding bovine serum albumin to the culture medium selectively increases the LVA Ca^{2+} currents in neuroblastoma cells, probably by removal of some inhibitory factors, among them the already mentioned arachidonic acid (Schmitt and Meves, 1994).

A possible new endogenous factor for modulation of Ca^{2+} channels which should be taken into account is *nitric oxide* (NO). At least in sympathetic neurones increase in Ca^{2+} currents has been observed after its intracellular liberation (Chen and Schofield, 1993). Conversely, in PC-12 phaeochromocytoma cells L- and N-type Ca^{2+} channel activity was inhibited by NO via a cGMP-mediated mechanism (Desole et al., 1994).

ONTOGENETIC DEVELOPMENT OF DIFFERENT Ca^{2+} CHANNELS

One way to understand the functional significance of the diversity of Ca^{2+} channels may be the investigation of their expression during ontogenetic development of the corresponding cells. Pioneering data in this respect were obtained in our group on rat DRG neurones. It has been shown that during postnatal development of sensory neurones quite complicated changes in the quantitative and qualitative expression of different voltage-operated ion channels do occur. Already at birth most neurones have TTX-sensitive Na^+ and HVA Ca^{2+} channels in their membrane; during postnatal development they retain their dominant position. However, another process takes

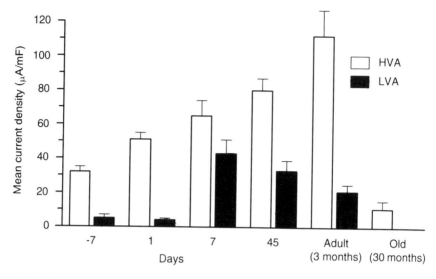

Figure 1.13. Changes in the mean densities of LVA and HVA Ca²⁺ currents in rat dorsal root ganglion neurones during prenatal and postnatal ontogenesis and ageing (combined from Kostyuk, 1992 and Kostyuk *et al.*, 1993)

place in parallel: a decrease in the proportion of neurones that show LVA Ca^{2+} channels and TTX-resistant Na$^+$ ones. At the age of 3 months, when the functional differentiation of sensory neurones is accomplished, about 60% of cells retained only TTX-sensitive Na$^+$ and HVA Ca^{2+} channels (Kostyuk *et al.*, 1986; Fedulova *et al.*, 1986; 1994).

These data prompted us to continue the analysis both backwards—to find out what kind of changes in channel expression occur during prenatal development—and forwards, during ageing. We found that the density of TTX-sensitive Na$^+$ and HVA Ca^{2+} channels in DRG neurones steadily increased during last 7 days of prenatal development. However, the density of LVA Ca^{2+} channels was quite low 7 days before birth and showed a maximum immediately after birth (Fedulova *et al.*, 1994).

Conversely, in aged rats (30 months old) no active LVA channels could be found in any cell (Kostyuk *et al.*, 1993). It should be stressed that kinetic characteristics of individual Ca^{2+} channels did not show significant changes during ontogenetic development of the cells. Only the steady-state inactivation of HVA I_{Ca} was shifted by 10–15 mV in a negative direction in cells from aged animals. A decrease in the sensitivity of the corresponding channels to phosphorylation by cAMP-dependent PK was also observed, in this case manifested by disappearance of the effects of intracellular administration of cAMP and ATP on the 'run-down' of I_{Ca}.

All these observations are summarized in Fig. 1.13 and indicate that during neuronal ontogenesis substantial changes in the expression of different types of Ca^{2+} channels occur; the expression of LVA channels is transient and occurs during cell maturation and differentiation, completely disappearing in old age. At the same time, the basic properties of the channels remain unchanged; some alterations in their functioning may be related to age-dependent changes in the intracellular milieu (elevation of $[Ca^{2+}]_i$, changes in the activity of phosphorylating and dephosphorylating enzymes, etc.).

These conclusions are in accord with most data obtained on other types of cells. In cultured embryonic sensory neurones from *Xenopus* LVA Ca^{2+} channels were expressed only in the first 20–40 h of culturing; obviously they were necessary during channel and receptor expression, outgrowth of cellular processes, etc. (Barish, 1991a). In rat and guinea-pig hippocampal pyramidal neurones LVA channels were found only in an immature state; they were absent in cells isolated from adult animals (O'Dell and Alger, 1991; Thompson and Wong, 1991). The same was true for neurones cultured from embryonic or adult rat neostriatum (Bargas *et al.*, 1991). In rat neocortical neurones in slices LVA Ca^{2+} currents were well expressed on the second postnatal day, but they completely disappeared on the twelfth postnatal day, when the density of HVA I_{Ca} continued to increase progressively (Tarasenko *et al.*, 1995). The ontogenesis of muscle cells seems to conform to the same rule: LVA Ca^{2+} channels are well expressed in embryonic cultured chick cardiomyocytes (Kawano and DeHaan, 1991) and skeletal muscle fibres (Adams and Beam, 1989; Kano *et al.*, 1991), but they disappeared when the growth rate of fibres reached zero (Xu and Best, 1992).

At the same time, there are certain differences in the time dependence of the expression of LVA and HVA Ca^{2+} channels in neurones from different brain structures. Thus, a significant LVA I_{Ca} could be recorded in hypothalamic, thalamocortical relay and Purkinje neurones isolated from adult rats (Akaike *et al.*, 1989; Coulter *et al.*, 1989; Kaneda *et al.*,1990). Among DRG neurones the expression of LVA channels in the adult state has been found to depend on the size of the cells: in medium-sized neurones, contrary to large ones, these channels are still well expressed, as can be seen from Fig. 1.14. Obviously, such differences reflect specific features of the activity of these neurones (see below). Some authors have reported that LVA Ca^{2+} channels may be better expressed in DRG neurones from adult than newborn rats (Lovinger and White, 1989), but this finding contradicts many other observations.

A very interesting finding is the possibility of evoking the expression of Ca^{2+} channels in cells where they are normally absent. Thus, in Schwann cells they appear in cases where the latter are co-cultured with embryonic DRG neurones; probably, a specific factor is released in the medium in this case or the channels may be transported from cell to cell in some way (Amedee *et al.*, 1991). Expression of Ca^{2+} channels could be induced also in cortical astrocytes; in this case the presence of substances known to increase the intracellular level of cAMP was necessary (Barres *et al.*, 1989). Obviously, the mechanisms of these effects should be analysed in more detail.

Less numerous are the attempts to clarify the developmental changes in expression of different subtypes of HVA Ca^{2+} channels. A convenient model for this purpose is the induced differentiation of clonal cells which start to grow neurites. In rat phaeochromocytoma cells subjected to nerve-growth factor (NGF) it has been shown that differentiation was followed by a large (about four-fold) increase in the density of ω-conotoxin-sensitive (N-type) I_{Ca}, whereas the density of L-type current became reduced (Usowicz *et al.*, 1990). This appears to support the conclusion about predominant expression of N-type channels during the development of presynaptic structures.

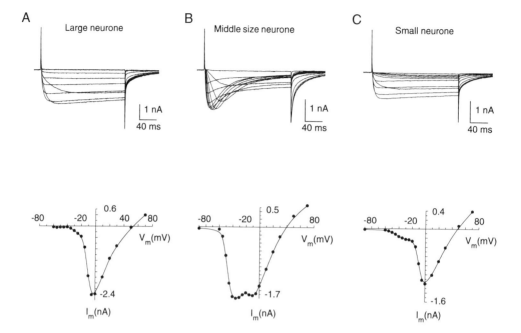

Figure 1.14. Ca^{2+} currents recorded from mouse dorsal root ganglion neurones with different soma diameters (Shmigol *et al.*, 1995a with permission of Elsevier Science Ltd). A, B and C represent families of I$_{Ca}$ recorded in response to increasing depolarizations from a holding potential of -80 mV and corresponding I–V curves in large, medium-size and small neurones

LIGAND-OPERATED Ca^{2+}-PERMEABLE CHANNELS

All eukaryotic cells sense the environment via specific membrane receptors, which translate incoming information into the intercellular language. From the conceptual point of view all receptors are classified as 'ionotropic' receptors (coupled with activation of transmembrane ionic transport) and 'metabotropic' receptors (which act via intracellular chemical messengers). The activation of both classes of receptor represent one of the key events in interneuronal synaptic transmission. The ionotropic receptors are, in fact, membrane channels opened by binding of specific chemical substances (ligands) to special receptor domains of the channel. Several subtypes of these channels form an additional pathway for Ca^{2+} entry into nerve cells. The ligand-operated channels are members of several gene families which encode glutamate, acetylcholine, adenine nucleotides, 5-HT, glycine and γ-aminobutyric acid receptors. The most important role in calcium signalling belongs to the excitatory neurotransmitter receptors (glutamate, acetylcholine and adenine nucleotide receptors), which we will discuss below.

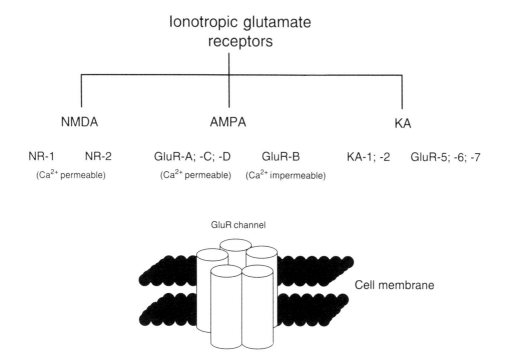

Figure 1.15. Classification and functional structure of glutamate receptors (from Burnashev, 1993b, with permission)

GLUTAMATE IONOTROPIC RECEPTORS

Glutamate-mediated neurotransmission seems to be one of the most important and abundant in the brain. Traditionally all glutamate receptors (GluRs) have been classified into three main groups in accordance with their preferential sensitivity to specific agonists. These three groups are (1) NMDA receptors; (2) AMPA-(α-amino-3-hydroxy-5-methylisoxazole-4-propionic acid) receptors and (3) kainate (KA) receptors. Members of GluR subfamilies contribute differently to the synaptic transmission in the brain: AMPA/KA receptors mediate fast excitatory postsynaptic potentials, while NMDA receptors are responsible for the slow component of postsynaptic excitation. Recent advances in molecular biology (reviewed by Burnashev, 1993a; Wisden and Seeburg, 1993) revealed that all GluRs are built from a number of subunits (see Fig. 1.15); which are assembled into a five-fold heteromeric channel structure. The elementary subunits comprise approximately 1000 amino acid residues and have four transmembrane regions, which actually form the channel; the transmembrane region TM2 is believed to form a channel pore (see Burnashev, 1993a). The very interesting feature of GluRs is the recently discovered post-translational RNA editing which may significantly alter the functional properties of the receptor.

The higher calcium permeability among GluRs has been demonstrated for NMDA channels. The detection of these channels has been delayed due to the fact that trypsin, which is usually used for isolation of brain neurones, irreversibly inactivates them

(Allen *et al.*, 1988). This permeability has been analysed by several groups (MacDermott *et al.*, 1986; Asher and Nowak, 1988; Mayer and Westbrook, 1987b). NMDA channels are less selective towards Ca^{2+} ions as compared with voltage-operated channels: P_{Ca}/P_{Na} is about 10 : 6. However, they are still about 70 times more permeable to Ca^{2+} than AMPA/KA GluRs, and acetylcholine-operated channels. The NMDA receptor ion channel has a conductance of approximately 50 pS and a mean open time of 5 ms. Like other glutamate-operated channels, they contain other binding sites for various ligands at which transmitters, cotransmitters and pharmacological agents can act and modulate channel function or modulate the effects of other ligands. They include two binding sites located in the extraneuronal domain which bind the allosteric modulator glycine and the divalent cation Zn^{2+} (Johnson and Asher, 1987; Peters *et al.*, 1987; Westbrook and Mayer, 1987) and two binding sites located in the transmembrane domain that bind Mg^{2+} and the anticonvulsant drug phenylcyclidine (Mayer *et al.*, 1984; Asher and Nowak, 1988; Huettner and Bean, 1988). The presence of an intrachannel site for binding Mg^{2+} is of special importance here, as it is responsible for potential dependence of channel functioning (Mayer and Westbrook, 1987a). The functional role of Ca^{2+} entry through NMDA channels is still under consideration. It may be important for membrane translocation and activation of PK-C, which in turn is responsible for phosphorylation of a series of membrane proteins including those involved in long-term changes of neuronal activity (cf. Zucker, 1989; Verhage *et al.*, 1994). Substantial and prolonged elevation of cytosolic Ca^{2+} concentration may also be the main reason for the well-known neurodegenerative processes and cell death induced by excessive extracellular concentrations of excitatory amino acids (for instance during brain ischaemia and anoxia—Rothman, 1984; Orrenius *et al.*, 1989).

The other two families of GluRs—AMPA and KA receptors—also appeared to be permeable to Ca^{2+} ions. Molecular cloning and expression studies of the non-NMDA GluRs have clearly demonstrated that their functional properties depend on the subunit composition. Assembling the GluR receptors in artificial expression systems as homo- or heteromeric channels comprised of GluR-A, -C and -D subunits resulted in the appearance of their Ca^{2+} permeability; however, introduction of the edited form of -B subunit determined a decrease in Ca^{2+} permeation. Therefore, the expression and post-translational editing of GluR-B subunit is a crucial step in the regulation of Ca^{2+} influx via glutamate ionotropic receptors. Indeed, single-cell PCR (polymerase chain reaction analysis of mRNA expression) experiments on neocortical neurones (Jonas *et al.* 1994) demonstrated that the relative (in respect to other subunits) expression of GluR-B-specific mRNA was about 10 times higher in pyramidal cells versus non-pyramidal neurones. Moreover, the expression of GluR-B subunit correlated well with the Ca^{2+} influx through glutamate receptors: GluR Ca^{2+} permeability (determined by reversal potentials of glutamate-activated whole-cell currents) was significantly higher in non-pyramidal that in pyramidal neocortical neurones. In cerebellar Purkinje neurones, despite a high expression of GluR-B subunit (as revealed by *in situ* hybridization—Keinanen *et al.* 1990) significant Ca^{2+} influx via non-NMDA GluR was observed (Brorson *et al.* 1994), suggesting the possible mosaic expression of GluR-B-containing and GluR-B-free glutamate receptor complexes within one cell. The importance of post-translational editing (Sommer *et al.*, 1991) of the B subunit (which also controls Ca^{2+} permeability of the appropriate receptor) in native neurones still remains unclear. Similarly to AMPA receptors the editing of the GluR-6 isoform of putative KA-gated channel considerably changes its Ca^{2+} permeability. Thus, mRNA editing might be a powerful mechanism which could be utilized by nerve cells in order to control the Ca^{2+} influx in glutamate-sensitive synaptic inputs.

The expression of Ca^{2+}-permeable GluRs in certain brain regions undergoes a developmental switch (Pellegrini-Giampietro *et al.* 1992): the highest expression of Ca^{2+}-permeable AMPA/KA GluRs in rat neocortex, striatum and cerebellum was observed at postnatal day 4; afterwards the number of Ca^{2+}-permeable GluRs declined. In hippocampus the number of Ca^{2+}-permeable channels increased between postnatal days 7 and 21, after which it also declined. The periods of increase in expression in Ca^{2+}-permeable GluRs correlate with periods of enhanced synaptic activity, and presumably the high expression of Ca^{2+}-permeable AMPA/KA GluRs may be important for brain development and formation of neuronal circuits.

NICOTINIC CHOLINORECEPTORS

Similarly to GluRs nicotinic cholinoreceptors belong to the extended gene family. Molecular cloning studies revealed a broad family of NChR subunits. Various combinations of these subunits form a functionally distinct palette of NChRs. From the physiological point of view NChRs are classified into three groups: one muscle-specific and two neuronal-specific, namely neuronal NChRs and bungarotoxin-sensitive NChRs. The muscle NChRs (see Karlin, 1993 for review) are composed of $\alpha 2$, β, γ (or ε) and δ subunits, while nerve NChRs are composed of seven α subunits ($\alpha 2$ to $\alpha 8$) and three β subunits ($\beta 2 - \beta 4$). In respect to $[Ca^{2+}]_i$ signalling the important point is that neuronal NChRs have about two times higher Ca^{2+} permeability as compared with muscle NChRs.

PURINORECEPTORS

The possible role of ATP as a synaptic transmitter and the existence of specific ATP or 'purinergic' receptors were suggested by Burnstock in the early 1970s (Burnstock, 1972). Further studies confirmed this idea, and clearly showed that ATP and its analogues act as an excitatory neurotransmitter in both the central and peripheral nervous system. The neuronal responses to adenine nucleotides are mediated via two major classes (Fig. 1.16) of purinoreceptors: P_1 (adenosine receptors) and P_2 (ATP/ADP) receptors. In the nervous system ATP is released as a cotransmitter (for example with noradrenaline in peripheral sympathetic terminals); the substantial release of ATP was also discovered from intact neurones and synaptosomal preparations.

The pharmacological classification of purinoreceptors has been extensively reviewed recently (Dubyak and El-Moatassim, 1993; Edwards, 1994; Fredholm *et al.*, 1994; Pintor and Miras-Portugal, 1994). In respect to $[Ca^{2+}]_i$ signalling the important issue is that practically all ionotropic ATP (or P_2) purinoreceptors displayed an appreciable Ca^{2+} permeability. In addition, activation of P_2 ionotropic receptors resulted in the generation of an inward cation current with a subsequent depolarization and opening of voltage-gated Ca^{2+} channels. Recently the P_4 (solely dinucleotide-sensitive) subclass of purinoreceptors coupled with a selective Ca^{2+}-permeable channel was

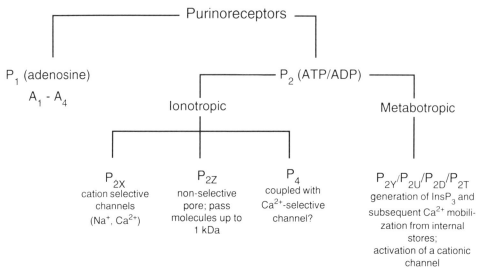

Figure 1.16. Classification of purinoreceptors

discovered in rat brain synaptosomes (Pintor and Miras-Portugal, 1994). Metabotrophic P_2 receptors are also coupled with generation of $[Ca^{2+}]_i$ signals either via triggering intracellular Ca^{2+} release (see Chapter 4) or via G protein-mediated activation of non-selective cationic channels which also may be involved in Ca^{2+} influx generation. Recently one of the member of ATP-gated ion channels family (corresponding presumably to P_{2x} receptor) has been molecularly cloned (Brake *et al.*, 1994, Valera *et al.*, 1994). This channel is permeable to Na^+, K^+ and Ca^{2+} and has a membrane topology different from other ligand-gated ion channels.

SECOND MESSENGER-ACTIVATED Ca^{2+}-PERMEABLE CHANNELS

A second group of Ca^{2+}-permeable channels comprises those activated from *inside* the cell by cyclic nucleotides. The first finding in this respect was made by Fesenko *et al.* (1985), who demonstrated that cGMP directly activates ionic conductance in excised patches of retinal rod plasma membrane. It turned out that the inward current through the corresponding channels in darkness is about 80% Na^+ and 15% Ca^{2+} (with the rest apparently carried by Mg^{2+}). However, because Na^+ is about 100 times more concentrated than Ca^{2+} in the extracellular space, the channel really prefers Ca^{2+} over Na^+ by 10 : 1 (Nakatani and Yau, 1988). The functional effects of these channels are rather complicated: as they close in light, they *diminish* the influx of Ca^{2+} in this condition, with efflux being unchanged; this causes a decline in the cytoplasmic Ca^{2+} concentration and activation of a complex negative-feedback mechanism responsible for light adaptation (cf. Yau, 1994). Similar channels were found in retinal cones, responsible for vision in bright light (Haynes and Yau, 1985). For both rod and cone channels, cGMP is the most effective ligand, consistent with its being the second messenger in phototransduction. cAMP can also open these channels, but at higher concentrations (about 50 times) (Yau, 1994).

Similar channels are also involved in olfactory transduction (Nakamura and Gold, 1987). As in photoreceptor channels, the olfactory channel is highly permeable to Ca^{2+}—a feature again important for sensory adaptation, which in this case involves a rise in cytoplasmic Ca^{2+} during odorant-induced channel opening (Restrepo et al., 1990; Reed, 1992). The olfactory channel requires much lower ligand concentrations, and cAMP here is only slightly less effective than cGMP. Unitary conductance of this channel is about 30 pS (Kurahashi and Kaneko, 1993) to 40 pS (Zufall et al., 1991).

Molecular cloning of these channels shows a domain on the cytoplasmic C-terminal segment with homology to the cyclic nucleotide-binding domains in the cGMP- and cAMP-dependent protein kinases. They consist of several copies of 63 kDa proteins and form six transmembrane segments, being homologous to the pore-forming region in voltage-gated channels (Kaupp, 1991); this may indicate a common ancestry between cyclic nucleotide-gated and voltage-gated channels.

Obviously, cyclic nucleotide-gated channels exist also in other neuronal structures, as well as in other tissues. Thus, the possibility to induce membrane conductance by intracellular injection of cAMP into snail neurones has been shown by our group (Kononenko et al., 1983, 1986) and by Sudlow et al. (1993). However, the corresponding channels may be of different structural type, as measurements of membrane current noise produced by their activity gave a very low single-channel conductance value (about 0.9 pS—Storozhuk et al., 1993).

Ca^{2+} RELEASE-ACTIVATED Ca^{2+} CHANNELS

Other types of Ca^{2+}-permeable ligand-operated channels may also exist in neuronal membranes. A quite peculiar one has been suggested on the basis of studies of intracellular Ca^{2+} release which indicated that plasmalemmal Ca^{2+} entry is in some way controlled by the exhaustion of an intracellular calcium pool. This new aspect of the interrelation between Ca^{2+} stores and membrane permeability led to the discovery of plasmalemmal Ca^{2+}-permeable channels controlled by the filling state of Ca^{2+} stores (Hoth and Penner, 1992, 1993; Penner et al., 1993). These channels appear to have high selectivity for Ca^{2+} ions and their single channel conductance was estimated to be as low as several femtosiemens (Zweifach and Lewis, 1993). At least three mechanisms have been suggested to explain the activation mechanisms of Ca^{2+} release-activated Ca^{2+} channels (CRAC). The most elaborate seems to be a hypothesis which postulated the generation of a diffusible messenger released by emptying of intracellular Ca^{2+} stores. This diffusible messenger (molecular weight approximately 500 Da) called CIF ('calcium influx factor') has been postulated to activate Ca^{2+} release-activated Ca^{2+} channels in macrophages, fibroblasts, Xenopus oocytes and astrocytes (Fasolato et al., 1994; Lückhoff and Clapham, 1994; Parekh et al., 1993; Randriamampita and Tsien, 1993). Alternatively, a G protein-mediated coupling between ER and plasmalemmal channels, as well as a direct interchange of Ca^{2+}-permeable channels between reticular and plasmalemmal membranes, have been suggested (see Fasolato et al., 1994 for review). However, while the existence of I_{CRAC} permeability has been shown in a variety of eukaryotic cells, in neurones it has not yet been demonstrated.

CONCLUSIONS

From all the data presented we may conclude that the members of a family of voltage-operated Ca^{2+} channels have common basic properties, indicating the presence of identical features in the structure of the channel-forming protein molecule (its α_1 subunit). The most essential subdivision of this family is between low- and high-voltage-activated (LVA and HVA) channels; their principal differences in the properties of natural and artificial gene expression and in the mechanisms of interaction with cytosolic processes. The group of LVA channels is quite homogeneous in their features; they do not seem to be susceptible to phosphorylation by intracellular protein kinases—a mechanism highly important for the functioning of HVA channels.

Contrary to LVA channels, HVA channels show immense variability in their properties, leaving little hope for strict classification based on kinetic characteristics, pharmacological sensitivity, etc. However, one should not be distressed by this fact and should not spend too much time in classifying, but use this feature for applied purposes to find ways for selective modification of Ca^{2+}-dependent cellular functions in different species, different tissues and different cells of the same tissue. This may be of major importance not only for medicine but even more so for effective analysis of the unprecedented role of Ca^{2+} ions in the living process.

2 Calcium Stores and Calcium Release Channels

GENERAL CHARACTERISTICS OF NEURONAL CALCIUM STORES

The second major source of calcium ions necessary for the development of $[Ca^{2+}]_i$ signal is associated with specialized intracellular structures which are able to accumulate, store and release calcium ions in response to appropriate stimuli. These structures are represented by distinct intracellular compartments, formed within endo(sarco)plasmic reticulum (ER); the compartments are equipped with calcium pumps (sarco(endo)plasmic reticulum calcium (SERCA) pumps, which underlie Ca^{2+} accumulation), low-affinity high-capacity Ca^{2+}-binding proteins (responsible mainly for Ca^{2+} storage) and Ca^{2+} release channels (which determine Ca^{2+} liberation from the store). The basic properties of calcium stores and mechanisms of intracellular calcium release in eukaryotic cells have been the subject of numerous reviews in recent years (Meldolesi *et al.*, 1990; Pietrobon *et al.*, 1990; Henzi and MacDermott, 1992; Pozzan *et al.*, 1994); here we will summarize the evidence concerning ER Ca^{2+} storage in nervous cells.

Neuronal ER is present in the form of rough ER (associated mostly with cisternae-like structures), smooth ER (formed by tubulae) and nuclear envelope. All these three subcompartments in fact form a discontinuous system, which has been revealed in a number of morphological studies (Broadwell and Cataldo, 1983, 1984). It is still unknown whether Ca^{2+} stores coincide with the entire ER or are restricted to specific modified portions of it.

Conceptually, calcium stores in neurones are separated into at least two types in respect to the mechanisms of Ca^{2+} liberation, which is controlled by two different second messengers, namely by inositol 1,4,5-trisphosphate (InsP3) or by Ca^{2+} ions (see Berridge, 1993; Ferris and Snyder, 1992; Pozzan *et al.*, 1994; Kostyuk and Verkhratsky, 1994) (Fig. 2.1). At the molecular level this heterogeneity is associated with the expression of two distinct subtypes of Ca^{2+} release channels: InsP3-gated and Ca^{2+}-gated channels, respectively. Markers which are specific for Ca^{2+} stores (SERCA pumps; Ca^{2+}-binding proteins) do not show striking heterogeneity of the ER in respect to its Ca^{2+}-handling capability; however, subtypes of Ca^{2+} release channels are often distributed quite unevenly within the ER networks.

A distinct spatial separation of both release mechanisms has been shown in many cases. In some *Aplysia* neurones a strong response to InsP3 injection has been observed only at distances 120–160 μm below the surface (Levy, 1992). In snail neurones Ca^{2+}-induced Ca^{2+} release was predominant in peripheral cytosol, whereas InsP3 evoked a Ca^{2+} release around the nucleus (Kostyuk and Kirischuk, 1993). The stores are not overlapping or only partially overlapping in adrenal chromaffin cells (Liu *et*

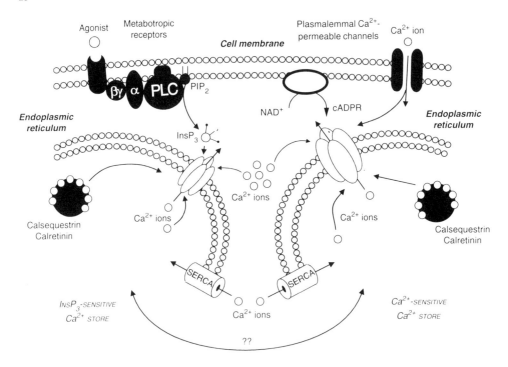

Figure 2.1. Conceptual scheme of Ca^{2+} liberation mechanisms from the internal calcium stores in eukaryotic cells (from Kostyuk and Verkhiatsky, 1994 with permission). Intracellular calcium stores are equipped with calcium (SERCA) pumps, Ca^{2+}-binding proteins (calsequestrin, calretinin, etc.) and two distinct sets of Ca^{2+} release channels. The activity of these channels is controlled by either $InsP_3$ ($InsP_3$-gated channels) or by cytoplasmic Ca^{2+} ions (Ca^{2+}-gated channels). Both types of channel also undergo feedback control by cytoplasmic Ca^{2+} being activated at low and moderate $[Ca^{2+}]_i$ and blocked at high $[Ca^{2+}]_i$. The activity of the Ca^{2+}-gated Ca^{2+} release channel might be also controlled by the newly discovered intracellular second messenger cyclic ADP-ribose (cADPR). The synthesis of cADPR from NAD^+ is triggered by ADP-ribosyl cyclase (ADPRC)

al., 1991; Robinson and Burgoyne, 1991). A distinct separation of both release mechanisms is obvious also from studies of their presence in different brain structures using immunohistochemical methods: in cortical cells $InsP_3$-gated channels were found in cell bodies and proximal dendrites, Ca^{2+}-gated ones in apical dendrites, etc. (Sharp *et al.*, 1993a, 1993b). Biochemical investigation of the distribution of the $InsP_3$- and Ca^{2+}- gated Ca^{2+} release channels in rat cerebellum microsomes shows that vesicles bearing the $InsP_3$-gated channel are separated from those bearing the Ca^{2+}-gated channel, which may suggest that the ER is not a homogeneous entity, and that Ca^{2+} stores are heterogeneous: $InsP_3$- and Ca^{2+}-sensitive Ca^{2+} release channels are segregated either to discrete intracellular organelles or to specialized ER subcompartments (Villa *et al.*, 1992, Nori *et al.*, 1993).

This clear separation of $InsP_3$- and Ca^{2+}-sensitive internal pools led to a several years discussion around the issue of whether the $InsP_3$-sensitive stores belong to the ER compartments or $InsP_3$-gated Ca^{2+} release channels are settled in a specialized organelle called a 'calciosome' (Rossier and Putney, 1991; Volpe *et al.*, 1988). However, a number of observations showing a functional overlap between two release mechanisms have appeared recently (Irving *et al.*, 1992a; Reber *et al.*, 1993). In addition, blockade of SERCA pumps by thapsigargin abolishes the InsP$_3$-mediated Ca^{2+} release in neural cells (Irving *et al.*, 1992b), suggesting therefore the ER origin of this pool. Careful and detailed analysis of the distribution of ER-related proteins in cerebellar Purkinje neurones revealed that both InsP$_3$- and Ca^{2+}-gated Ca^{2+} release channels as well as SERCA pumps and Ca^{2+}-binding proteins are ER-resident proteins which are present in ER compartments that may be anatomically segregated (Takei *et al.*, 1992; Villa *et al.*, 1991; Walton *et al.*, 1991). It seems that both types of calcium store are actually coupled with ER and they may or may not communicate with each other in various types of cells. It should be noted that at least in chromaffin cells the presence of a third type of store, highly sensitive to both InsP$_3$- and caffeine-ryanodine (selective probes for Ca^{2+}-gated channels), has been postulated (Stauderman and Murawsky, 1991; Stauderman *et al.*, 1991; Zacchetti *et al.*, 1991).

Second messengers regulate the open probability of appropriate Ca^{2+} release channels, thus changing the conductance of the ER membrane for Ca^{2+}. The availability of Ca^{2+} stores for Ca^{2+} release is controlled by both ER membrane Ca^{2+} conductance and the amount of releasable Ca^{2+} inside the ER lumen. The concentration of releasable Ca^{2+} is determined by the activity of SERCA pumps and can also involve the activation of additional Ca^{2+} influx from extracellular space via Ca^{2+} release-activated Ca^{2+} channels (Hoth and Penner, 1992). The direct refilling of Ca^{2+} stores from the extracellular space (Putney, 1986) or the preferential location of SERCA-rich parts of ER in close proximity with plasmalemmal Ca^{2+} channels (Reber *et al.*, 1993) have also been suggested.

ER Ca^{2+} ACCUMULATION: SERCA PUMPS

Most eukaryotic cells coexpress plasmalemmal Ca^{2+} pumps and the SERCA pumps. Up to now at least three different mammalian SERCA genes have been described, and it appears that SERCA 1 pumps are localized almost exclusively in fast-twitch skeletal muscles, while SERCA 2 are widespread in various tissues; the significance of the SERCA 3 pumps is less clear (Brandl *et al.*, 1986; Korczak *et al.*, 1987; Burk *et al.*, 1989). The SERCA 1 pump exists in two isoforms, resulting from alternative splicing; SERCA 1b isoform is present in neonatal tissues, and during development it is replaced with SERCA 1a (Brandl *et al.*, 1986). SERCA 2 proteins also exist in two distinct isoforms: SERCA 2a, which is predominantly expressed in cardiac and smooth muscle, and SERCA 2b, which seems to be the major form in brain tissue (Plessers *et al.*, 1991). It seems that SERCA pumps are differentially regulated by cytoplasmic and intraluminal Ca^{2+}: the increase of [Ca^{2+}]$_i$ activates Ca^{2+} pumping into the ER, while increase of luminal free Ca^{2+} content inhibits SERCA pumps. SERCA pumps are effectively and selectively blocked by thapsigargin in nanomolar concentrations (Thastrup *et al.*, 1990; Lytton *et al.*, 1991) and by micromolar concentrations of cyclopyasonic acid (Seidler *et al.*, 1989). Recently, 4-aminopyridine also was found to be a relatively specific inhibitor of the SERCA pump (Ishida and Honda, 1993).

The functional topology of all SERCA pump isoforms is quite similar (MacLennan *et al.*, 1985; Toyoshima *et al.*, 1993): they have a huge cytoplasmic domain, the intramembrane portion, comprised of 10 putative membrane-spanning domains and a small luminal domain. Transmembrane domains M4, M6 and M9 are critically important for Ca^{2+} transport, as shown by specific mutations (Clarke *et al.*, 1989a, 1989b). Transmembrane Ca^{2+} transfer starts from the binding of two Ca^{2+} ions to the high-affinity site on the cytoplasmic portion of the SERCA pumps, with subsequent ATP-dependent phosphorylation and conformational change of the pump molecule which caused Ca^{2+} translocation to the luminal domain. Further on, Ca^{2+} is released inside the ER lumen from the low-affinity binding site on the luminal part of the SERCA pump.

ER CALCIUM STORAGE: Ca^{2+}-BINDING PROTEINS

The ability of internal calcium pools to accumulate and store Ca^{2+} ions is determined mainly by the existence of intraluminal low-affinity, high-capacity Ca^{2+}-binding proteins. Although the ER contains a number of proteins with Ca^{2+}-binding capabilities, the most important are calsequestrin and calreticulin. Both of them have a high capacity (25–50 M Ca^{2+} per mole of protein) and a low affinity, with K_D for Ca^{2+} in the range of 1–4 mM (see Pozzan *et al.*, 1994 for review). Calsequestrin (molecular weight 43–45 kDa) is present in two major isoforms, skeletal and cardiac; these isoforms are the product of two distinct genes and show 65% homology. So far, in nervous tissue calsequestrin was found only in avian cerebellar Purkinje neurones (e.g. Takei *et al.*, 1992). In contrast, members of the calreticulin family (molecular weight ~46 kDa) are widely expressed in nervous cells (Michalak *et al.*, 1992). The nature of calreticulin diversity (different genes/alternative splicing, etc.) is not yet understood. Neuronal ER appears to contain a significant density of calreticulins forming an intraluminal matrix, which actually serves as a Ca^{2+} reservoir.

Another class of possible Ca^{2+}-binding proteins are the recently discovered reticuloplasmins (endoplasmin, BiP, protein disulphide isomerase (PID), which also possess low Ca^{2+} affinity (K_D ~1 mM). However, it is still unclear whether reticuloplasmins are indeed involved in Ca^{2+} storage within ER lumen, or whether they participate in the turnover of other intra-ER proteins (Pozzan *et al.*, 1994).

Calcium storage within the ER lumen may also be achieved by integral proteins of the ER membrane (calnexin and signal sequence receptor) which protrude into the ER lumen. A newly discovered ER protein, reticulocalbin, which has four Ca^{2+} high-affinity sites, may also be involved in the handling of intra-ER Ca^{2+} ions.

ER CALCIUM RELEASE: Ca^{2+} RELEASE CHANNELS

Calcium release channels of the ER belong to ligand-gated Ca^{2+}-permeable channels and include two distinct protein subclasses encoded by two gene families. These channels are activated by two intracellular messengers, namely $InsP_3$ and Ca^{2+} ions, being thus classified as $InsP_3$-gated and Ca^{2+}-gated channels. From the functional point of view Ca^{2+}-gated channels are responsible for the generation of Ca^{2+}-induced Ca^{2+} release (CICR), while InsP3-gated channels are responsible for the development of the InsP3-induced Ca^{2+} release (IICR). In fact, this discrimination remains somewhat semantic, particularly taking into account depolarization-induced Ca^{2+} release in skeletal muscle or dual regulation of InsP3-gated Ca^{2+} release channels by both InsP3 and cytoplasmic Ca^{2+} concentration. However, for clarity we will term Ca^{2+}-gated Ca^{2+} release channels as CICR channels and InsP3-gated channels as IICR channels.

Ca^{2+}-GATED Ca^{2+} RELEASE CHANNELS

Molecular architecture

The purification and characterization of CICR channels was greatly facilitated after the discovery of the plant alkaloid ryanodine (Jenden and Fairhurst, 1969), which appeared to be a selective and specific probe for these channels. Using specific binding of ryanodine, CICR channels were isolated from various tissues. Due to the high selectivity of Ca^{2+} release channels to ryanodine they have been termed and are now commonly known as a ryanodine receptors (RYRs). It is widely accepted now that RYRs/CICR channels belong to a protein family encoded by at least three distinct genes.

Using binding with [^{3}H]ryanodine, CICR channels which retain their functional activity were purified from mammalian skeletal and cardiac muscle, and later from mammalian brain (see Meissner, 1994; Furuichi et al., 1994b for review). Density gradient centrifugation of the solubilized protein revealed a 30 S protein complex, which consists (as was found using gel electrophoresis) of 560 kDa monomers. Such a structure was consistent for RYRs obtained from all tissues. Expression of mRNA or cDNA encoding RYRs in an artificial system suggests that 560 kDa protein is sufficient to form a functional channel with conserved sensitivity to ryanodine, caffeine and Ca^{2+}.

The functional CICR channel is a tetramer, which was demonstrated by scanning transmission electron microscopy studies. The CICR channel complex was found to be a four-leaf clover structure with plane dimensions of 27×27 nm and a central hole of ~2 nm in diameter. This structure seems to span the ER membrane and has a length of 14 nm (Radermacher et al., 1992).

The primary structure of CICR channels was determined using cDNA cloning and sequencing. The molecular cloning revealed the existence of several different RYRs/CICR channel isoforms (see Fig. 2.2) encoded by three distinct genes. These isoforms correspond to the skeletal (or RYR1), cardiac (RYR2) and brain (RYR3) subtypes of the CICR channel. The cDNAs for RYR1 and RYR2 isoforms of Ca^{2+} release channels have been cloned from rabbit and human (Takeshima et al., 1989; Zorzato et al., 1990; Otsu et al., 1990) preparations, and functional expression of Ca^{2+}-gated Ca^{2+} release channels was achieved in a model cellular system transfected by cDNA (Chen et al., 1993).

The cardiac isoform of the CICR channel appeared to be the most abundant, being expressed not only in the heart, but also in many other tissues; expression of the skeletal muscle isoform is restricted almost exclusively to skeletal myocytes (although recently evidence has appeared indicating relatively high expression of the RYR1 isoform in cerebellar Purkinje neurones (Kuwajima et al., 1992). The third subtype of

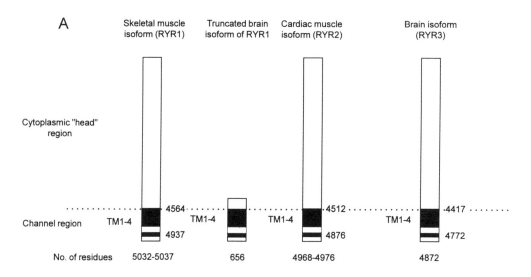

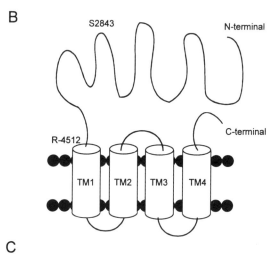

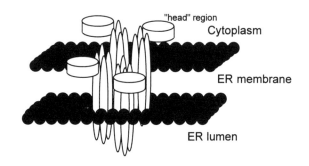

CICR channel (RYR3) was first detected in an epithelial cell line treated with transforming growth factor $\beta1$ (Giannini *et al.*, 1992); later its expression was also demonstrated in a variety of brain regions (Hakamata *et al.*, 1992). All three CICR channels show high homology, with 66–70% identity in the primary structure.

The skeletal muscle isoform of the CICR channel from rabbit preparation is comprised of 5037 amino acids (Takeshima *et al.*, 1989), while the same isoform found in human skeletal muscle is five amino acids shorter (5032 residues) (Zorzato *et al.*, 1990). The CICR channel has a long cytoplasmic N-terminal which forms a 'head' of the channel, and a C-terminal which anchors the channel in the ER membrane. Near the C-terminal 4–12 transmembrane domains, which actually form the channel pore, are located. Several (at least three) high-affinity Ca^{2+}-binding sites, as well as a number of low-affinity Ca^{2+}-binding sites, have been also localized.

The large cytoplasmic portion was postulated to form a 'foot' structure, which connects the ER channel with plasmalemmal voltage-operated Ca^{2+} channels and underlies the depolarization-triggered activation of the skeletal isoform of the CICR channel.

The cardiac isoform of the CICR channel (determined by cDNA cloning—Otsu *et al.*, 1990; Nakai *et al.*, 1990) consists of 4969–4976 amino acid residues, and its primary structure is 66% homologous to that of skeletal isoform; similarly the functional cardiac CICR channel has a quarterfold structure. The cardiac isoform also has a large cytoplasmic N-terminal, however, it lacks the 'foot' structure, thus functioning as an exclusively Ca^{2+}-gated channel.

In addition to these two types of Ca^{2+}-gated Ca^{2+} release channels, the third type of Ca^{2+} release channel was identified recently and was shown to be a novel gene product (Hakamata *et al.*, 1992; Sorrentino and Volpe, 1993). The brain isoform of CICR channel (RYR3) was cloned from rabbit brain. The brain isoform has 4872 amino acids; and its sequence is 67% identical to the skeletal isoform and 70% identical to the cardiac isoform of CICR channel (Hakamata *et al.*, 1992). The most distinct functional feature of the RYR3 is its insensitivity to caffeine (Giannini *et al.*, 1992).

Recently the truncated form of the skeletal subtype of CICR channel, which comprises only 656 amino acids, has been found in rabbit brain (Takeshima *et al.*, 1993). This short isoform of the ryanodine receptor contains transmembrane domains as well as Ca^{2+}-binding sites and presumably may form a functional Ca^{2+} release channel.

Functional characterization

Apart from the structural variability between the three CICR channels isoforms, they also show distinct differences in mechanisms of activation. The skeletal muscle Ca^{2+}

Figure 2.2. Molecular architecture of Ca^{2+}-gated Ca^{2+} release channel/ryanodine receptor isoforms. (A) Schematic representation of the primary structure of three major forms of CICR channels/ryanodine receptors. The channel domain is denoted by grey shading; the pore region is presumably located between putative transmembrane domains 3 and 4. (B) Schematic topology of a monomer of the CICR channel/ryanodine receptor. The large cytoplasmic portion contains ~80% of the molecule and protrudes into the cytoplasm. (C) Topology of the functional tetrameric CICR channel/ryanodine receptor

release channel (RYR1) is coupled directly to the plasmalemmal high-voltage-activated (L-type) Ca^{2+} channels through the 'foot' structure, thus forming a functionally active structure—the 'triade'. In skeletal muscle the plasmalemmal depolarization directly activates Ca^{2+} release from sarcoplasmic reticulum, due to the fact that plasmalemmal Ca^{2+} channels serve as a voltage sensor, transducing the activating signal directly to the Ca^{2+} release channel via the foot structure (Rios and Pizarro, 1991). Therefore, the skeletal muscle Ca^{2+} stores possess the depolarization-induced mechanisms of Ca^{2+} release. In contrast, cardiac and brain isoforms of CICR channels are not connected with the plasmalemma, and they require an increase in $[Ca^{2+}]_i$ as an appropriate stimulus.

All isoforms of Ca^{2+}-gated Ca^{2+} release channels belong to cation-selective channels which are characterized by a very high conductance for both monovalent (up to 600–750 pS for Na^+ and K^+) and divalent (100–150 pS for Ca^{2+}) cations. The conductance and basic properties of single Ca^{2+} release channels were initially estimated on sarcoplasmic vesicles from skeletal (Smith *et al.*, 1986) and cardiac (Rousseau *et al.*, 1986) muscles as well as on specially designed 'sarcoballs' from native skeletal muscle (Stein and Palade, 1988). Similarly the initial recordings of single-channel properties of Ca^{2+}-gated Ca^{2+} release channels have been performed on brain microsomes (Ashley, 1989).

Properties of elementary currents through Ca^{2+}-gated Ca^{2+} release channels have been studied on purified channels, incorporated into planar membranes. The single-channel behaviour for the Ca^{2+}-gated Ca^{2+} release channel isolated from various tissues appeared to be quite similar (Ashley, 1989; Anderson *et al.*, 1989; Herrman–Frank *et al.*, 1991; see also Meissner, 1994 for review); all of them are highly selective for cations over anions. Divalent cations pass the channel in the order $Ba^{2+} > Ca^{2+} > Sr^{2+} > Mg^{2+}$. Both microsomal and purified Ca^{2+} release channels display multiple (usually three to four) conductance levels, the most frequently observed single-channel conductance being 100–150 pS (at 50 mM of Ca^{2+} from the *trans* side). Multiple conductances were also found, while monovalent cations were used as the main conducting ions (Smith *et al.*, 1988). These multiple conductances may indicate either the functional assembling of four individual monomers of the channel each with its own single conductance, or several discrete conductance states within a single conducting pore formed by the RYR tetramer. The kinetic properties of the CICR single-channel currents are also quite variable: the channel can be opened as a single event as well as bursts of openings; elementary opening times vary between hundreds of microseconds and tens of milliseconds.

The open probability of the CICR channels is regulated by cytoplasmic Ca^{2+} concentration, as well as by other divalent cations and adenine nucleotides. Both Ca^{2+} efflux from sarcoplasmic reticulum (SR) or ER vesicles and open probability of purified CICR channels possess a bell-shaped activation curve by cytoplasmic (which corresponds to *cis* Ca^{2+} in bilayer experiments) calcium. The mean open probability (P_o) of the Ca^{2+}-gated Ca^{2+} release channel is close to zero at nanomolar free Ca^{2+} at the *cis* side; P_o increases substantially at a $[Ca^{2+}]_i$ between 0.1 and 1 μM, while higher levels of $[Ca^{2+}]_i$ ($> 10\ \mu M$) inhibit channel opening. This dual control of calcium release channel by cytoplasmic calcium was found for both RYR1 and RYR2 isoforms (Smith *et al.*, 1986; Bezprozvanny *et al.*, 1991). Such a bell-shaped regulation suggests the existence of at least two Ca^{2+} binding sites responsible for channel gating in the structure of the CICR channel molecule. Other divalent cations also affect CICR channel opening. Cytoplasmic Sr^{2+} activates the CICR channel, whereas Ba^{2+} and Mg^{2+} inhibit CICR channel opening, as well as Ca^{2+}-induced Ca^{2+} release.

Regulation of channel activity

Adenine nucleotides (AMP-PCP, AMP, ADP, cADP, adenosine and ATP) also activate CICR channels in the absence of Ca^{2+} ions, and strongly potentiate Ca^{2+}-dependent activation, presumably due to specific binding to the adenine regulatory site (located at residues 4345–4350 in the RYR2 isoform of the CICR channel (Otsu *et al.*,1990). Among them ATP is the most potent activator of the CICR channel. The maximal potentiating effect of ATP was observed at millimolar concentrations (Meissner, 1994).

Apart from these known adenine nucleotides, the newly discovered endogenous substance cyclic ADP-ribose (cADPR) appears to be a candidate for a specific intracellular second messenger controlling the availability of cardiac and brain Ca^{2+}-gated Ca^{2+} release channels (see chapter 4), although it is still unclear whether cADPR binds to its own site or interferes with the adenine regulatory site. In addition to cADPR, another endogenous substance—palmitoyl carnitine, the fatty acid meta-bolite—has been reported to directly activate Ca^{2+}-gated Ca^{2+} release channels from skeletal muscle SR at micromolar concentrations (El-Hayek *et al.*, 1993). Palmitoyl carnitine increased the open time of Ca^{2+} release channels incorporated into planar bilayers by factor of seven. It was suggested that in this way metabolism of fatty acids can modulate $[Ca^{2+}]_i$ in myocytes; moreover, this pathway could be involved in the development of muscle disorders in palmitoyl transferase II-deficient patients.

The activation of the Ca^{2+}-gated Ca^{2+} release channel is affected by caffeine and ryanodine. Caffeine (<5 mM) was found to shift the Ca^{2+} activation curve towards the lower $[Ca^{2+}]_i$ concentrations; at caffeine concentrations > 5 mM it opens the CICR channel in a Ca^{2+}-independent way (Sitsapesan and Williams, 1990). Ryanodine also demonstrates dual action on the CICR channel: at low concentrations (<10 μM) it locks the channel in the subconductance state and brings the channel opening probability to one, whereas at higher concentrations (~100 μM) ryanodine blocks channel openings. This dual regulation by ryanodine is consistent with biochemically determined two ryanodine-binding sites with high (K_D ~5-10 nM) and low (K_D ~3 μM) affinities.

The elementary CICR channel currents are also influenced by pH (inhibition of channel openings upon pH lowering) as well as by anion composition and ionic strength of solutions (see Meissner, 1994 for review). Recently the regulation of Ca^{2+}-gated Ca^{2+}-release channel openings by intraluminal calsequestrin was discovered (Kawasaki and Kasai, 1994), therefore suggesting a direct link between ER Ca^{2+} release channels and ER matrix. The opposite feedback was also suggested: based on investigations performed on SR vesicles Ikemoto *et al.* (1991) postulated that Ca^{2+} release triggers a signal leading to the dissociation of bound calcium from calsequestrin, thus supplying additional Ca^{2+}-releasable ions.

The functional activity of CICR channels is also regulated by phosphorylation. The preferred site for Ca^{2+}/calmodulin-dependent phosphorylation in the cardiac isoform of the CICR channel occurred at serine residue 2809; phosphorylation at this site was

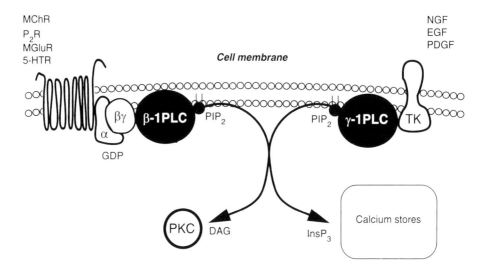

Figure 2.3. General pathways of InsP$_3$ generation in eukaryotic cells. The synthesis of InsP$_3$ is controlled by two classes of plasmalemmal receptors, namely by seven-spanning metabotropic receptors (glutamate: mGluRs 1–6; M-cholinoreceptors: MChR, predominantly M$_3$ subtype; purinoreceptors: P$_{2Y}$ and P$_{2U}$; serotonin receptors: 5-HTR) and by tyrosine kinase (TK; coupled with growth factor receptors). Both metabotropic receptors and tyrosine kinase control the activity of certain isoforms of phospholipase C (PLC; β-1PLC isoform for metabotropic receptors and γ-1 PLC isoform for tyrosine kinase). Metabotropic receptors are coupled with PLC by intramembrane transducing G proteins (composed of α and βγ subunits). PLC hydrolyses membrane-associated PIP$_2$, forming InsP$_3$ and DAG. DAG controls the activity of intracellular protein kinase C (PKC) while InsP$_3$ acts via Ca^{2+} ion liberation from the internal stores

reported to activate the channel (Witcher *et al.*, 1991). Dephosphorylation of the skeletal muscle isoform of the CICR channel by endogenous Ca^{2+}-dependent protease calpain inhibits its openings. In addition both skeletal and cardiac isoforms are inhibited by calmodulin, which directly interacts with channel protein.

INSP$_3$-GATED Ca^{2+} RELEASE CHANNELS

InsP$_3$-gated ER channels are activated by second messenger InsP$_3$, which is produced by phospholipase C. This enzyme is a part of the phosphoinositide signal transduction cascade, represented by two major pathways (Fig. 2.3). Firstly these are plasmalemmal 'metabotropic' receptors which have the common seven-membrane-spanning segments structure, and are linked to the β1 isoform of phospholipase C. These receptors are represented by isoforms of metabotropic glutamate (mGluR1–6), metabotropic purinoreceptors, muscarinic-cholinoreceptors and serotonin (5-hydroxytryptamine, 5-HT) receptors. The second major pathway is associated with tyrosine kinase receptors, coupled with the γ1 subtype of phospholipase C. These receptors are involved in signal transduction activated by numerical growth factors (e.g. nerve, epidermal or platelet-derived growth factors).

Having been activated, phospholipase C triggers the hydrolysis of the membrane-associated phosphatidylinositol bisphosphate (PIP2), producing inositol 1,4,5-trisphosphate (InsP3) and diacylglycerol (DAG), which both represent the phosphoinositide second messenger system. While DAG affects the activity of protein kinase C, InsP3 triggers Ca^{2+} liberation from the ER stores via activation of the InsP3-gated Ca^{2+} release channel.

InsP3-gated Ca^{2+} release channels, like CICR channels, belong to a distinct gene family, and so far at least three isoforms of IICR channel have been fully characterized, and one form (discovered by polymerase chain reaction technique on brain tissue) remains as yet uncharacterized at the molecular level. Further variability in the IICR channel family arise from alternative splicing in several regions which produces several additional subtypes.

Molecular architecture

The structure of InsP3-gated Ca^{2+} release channels is quite similar to Ca^{2+}-gated release channels, although InsP3 channels are substantially smaller. The InsP3-gated Ca^{2+} release channel is also thought to be a homotetramer (the molecular weight of single monomer is in the region of 260 kDa) with four transmembrane regions.

Historically, InsP3 receptors were first discovered as so-called P_{400} proteins in Purkinje neurones (Mikoshiba et al., 1985) and later their identity with InsP3-gated Ca^{2+} release channels was shown (Maeda et al., 1989; Maeda et al., 1990). Subsequently, InsP3-gated Ca^{2+} release channels were detected in SR (Ehrlich and Watras, 1988). They were half-maximally activated by 15 μM InsP3 and blocked by ruthenium red and La^{3+} (Suarez-Isla et al., 1991). Later they were also purified from the brain of mammals and their amino acid sequence has been determined.

The most abundant isoform of the IICR channel is the so-called InsP3R1 isoform which was cloned from mammalian brain and comprises 2749 amino acid residues (Mignery et al., 1990; for the structure of InsP3-gated channels see also the review by Furuichi et al. ,1994b). This form is in fact a subject for alternative splicing in two regions, so it actually represents a whole group of IICR channels. Similarly to the RYRs/CICR channels, InsP3-gated channels have a large cytoplasmic 'head' part, which contains the InsP3-binding site (Fig. 2.4), a relatively small channel-forming part (residues 2276-2589) represented by six membrane-spanning domains and the so-called modulatory and transducing domain, which appears to be a site for action of various modulatory molecules. This part of the InsP3-gated channel is believed to transduce signals arising from the ligand-binding to the channel domain, finally converting it into the channel opening. Other intracellular messenger molecules, such as cAMP-dependent protein kinases, calmodulin and adenine nucleotides, also have targets on the modulatory and transducing domain, affecting the functional properties of the InsP3-gated channel. This domain also has a Ca^{2+}-binding site located between residues 1961 and 2219, which presumably is involved in Ca^{2+} control of the InsP3 receptor.

The second isoform of the InsP3-gated channel, InsP3R2, has been cloned from mammalian brain and human cell lines (Sudhof et al., 1991; Furuichi et al., 1994b). It comprises 2701 amino acids and displays 70% homology with InsP3R1. The affinity of the ligand-binding site of the InsP3R2 is somewhat higher as compared with InsP3R1.

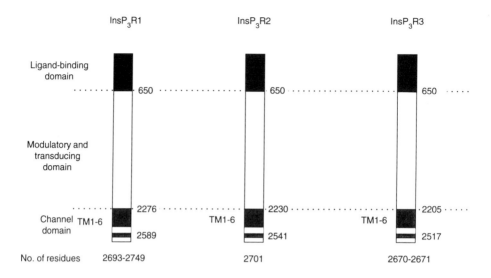

Figure 2.4. Molecular architecture of InsP$_3$-gated Ca^{2+} release channel isoforms. Schematic representation of the primary structure of three major forms of CICR channels/ryanodine receptors. The channel domain is denoted by grey shading; the pore region is located between putative transmembrane domains 3 and 4

The third isoform, InsP$_3$R3, contains 2670 or 2671 amino acid residues and it was cloned from rat and human cell lines (Blondel *et al.*, 1993; Furuichi *et al.*, 1994b). This isoform (or at least a truncated part of it) was shown to bind not only InsP$_3$ but also InsP$_4$ and InsP$_6$. The functional InsP$_3$-gated Ca^{2+} release channel is composed from four monomers, and demonstrates the similar tetra-leaf structure as was found for RYRs.

Functional properties

The single-channel properties of the neuronal InsP$_3$-gated Ca^{2+} release channels have been studied in purified cerebellar microsomal proteins, incorporated into lipid membranes. The conductance of InsP$_3$-gated release channels has been estimated at 10-26 pS, being thus four times smaller compared with the Ca^{2+}-gated Ca^{2+} release channel; they also show multiple conductance states (about four) (Bezprozvanny *et al.*, 1991; Maeda *et al.*, 1991). Binding of InsP$_3$ to the channel causes its opening; however, in addition to InsP$_3$ the activity of IICR channels is regulated by cytoplasmic Ca^{2+}. This regulation appears to be biphasic: at a constant InsP$_3$ level Ca^{2+} concentrations below 300 nM enhance channel activity, while higher Ca^{2+} concentrations inhibit channel openings (Bezprozvanny *et al.*, 1991; Iino and Tsulioka, 1994). This means that at constant cytosolic InsP$_3$ concentrations a local increase of [Ca^{2+}]$_i$ may trigger Ca^{2+} release from InsP$_3$-sensitive stores, thus converting IICR into CICR. The increase of [Ca^{2+}]$_i$ to levels higher than 1 μM causes a sharp decrease of the open probability of the cerebellar InsP$_3$-gated Ca^{2+} release channel (Bezprozvanny *et al.*, 1991). Interestingly, the kinetics of the potentiating and inhibitory effects of Ca^{2+} ions appear to be different: the stimulating effect develops very fast, while the onset of the suppressing effects of high Ca^{2+} concentrations is much slower (Iino and Tsulioka, 1994). The molecular mechanism of the Ca^{2+}-mediated regulation of $InsP_3$-gated channels is still unclear; however, it has been shown that Ca^{2+} ions at 100 nM concentration enhance the affinity of the $InsP_3$-binding site, while at high Ca^{2+} concentration the low-affinity site for $InsP_3$ (which does not open the channel) is activated (Migneri et al., 1992). It has also been demonstrated that at concentrations greater than 300 nM Ca^{2+} ions inhibit $InsP_3$ binding to its receptor (Worley et al., 1987). This immediate $[Ca^{2+}]_i$-dependent feedback has been suggested as an important determinant of the time course of Ca^{2+} release (Iino and Endo, 1992). Interestingly, the Ca^{2+}-dependent modulation of $InsP_3$ binding to the IICR channel disappears while purifying the $InsP_3$-gated channel (Supattapone et al., 1988). Later the involvement of the specific Ca^{2+}-binding protein (calmedin) in the Ca^{2+}-induced modulation of $InsP_3$ binding was demonstrated (Danoff et al., 1988).

Luminal Ca^{2+} also has been proposed to regulate the sensitivity of IICR channels to $InsP_3$ and perhaps thereby contribute to the mechanisms responsible for regenerative intracellular Ca^{2+} signals. The increase of luminal Ca^{2+} concentration was reported to facilitate $InsP_3$ binding to ER channels (Oldershaw and Taylor, 1993). The efficacy of $InsP_3$-mediated Ca^{2+} release increases when releasable Ca^{2+} content in stores is higher; and vice versa, when stores are empty $InsP_3$-gated Ca^{2+} release channels are reluctant to open, therefore allowing Ca^{2+} accumulation (Nunn and Taylor, 1992; Taylor, 1992).

Another interesting feature of the IICR is the so-called 'quantal' Ca^{2+} liberation from the $InsP_3$-releasable stores. While monitoring Ca^{2+} release it was found that submaximal concentration of $InsP_3$ releases only part of the Ca^{2+} accumulated in the store. Successive application of higher concentrations of $InsP_3$ would induce greater calcium release (Muallem et al., 1989; Taylor and Potter, 1990). In contrast, experiments on single purified IICR channels did not reveal any prominent desensitization of the receptor; it has been found that the open probability of the channels simply increased with increasing $InsP_3$ concentration. Therefore, assuming $InsP_3$-gated channels will be constantly open in the presence of $InsP_3$, the stores must be eventually depleted regardless of the agonist concentration. Contrary to this assumption, submaximal concentrations of $InsP_3$ are able to release only a fraction of stored Ca^{2+}. Such behaviour may be explained in terms of an additional mechanism which controls the availability of the $InsP_3$-gated channel. Several hypotheses have been proposed (Missiaen et al., 1994; Bootman, 1994), including possible desensitization of the $InsP_3$ receptor, subcompartmentalization of the ER stores into distinct parts bearing receptors with different affinity to $InsP_3$ and finally Ca^{2+} control of IICR channel availability. Bearing in mind that both intraluminal and cytoplasmic Ca^{2+} affects IICR channel openings, the last hypothesis seems to be preferable.

It seems that $InsP_3$-gated Ca^{2+} release channels can also be modulated by phosphorylation/dephosphorylation: the cerebellar $InsP_3$ receptor appears to be a substrate for Ca^{2+}-activated neutral protease (calpain) (Magnusson et al., 1993). Activation of the $InsP_3$ receptor, by causing an increase in $[Ca^{2+}]_i$, might result in degradation of the $InsP_3$-binding part of the receptor, therefore developing a negative feedback. In addition, purified $InsP_3$ receptors can be phosphorylated by cAMP-dependent protein kinase, protein kinase C (PK-C) and Ca^{2+}-calmodulin-dependent protein kinase (Ferris and Snyder, 1992; Marshall and Taylor, 1993). Indeed, the

PK-C-dependent downregulation of the InsP$_3$-mediated Ca^{2+} release mechanism was demonstrated in chick sensory neurones (Mironov, 1994b).

An important recent finding is a blocking effect of caffeine in InsP$_3$-gated channels from cerebellar microsomes. At a concentration of 5 mM it increased the closed time of the channel 3.3-fold, with little effect on the mean open time. Increase in InsP$_3$ to 20 μM partially reversed the effect (Bezprozvannaya et al., 1994). Furthermore, caffeine was reported to block InsP$_3$ production in mouse pancreatic acinar cells, which might be another pathway for influencing IICR (Toescu et al., 1992). Thus the action of caffeine on Ca^{2+} release must be considered with some caution. A similar warning has appeared recently concerning the validity of fura-2-based measurements of InsP$_3$-mediated Ca^{2+} release: it was demonstrated (Richardson and Taylor, 1993) that InsP$_3$ binding to the cerebellar Ca^{2+} release channel was competitively inhibited by fura-2 (with IC$_{50}$ ~120 μM) as well as BAPTA (IC$_{50}$ ~340 μM) and ethylenediaminetetraacetic acid (EDTA) (IC$_{50}$ ~8.7 mM).

PHARMACOLOGICAL MODULATORS OF Ca^{2+} RELEASE CHANNELS

The ER Ca^{2+} release channels are the targets for various pharmacological substances which are summarized in Table 2.1.

Pharmacology of CICR channels/RYRs

Ryanodine

Ryanodine is a plant alkaloid (Jenden and Fairhurst, 1969) which binds specifically to the Ca^{2+}-gated Ca^{2+} release channels of SR and ER and substantially modulates its function (Fill and Coronado, 1988; Nagasaki and Fleishner, 1988; see also review by Ogawa, 1994). The binding of ryanodine to the channel is reported to be use-dependent: ryanodine preferentially binds to the open channel (Nagasaki and Fleishner, 1988). Following binding, ryanodine in 1-10 μM concentrations locks the channel in a subconductance state (with a preferential conductance of around 40 ps Rousseau et al., 1987) that causes the inhibition of both Ca^{2+}- and caffeine-mediated calcium release due to the prevention of Ca^{2+} accumulation by internal stores; or, at higher concentrations (around 50 - 100 μM) induces blockade of the Ca^{2+}-activated Ca^{2+} release channel (McPherson et al., 1991). For skeletal and heart muscles positive cooperativity of ryanodine binding to the Ca^{2+} release channel has been reported; the Ca^{2+} release channel appears to have two ryanodine-binding sites with K_D 5-10 nM and ~3 μM, respectively. Ryanodine binding to the high-affinity site stabilizes channels in the open state, while occupation of the low-affinity site locks the channels in the closed state (McGrew et al., 1989). In both peripheral and central neurones ryanodine treatment completely and irreversibly blocked the caffeine-induced [Ca^{2+}]$_i$ transients. In cultured bovine chromaffin cells ryanodine at concentrations of 0.4 - 50 μM suppressed caffeine-mediated [Ca^{2+}]$_i$ elevation and catecholamine secretion (Teraoka et al., 1991). At similar concentrations (0.1-100 μM) ryanodine inhibited caffeine-evoked [Ca^{2+}]$_i$ transients in cultured rat sensory (Usachev et al., 1993), hippocampal, neocortical and nucleus cuneatus (Shmigol et al., 1994a) neurones as well

Table 2.1. Pharmacology of Ca^{2+} release channels

Substance	Channel isoform	Effective concentration	Action	References
RyRs/CICR channels				
Endogeneous modulators				
cADPR	RYRs2,3	$K_D \sim 18$ nM	↑	Galione (1993, 1994)
Fatty acid metabolites	RYR1	10μM	↑	El-Hayek et al. (1993)
Exogeneous modulators				
Caffeine[a]	RyRs1,2	5–50 mM	↑	Sitsapesan and Williams (1990)
Ryanodine	RyRs1–3	< 10μM	↑	Sorrentino and Volpe (1993)
		10–100μM	↓	Ogawa (1994)
Procaine	RYRs1,2	1–5 mM	↓	Volpe et al. (1993)
Ruthenium red	RYRs1,2	10–100 μM	↓	Smith et al. (1988b)
Dantrolene	RYRs1,2	10–100μM	↓	Danko et al. (1985)
Brittotus hottentota toxin	RYR1	20–30 nM (K_D)	↑	Valdivia et al. (1991)
Imperatoxin 10.5 kDa	RYRs1,2	10 nM (EC$_{50}$)	↑	Valdivia et al. (1992)
Imperatoxin 8.7 kDa	RYRs1,2	6 nM (EC$_{50}$)	↑	
Digitoxin	RYR2	12.5 nM (K_D)	↑	Hymel et al. (1994)
Doxorubicin	RYR2	10 μM	↑↓	Ondrias et al. (1990)
InsP$_3$-gated (IICR) channels				
Heparin[b]	All types	1–10 μM	↓	Hill et al. (1987)
Timerosal[b]	All types	1–10 μM	↑	Tanaka and Tashjian (1994), Bird et al. (1993)
Adenophostin A,B	All types (?)	< 1 μM	↑	(Takahashi et al. (1993)

[a] May also inhibit InsP$_3$-gated channels.
[b] May also activate CICR channels.

as in mouse cortical neurones (Tsai and Barish, 1991; see also chapter 4). Recently basic ryanodine derivatives (amino- and guanidino-acrylryanodines) with enhanced affinity for SR Ca^{2+} release channels have been also described (Gerzon et al., 1993).

Ruthenium red

Ruthenium red has been reported to block opening of the purified muscle SR as well as cerebellar ER Ca^{2+}-gated Ca^{2+} release channels incorporated into lipid bilayers (Bezprozvanny et al., 1991; Smith et al., 1988). Ruthenium red effectively inhibited caffeine-induced $[Ca^{2+}]_i$ elevation in Purkinje neurones in slices (Kano et al., 1995); however, in bullfrog sympathetic neurones ruthenium red failed to inhibit caffeine-induced calcium release (Marrion and Adams, 1992). Ruthenium red, however, inhibits not only ER Ca^{2+} release channels but also mitochondrial Ca^{2+} transport (cf. Thayer and Miller, 1990).

Procaine

The local anaesthetic procaine is known to inhibit reversibly the Ca^{2+}-activated Ca^{2+} release in muscle fibres (Konishi and Kurihara, 1987) and in bullfrog sympathetic neurones (Marrion and Adams, 1992). In mammalian sensory and hippocampal neurones, similarly to the above-mentioned cells, procaine also caused an inhibition of caffeine-induced calcium release from internal stores (Usachev et al., 1993; Shmigol et al., 1994a).

Dantrolene

Dantrolene sodium is another compound known to be an effective modulator of caffeine-sensitive intracellular calcium stores. It has been reported that dantrolene sodium blocked Ca^{2+}-induced Ca^{2+} release from SR vesicles and caused inhibition of Ca^{2+} liberation from internal calcium stores in muscle fibres (Ohta and Ohga, 1990) and nerve cells (Thayer et al., 1988; Usachev et al., 1993).

Neurotoxins

Recently several new toxins reported to interact with Ca^{2+}-gated Ca^{2+} release channels have been purified and their activity was tested on SR Ca^{2+} release channels. A toxin with a molecular weight of 5–8 kDa purified from venom of the scorpion *Brithotus hottentota* opens Ca^{2+}-gated Ca^{2+} release channels with a K_D of 20-30 nM (Valdivia et al., 1991), while two other toxins obtained from the venom of the scorpion *Pandinus imperator* (imperatoxins) with molecular weights of 10.5 and 8.7 kDa exert a dual action on these channels: the first blocks them with an ED_{50} of ~10 nM, while the second activates them with an ED_{50} of 6 nM (Valdivia et al., 1992).

Cardiac glycosides

Surprisingly, one of the oldest known cardiac glycosides—digitoxin—appeared to bind with a K_D of ~12.5 nM to cardiac Ca^{2+}-gated Ca^{2+} release channels; moreover digitoxin caused Ca^{2+} release from cardiac Ca^{2+} stores (Hymel et al., 1994).

Doxorubicin

The action of another modulator—doxorubicin (Adriamycin, the well-known chemotherapeutic substance)—has been described in cardiac SR Ca^{2+} release channels (Ondrias et al.,1990). Treatment with doxorubicin caused initial activation of Ca^{2+}-gated Ca^{2+} release channels which changed to irreversible inhibition after several minutes incubation with doxorubicin.

Pharmacology of InsP$_3$-gated Ca^{2+} release channels

Two competitive antagonists of the InsP$_3$-gated channel have been described so far, namely heparin (Hill et al., 1987) and (possibly) decavanadate (Strupish et al., 1991), which are believed to compete with InsP$_3$ for binding site. Heparin effectively blocks the opening of cerebellar InsP$_3$-gated channels at micromolar concentrations (Bezprozvanny et al., 1991; Bezprozvanny and Ehrlich, 1993). Unfortunately, heparin can no longer be attributed as an absolutely selective blocker of the InsP$_3$-gated Ca^{2+} release channel: it was discovered recently that heparin activates CICR from SR vesicles and opens Ca^{2+}-gated Ca^{2+} release channels incorporated into bilayers (Ehrlich et al., 1994). The cross-sensitivity of Ca^{2+} release channels to heparin and caffeine substantially complicates the achievement of a clear separation between them under physiological conditions.

In addition, InsP$_3$-gated channels are reported to be inhibited by specific antibody 18A10 created against mammalian InsP$_3$ receptors. This antibody presumably interacts with the N-terminal portion of the InsP$_3$ receptor, and it effectively suppresses InsP$_3$-mediated Ca^{2+} release in cerebellar microsomes (see Myazaki, 1994 for review).

Another group of substances which can modulate InsP$_3$-gated Ca^{2+} release channels are the sulphydryl reagents. Initially, it was reported that one such reagent—timerosal—sensitizes the CICR mechanism and evokes spontaneous Ca^{2+} oscillation in hamster eggs (Swann, 1991); subsequently, however, other authors have reported that timerosal cannot distinguish between Ca^{2+}-sensitive and InsP$_3$-sensitive calcium stores (Tanaka and Tashjian, 1994). Recently two new, very potent (Ca^{2+}-releasing activity about 100 times higher as compared with InsP$_3$) agonists of the InsP$_3$-gated channels, adenophostin A and B, were obtained from fungi metabolites (Takahashi et al., 1993).

DISTRIBUTION OF Ca^{2+} RELEASE CHANNELS IN NERVOUS TISSUE

Using various types of morphological approaches (including immunocytochemistry and autoradiography) an uneven distribution of Ca^{2+}- and InsP$_3$-gated Ca^{2+} release channels has been found in the nervous system of mammals. All three isoforms of CICR channels have been found in the brain; however, the cardiac isoform appeared to be predominant. So far the RYR1 isoform of the CICR channel has been discovered only in cerebellar Purkinje neurones of mouse (Kuwajima *et al.*, 1992) and chick (Ouyang *et al.*, 1993). The precise localization of the truncated (656 residues) form of the RYR1 discovered in rabbit brain (Takeshima *et al.*, 1993) is not yet determined. In contrast, RYR2 isoform is expressed throughout the brain, including cerebral cortex, hippocampus, cerebellum, olfactory bulb, thalamus, hypothalamus, etc., with the highest expression in CA3/4 hippocampal regions, gyrus dentatus and cerebral cortex (Sharp *et al.*, 1993b; Sharp *et al.*, 1993a). In guinea-pig and rat cerebellum, RYR2 immunoreactivity was restricted to the soma and proximal dendrites of Purkinje cells. In the medulla, neurone somata in the hypoglossal nucleus were stained in both species, but in the dorsal motor nucleus of the vagus somata were stained in guinea-pigs but not in rats (Sah *et al.*, 1993). RYR3 isoform of CICR channels are predominantly localized in the CA1 region of the hippocampus, in striatum and dorsal thalamus (Furuichi *et al.*, 1994b). The immunoreactivity probes, however, are not extremely specific against various isoforms of RYRs/CICR channels, which led to some controversial results. Recently Furuichi and his coworkers (Furuichi *et al.*, 1994a) performed a comprehensive analysis of the distribution of RYRs isoform mRNA in rabbit brain using *in situ* hybridization with RYRs isoform-specific cDNA fragments. They confirmed that the most abundant mRNA belongs to the cardiac isoform of CICR channel (RYR1); however, mRNA of the skeletal isoform (RYR2) also appeared to be present in many brain regions, the highest expression being in cerebellar Purkinje and CA1 hippocampal neurones and with reasonable expression in some other regions. Certainly, the existence of mRNA does not necessarily mean the existence of a functionally active channel, the expression of skeletal RYRs and correspondingly of depolarization-induced Ca^{2+} release in nerve cells has to be taken into account in future experiments. The mRNA for the brain isoform of CICR channel (RYR3) was mainly restricted to CA1 hippocampal neurones, basal ganglia and dorsal thalamus. Interestingly, the mRNA for all three forms coexist in certain neurones, particularly in CA1 hippocampal neurones, which shows the high expression of all three mRNAs. This might be important for spatial aspects of $[Ca^{2+}]_i$ signalling, especially assuming the existence of ER subcompartments bearing different RYRs isoforms, which may determine their differential sensitivity to physiological stimulation.

The major type of InsP$_3$-gated Ca^{2+} release channel, namely InsP$_3$R1, is expressed throughout the brain, with predominant localization in cerebellar Purkinje cells, striatum, the CA1 region of the hippocampus and in cerebellar cortex. Expression of InsP$_3$R1 was also found in the vertebrate retina. InsP$_3$R2 was found to be highly expressed in brain glial cells and, to a lesser extent, in the spinal cord. The third isoform of the IICR channel, InsP$_3$R3, was found to be expressed in soma and axons of cerebellar granule cells, in synaptic terminals in thalamus, in the locus coeruleus and anterior olfactory nucleus (see Furuichi *et al.*, 1994b for references).

At the cellular level, both Ca^{2+}-gated and InsP$_3$-gated Ca^{2+} release channels are present in dendrites, cell bodies and synaptic terminals (Lai *et al.*, 1992), although the differential localization of CICR and IICR channels was found not only between different brain regions, but also within one cell. In the cortex, InsP$_3$-gated channels are found in pyramidal cell bodies and proximal dendrites, whereas ryanodine receptors are located predominantly in long, thin apical dendrites of pyramidal cells. In deep cerebellar nuclei, ryanodine receptors are located in cell bodies that appear devoid of

InsP$_3$-receptors, whereas InsP$_3$ receptors are enriched in terminals surrounding cell bodies. Electron microscopy in the hippocampus reveals ryanodine receptors in axons, dendritic spines, and dendritic shafts near dendritic spines, while InsP$_3$-receptors are primarily identified in dendritic shafts and cell bodies (Sharp *et al.*, 1993a, 1993b).

Functionally, both caffeine-mediated and InsP$_3$-mediated [Ca^{2+}]$_i$ release has been detected in all regions of neurones, including soma and neurites. However, the Ca^{2+}-gated and InsP$_3$-gated Ca^{2+} release channels can be unhomogeneously distributed within subcellular compartments. For instance, the ER localized in the dendritic spines of Purkinje neurones is primarily equipped with InsP$_3$-gated Ca^{2+} release channels but lacks both Ca^{2+}-gated release channels and the Ca^{2+} storage protein calsequestrin, whereas the juxtaspinal regions of dendrites are rich in all these components (Takei *et al.*, 1992). Antibodies against the cardiac type of Ca^{2+}-gated Ca^{2+} release channel stained mainly the somata of Purkinje neurones (Kuwajima *et al.*, 1992; Takei *et al.*, 1992). Within the spines [Ca^{2+}]$_i$ changes of intracellular origin are therefore probably different in mechanism (exclusively InsP$_3$-dependent) from those in the dendritic stalk.

CONCLUSIONS

Neural cells are equipped with specifically organized internal calcium stores, which are able to accumulate, store and release Ca^{2+} ions in response to appropriate stimulation. At the cellular level, these stores are connected to ER structures containing Ca^{2+}-binding proteins, SERCA pumps and Ca^{2+} release channels; they have been discovered in almost all parts of neuronal cells, including soma, axons, nerve terminals, dendrites and dendritic spines. At the molecular level Ca^{2+} release channels in fact represent a huge family of ER Ca^{2+}-permeable channels with different features and preferential sensitivity to either InsP$_3$ or Ca^{2+} ions. In addition, InsP$_3$ receptors are dually regulated by both cytosolic InsP$_3$ and Ca^{2+}. The distinct, unhomogeneous distribution of various subtypes of Ca^{2+} release channels within the brain regions and within single neurones is obviously very important for the formation of spatially and temporally organized [Ca^{2+}]$_i$ signals.

3 Temporal and Spatial Organization of Calcium Signal in Nerve Cells

Different stimuli which act on neuronal cells affect the cytoplasmic calcium concentration, thereby generating a $[Ca^{2+}]_i$ signal. As has already been mentioned at the beginning of this book, the temporal characteristics of the cytoplasmic calcium signal are determined by (1) the amount of calcium entering the cytoplasm via plasmalemmal channels and the amount of calcium released from the stores; (2) cytoplasmic calcium buffering by fast Ca^{2+} chelators; (3) calcium uptake by intracellular organelles; and (4) calcium extrusion into the extracellular space. Here we will summarize the current data concerning the basic features of the mentioned components of the calcium signal generation chain.

DEPOLARIZATION-TRIGGERED Ca^{2+} SIGNALS

The most abundant stimulus which practically always induces a prominent elevation of intracellular Ca^{2+} in nerve cells is the depolarization of the cellular membrane. This depolarization opens plasmalemmal voltage-operated Ca^{2+} channels, which deliver Ca^{2+} ions in the form of a transmembrane calcium current. These Ca^{2+} ions in turn may trigger Ca^{2+}-induced Ca^{2+} release, which further amplifies the depolarization-induced $[Ca^{2+}]_i$ signal. Fig. 3.1 shows examples of $[Ca^{2+}]_i$ transients measured simultaneously with transmembrane calcium currents in mammalian peripheral and central neurones. It is quite obvious that while the depolarization and, respectively, transmembrane calcium current develop in a millisecond time range, the $[Ca^{2+}]_i$ transients last for several seconds. This time dissociation between I_{Ca} and $[Ca^{2+}]_i$ transient is quite a consistent observation for many neuronal types (Mironov et al., 1993; Llano et al., 1994; Shmigol et al., 1995b; Hua et al., 1993; Thayer and Miller, 1990). It may equally well reflect either Ca^{2+} redistribution within the cellular cytoplasm or the amplifying effect of CICR, triggered by calcium entry (see below). Calcium removal from the bath also abolished depolarization-induced $[Ca^{2+}]_i$ transients, indicating that I_{Ca} and $[Ca^{2+}]_i$ elevation are causally related. Further evidence for such a relation comes from a comparison of the voltage dependence of peak I_{Ca} with the voltage dependence of the peak $[Ca^{2+}]_i$ transient (Fig. 3.1): the $[Ca^{2+}]_i$ transient usually mirrors the I-V curve of the calcium current.

Various subtypes of calcium channels obviously contribute differently to the delivery of Ca^{2+} ions into the cytoplasm during the natural electrical activity of nerve cells. Fig. 3.2 shows examples of $[Ca^{2+}]_i$ transients, recorded from the fura-2/AM loaded granule neurone in acutely prepared cerebellar slice in response to increasing

59

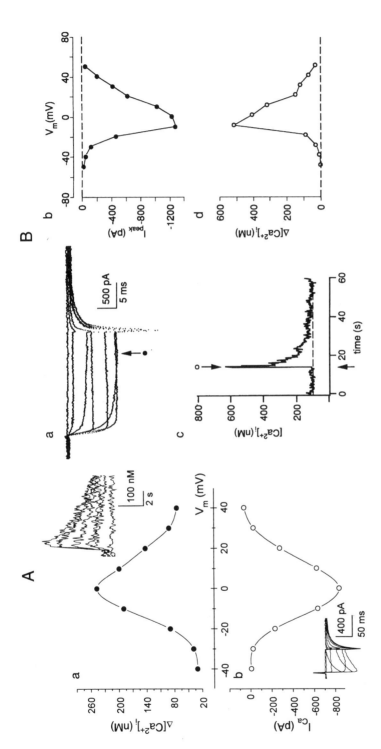

Figure 3.1. Calcium current-induced [Ca^{2+}]$_i$ transients in rat sensory neurones (A) (from Shmigol *et al.*, 1995b) and rat cerebellar Purkinje neurones (B) (Kano, Schnegenburger and Verkhratsky own observations). Calcium currents were measured using whole-cell voltage-clamp patch-clamp technique. Simultaneously the patch pipette was used to deliver [Ca^{2+}]$_i$-sensitive dyes indo-1 (A) or fura-2 (B) into the cytosol. [Ca^{2+}]$_i$ was recorded using photomultipliers attached to the fluorescent microscope. This technique allowed recording of the I$_{Ca}$ I–V curve (Ab and Bb) and the relation between depolarization and amplitude of [Ca^{2+}]$_i$ elevation (Aa and Bd). In A calcium currents and [Ca^{2+}]$_i$ transients used for constructing their voltage dependence curves are shown in the insets

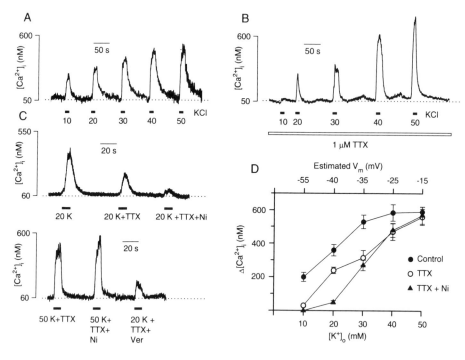

Figure 3.2. Depolarization-induced $[Ca^{2+}]_i$ transients recorded from granule neurone in cerebellar slice (Kirischuk *et al.*, 1995e with permission). Granule neurones were loaded with fura-2/AM; after the end of the experiment cells were approached using a patch pipette in order to determine (i) the resting membrane potential and (ii) the background fluorescence (the latter was measured after 10 min dialysis with fura-2-free intrapipette solution). The neurones were challenged by increasing KCl concentrations in the Na^+-containing external solution (A) and in the presence of 1 mM TTX in order to inhibit Na^+ currents (B). $[Ca^{2+}]_i$ responses evoked by different degrees of depolarization (i.e. by different KCl concentrations) demonstrated distinct sensitivity to pharmacological blockade: $[Ca^{2+}]_i$ transients triggered by moderate depolarization (20 mM KCl) were blocked by 50 μM Ni^{2+} ions; $[Ca^{2+}]_i$ transients triggered by 50 mM KCl were insensitive to Ni^{2+}, but verapamil (100 μM) blocked them substantially (C). In (D) the mean amplitudes of $[Ca^{2+}]_i$ transients evoked by application of increasing concentrations of KCl were measured in controls, in the presence of 1 mM TTX and in the presence of both TTX and Ni^{2+} (50 μM). The estimated V_m was taken from whole-cell current-clamp recordings from neurones in the same slice challenged by different concentrations of KCl

depolarizations. In this experiment the different degrees of depolarization were achieved by titration of the cells with increasing concentrations of extracellular K^+ ions. It is quite obvious that while recording in normal Tyrode solution (Fig. 3.2A) the amplitude of $[Ca^{2+}]_i$ transient increases very steeply with depolarization: even a small depolarization induces nearly maximal response. This is a characteristic situation for the unclamped cell that reflects the generation of Na^+-driven action potentials, which amplify the degree of depolarization. Fig. 3.2B shows similarly activated $[Ca^{2+}]_i$ transients recorded, however, in the presence of 1 mM tetrodotoxin, which inhibited Na^+ permeability and action potential generation. In this case the dependence of $[Ca^{2+}]_i$ transient amplitude versus membrane potential looks much smoother, reflecting gradual activation of plasmalemmal Ca^{2+} channels with depolarization. At different potentials distinct subsets of plasmalemmal Ca^{2+} channels are responsible for $[Ca^{2+}]_i$ transient generation. At small depolarizations $[Ca^{2+}]_i$ transients appeared to be sensitive to blockers of T-channels (Ni^{2+} ions), whereas at high depolarizations blockers of HVA Ca^{2+} channels became effective (Fig. 3.2C).

Certainly, this experiment reflects an artificial situation, and physiologically activated action potentials presumably will involve various types of Ca^{2+} channels in a different manner. However, our understanding of the relative importance of Ca^{2+} fluxes through different types of Ca^{2+} channels in physiological conditions is very limited. Scroggs and Fox (1992a) on the basis of solely electrophysiological analysis of rat DRG neurones suggested that during naturally evoked action potentials the major role in Ca^{2+} delivery to the cytoplasm belongs to the LVA T channels. However, Piser and co-authors demonstrated that up to 80% of action potential-induced $[Ca^{2+}]_i$ elevation in rat DRG neurones were blocked by ω-conotoxin GVIA, while nitrendipine had little effect (Piser et al., 1994). This result suggests the leading role of N-type calcium channels in Ca^{2+} entry to the cytoplasm during natural electrical activity. Barish (1991a) analysing $[Ca^{2+}]_i$ signals in response to small depolarizations of *Xenopus* spinal neurones demonstrated that both T and N channels are involved in the generation of Ca^{2+} influx.

CYTOPLASMIC CALCIUM BUFFERING

After entering the cell through Ca^{2+}-permeable channels either from the extracellular space or from intracellular stores, Ca^{2+} ions immediately face the strongest challenge from a wide complex of mechanisms trying to exclude them from their possible physicochemical activity. They include direct binding by cytosolic buffers, expulsion back to the extracellular space by plasmalemmal transporting systems (Ca-ATPase, Na^+/Ca^{2+} exchange) and reabsorption into intracellular stores. These mechanisms have different affinity and different kinetic characteristics, and their separation and analysis depend entirely on the availability of technical possibilities for recording intracellular changes of free Ca^{2+} with adequate time and space resolution. This is especially important for the evaluation of the first of the mentioned steps—binding by cytosolic buffers—which obviously takes place with much faster time constants (in the millisecond range) compared with mechanisms involving energy-consuming ion-transporting systems.

The major part of Ca^{2+} ions entering the cell is almost instantly buffered by cytoplasmic calcium-binding sites. Only a small amount of calcium which penetrated into the cytosol shows up as free Ca^{2+} (cf. Gorman and Thomas, 1980). An extensive analysis of such binding has been made recently on chromaffin cells using digital imaging and photometry in conjunction with the fluorescent indicator fura-2 (Neher and Augustine, 1992). Dialysis of the cell with the indicator through a patch pipette caused concentration-dependent changes in the depolarization-induced Ca^{2+} signal, decreasing its amplitude and slowing the recovery time. These changes were used to estimate the properties of the endogenous cytoplasmic Ca^{2+} buffer with which fura-2 competes for Ca^{2+}. It was established that the endogenous buffer capacity in these cells

(K_s = bound Ca^{2+}/free Ca^{2+}) is about 75. It is created mostly by some immobile molecules, since it did not decrease substantially even during long-lasting dialysis of the cell, and has a low affinity for Ca^{2+} ions, because it did not saturate even with 1 mM Ca^{2+} inside the cell. They obviously represented by Ca^{2+}-binding proteins which belong to the so-called EF-hand family, where EF corresponds to a Ca^{2+}-coordinating helix-loop-helix sequence (Pochet *et al.*, 1990; Heizmann and Hunziker, 1991). Possible candidates are calmodulin, calreticulin, parvalbumin and calbindin D_{28K}. Intracellular administration of calbindin D_{28K} and parvalbumin into rat sensory neurones did not significantly alter the basal $[Ca^{2+}]_i$ but substantially reduced the peak amplitude of the Ca^{2+} signal obtained by membrane depolarization, decreased its rate of rise and altered the kinetics of decay to a single slow component, calbindin being more effective (Chard *et al.*, 1993). However, Neher and Augustine have considered calmodulin as more compatible with the physiological characteristics of cytosolic Ca^{2+} buffering, while parvalbumins are not (because their Ca^{2+} affinities are in the submicromolar range). In addition, cytosolic buffer capacity can be mediated by ATP, which seems to be able to bind a significant amount of Ca^{2+} ions; in this case they represent mobile intracellular buffers which could be functionally important by supporting cytoplasmic diffusion of Ca^{2+} ions and facilitating the spreading of Ca^{2+} signals (Zhou and Neher, 1993b).

Despite the presence of this rapid buffering capacity, Ca^{2+} ions entering the cell during depolarization still produced in these cells substantial spatial gradients, being highest in the vicinity of the plasmalemma and declining towards its centre. Model calculations indicate that in the immediate vicinity of the channels the concentration of free Ca^{2+} would be especially high – in the micromolar region (Augustine and Neher, 1992b). However, direct measurements of such a gradient would need a resolution and sensitivity substantially better than those available now.

Although chromaffin cells are close relatives of neurones, direct analysis of calcium buffering in nerve cells was necessary. In our group this has been done using a different technical approach which can be called 'Ca-clamp' (Belan *et al.*, 1993a, b). In this technique the intracellular free Ca^{2+} concentration has been fixed at different physiologically significant levels in large snail neurones by a feedback system between the fluorescent signal of the fura-2 probe loaded into the cell and ionotphoretic injection of Ca^{2+} ions through a $CaCl_2$-loaded microelectrode. The membrane potential of the neurone has also been clamped. Clamping of $[Ca^{2+}]_i$ at a new increased level was accompanied by a transient of the Ca^{2+}-injecting current corresponding to injection of 36 ± 20 μM Ca^{2+} for a change in resting level of 0.1 μM. Obviously, this transient represents the filling of a fast cytosolic buffer which has to be done before reaching a new increased level of $[Ca^{2+}]_i$. Taking into account that some additional capacity is added by fura-2, the endogenous buffer capacity here equals about 300; this is much higher than in chromaffin cells. Examples of such transients and the relation between injected Ca^{2+}-carrying currents and changes in intracellular free Ca^{2+} are presented in Fig. 3.3. As in the case of chromaffin cells, the buffering system seems to be far from saturation during such physiological changes in $[Ca^{2+}]_i$.

The 'Ca²⁺-clamp' technique has some disadvantages, mainly because of instability of Ca^{2+}-injecting electrodes; nevertheless this cannot explain the large difference between the values obtained for neurones and chromaffin cells. Even higher values for

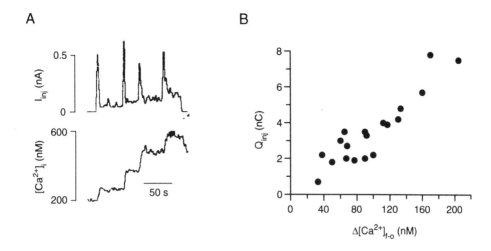

Figure 3.3. Measurements of Ca^{2+} buffering in snail neurones by 'Ca^{2+}-clamp' technique (from Belan *et al.*, 1993a; reproduced by permission of The Physiological Society). (A) Clamping of $[Ca^{2+}]_i$ at four successively increasing levels (lower record) and corresponding transients of the Ca^{2+}-injecting current (upper record). (B) Dependence of charge transferred during injection current transients (Q_{inj}) and change in clamped $[Ca^{2+}]_i$ level determined as the difference between its final and original values

buffering capacity of identified snail neurones have been obtained recently by using an approach very similar to that used in the latter case (Müller T.H. *et al.*, 1993). The only difference was that nerve cells were not dialysed but injected with different amounts of fura-2. The value of K_s was estimated to be about 480 without variations with the amount of Ca^{2+} influx, indicating that the buffer shows no saturation up to micromolar concentrations of Ca^{2+} in the cytosol. The spatial gradients of $[Ca^{2+}]_i$ here were even more pronounced and did not equilibrate until most of the injected Ca^{2+} had been removed. Similar experiments performed on isolated nerve endings from rat neurohypophyseal cells gave an estimated K_s value of ~175 (Stuenkel, 1994). The highest buffer capacity so far has been claimed for cerebellar Purkinje neurones: the estimated K_s value was about 4700 (Llano *et al.*, 1994).

These differences in the buffer capacity may indicate diversity of cytosolic properties in different types of cells. On the other hand, cell conditions during measurement also should be taken into account: intracellular dialysis through the pipette may affect the properties of endogenous buffers. Obviously, special studies of the cytosolic buffering in different types of nerve cells would be quite important, taking into account that the spectrum of Ca^{2+}-binding proteins is also very variable in different neurones (cf. Baimbridge *et al.*, 1992; Andressen *et al.*, 1993) and, moreover, Ca^{2+}-binding proteins are differently expressed in various neurone subpopulations. The changes in buffering properties during ontogenesis and especially during ageing might also be very interesting: there are data that in some brain structures (hippocampus) a substantial loss of such proteins as calbindin and calretinin occurs with ageing, while in others (cerebellum) this is not the case (Villa *et al.*, 1994).

Ca^{2+}-INDUCED Ca^{2+} RELEASE IN NEURAL CELLS

Calcium induced Ca^{2+} release plays a defined and very important role as an amplifier of $[Ca^{2+}]_i$ signal in a variety of excitable cells. Most of the current knowledge concerning the CICR mechanism came from experiments on muscle cells where CICR plays a crucial role in initiation of the contraction (see Wier, 1990 for review). In myocytes, plasmalemmal Ca^{2+} influx is responsible for only 10-20% of actual $[Ca^{2+}]_i$ signal; the rest is due to internal Ca^{2+} release. In neural cells the role and importance of the CICR mechanism is less clear. As was mentioned above, the CICR mechanism is associated with the activity of Ca^{2+}-gated Ca^{2+} release channels incorporated into the membrane of the ER. Using various modulators of these channels it appeared possible to describe major physiological properties of CICR in nerve cells.

CAFFEINE PROBING FOR CICR MECHANISM IN NEURONES

Caffeine is one of the most popular and convenient tools for studying the properties of Ca^{2+}-sensitive Ca^{2+} stores. It belongs to methylxanthines, which have a number of well-defined pharmacological effects, related to the blockade of adenosine receptors, inhibition of phosphodiesterases etc. From the pharmacological point of view methylxanthines are effective stimulators of the central nervous system (see Daly, 1993 for review).

An additional feature of caffeine and several other methylxanthines (theophylline and IBMX) which is important for investigations of $[Ca^{2+}]_i$ signalling is their ability to activate Ca^{2+}-gated Ca^{2+} release channels, thus inducing Ca^{2+} liberation from internal stores. The discovery of caffeine as a potent Ca^{2+} mobilizer from the internal stores came from investigations of caffeine-induced contractures in skeletal and cardiac muscle (e.g. Blinks *et al.*, 1972). Later on, direct recordings of $[Ca^{2+}]_i$ demonstrated that caffeine induces an elevation of cytoplasmic calcium concentration in muscle cells; this elevation persists in Ca^{2+}-free extracellular solution, thus suggesting its origination from intracellular structures (cf. Ganitkevitch and Isenberg, 1992).

The effects of caffeine were investigated in parallel on neuronal cells. Neering and McBurney (1984) first discovered $[Ca^{2+}]_i$ transients (measured by means of arsenaso III fluorescence) induced by millimolar concentrations of caffeine in mammalian sensory neurones. Further experiments demonstrated the existence of caffeine-sensitive Ca^{2+} release mechanism in various types of nerve cells (Table 3.1).

It is generally accepted that methylxanthines interact with Ca^{2+}-gated Ca^{2+} release channels of the ER, making them more sensitive to Ca^{2+}, so that the Ca^{2+} release mechanism can be activated even at resting levels of $[Ca^{2+}]_i$. Within this framework (schematically represented in Fig. 3.4A) it can be argued that the responsiveness of caffeine-sensitive internal calcium stores is determined by (1) the number of activated CICR channels and (2) the electro-driving force for Ca^{2+} ions between the ER lumen and the cytoplasm, i.e. by releasable Ca^{2+} content of internal stores.

Fig. 3.4B,C demonstrates examples of methylxanthine-induced $[Ca^{2+}]_i$ transients measured in peripheral and central neurones. Caffeine (as well as IBMX and theophylline)-induced calcium elevation persisted while suprefusing the cell with Ca^{2+}-free solution, thus indicating the intracellular source of Ca^{2+} ions.

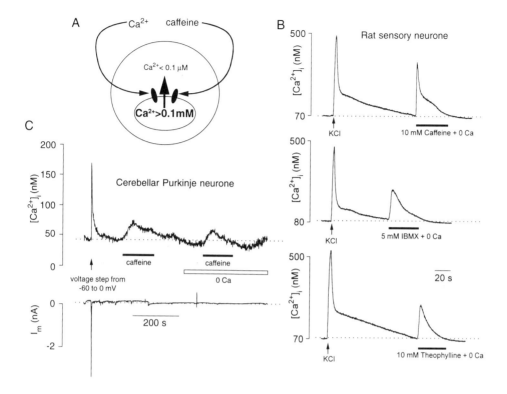

Figure 3.4. Caffeine-induced Ca^{2+} release from ER stores in mammalian neurones (A) The conceptual scheme of caffeine/Ca^{2+}-triggered Ca^{2+} release. The Ca^{2+} concentration gradient between ER lumen and cytoplasm underlies the generation of the electro-driving force which permits Ca^{2+} efflux from the stores. Caffeine sensitizes the CICR channel to Ca^{2+} allowing opening of the channel and Ca^{2+} liberation from the stores (B) Comparison of depolarization (by means of cell exposure to 50 mM KCl) and methyxanthine-induced Ca^{2+} transients recorded from indo-1/AM-loaded rat DRG neurones. Note that methyxanthines produce a $[Ca^{2+}]_i$ response in the absence of Ca^{2+} ions in the external milieu (from Usachev and Verkhratsky, 1995 by permission of Churchill Livingstone). (C) An example of depolarization (in response to voltage step from -60 mV to 0 mV) and caffeine-triggered $[Ca^{2+}]_i$ transients recorded from voltage-clamped, fura-2-loaded Purkinje neurone in rat cerebellar slice (from Kano *et al.*, 1995 by permission of The Physiological Society)

Caffeine-induced $[Ca^{2+}]_i$ transients in peripheral neurones

General properties

Effects of caffeine on $[Ca^{2+}]_i$ in peripheral neurones were studied on freshly isolated and cultured sensory and sympathetic neurones from both non-mammalian and mammalian preparations (Neering and McBurney, 1984; Kostyuk *et al.*, 1989; Friel and Tsien, 1992a; Lipscombe *et al.*, 1988; Thayer *et al.*, 1988; Marrion and Adams, 1992; Usachev *et al.*, 1993; Usachev and Verkhratsky, 1995, see also Table 3.1). The major properties of caffeine-evoked $[Ca^{2+}]_i$ transients appeared to be quite similar in these preparations. Superfusion of peripheral neurones by solutions containing 10-20 mM

Table 3.1. Caffeine-induced [Ca^{2+}]$_i$ transients in nerve cells

Preparation/neurone type	Amplitude of caffeine-induced [Ca^{2+}]$_i$ transient	Pharmacological inhibition	References
Peripheral neurones			
Acutely isolated/snail (*Helix pomatia*) neurones	~800–1000	Procaine (1 mM)	Kostyuk *et al.* (1989)
Culture/neuroblastoma × glioma hybrid cell line	525 ± 95		Robbins *et al.* (1992)
Culture/bull-frog /sympathetic neurones	~270 nM (resting [Ca^{2+}]$_i$ 84 ± 6 nM; peak caffeine-induced [Ca^{2+}]$_i$ transient 353 ±33nm)	Ryanodine (10 μM) Procaine (5 mM)	Marrion and Adams (1992)
Culture/bull frog/sympathetic neurones	439 ± 20 nm	Ryanodine (1 μM)	Friel and Tsien (1992a)
Culture/rat/sympathetic neurones	357 ± 26 nM	Ryanodine (1 μM) Dantrolene Na (10 μM)	Thayer *et al.* (1988)
Culture/rat/superior servical ganglia	30 (1 mM caffeine) 150 (3 mM caffeine) 450 (10 mM caffeine)		Trouslard *et al.* (1993)
Culture/rat/DRG	80 (2 mM caffeine) 270 (10–20 mM caffeine)	Ryanodine (10 μM) Dantrolene Na (10 μM) Procaine (5 mM) Ba^{2+} ions (0.5 mM)	Usachev *et al.* (1993)
Acutely isolated/rat/DRG	200–400 (caffeine, IBMX, teophylline)	Ryanodine (100 μM)	(Usachev and Verkhratsky (1995)

Preparation	Value	Agents	Reference
Short-term culture/chick/DRG	318 ± 181[b]	Thapsigargin (2 μM), Ryanodine (2 mM), Procaine (1 mM), Ruthenium red (10 kM)	Mironov et al. (1993), Mironov (1994b)
Acutely isolated/mouse/DRG neurones	200–400	Thapsigargin (20–50 nM), Procaine (1 mM), Ryanodine (100 kM)	Shmigol et al. (1994b, 1995a)
Central neurones			
Culture/*Xenopus*/spinal cord	457 ± 221	Ryanodine	Barish (1991)
Culture/rat/septum	85 ± 14 nM	Thapsigargin (2 μM)	Bleakman et al. (1993)
Culture/rat/cerebellum	269 ± 41 nM[a]	Ryanodine (10 μM)	Brorson et al. (1991)
Culture/rat/hippocampus	29 ± 2[a], 182 ± 14[a]	Ryanodine (100 μM), procaine (5 mM)	Shmigol et al. (1994a)
Culture/rat/neocortex	35 ± 9[a]	Ryanodine (100 μM), procaine (5 mM)	Shmigol et al. (1994a)
Culture/rat/nucleus cuneatus	261 ± 40[a], 23 ± 2[a]	Ryanodine (100 μM), Procaine (5 mM)	Shmigol et al. (1994a)
Culture/rat/cerebellar granule neurones	100–200	Ryanodine (10 μM), thapsigargin (0.1–1 μM)	Irving et al. (1992a)
Slice/rat/cerebellar Purkinje neurones	0–250[b]	Ryanodine (10 μM), ruthenium red (10 μM)	Kano et al. (1995)
Slice/mouse/cerebellar granule neurones	30–200[a]	Thapsigargin (50 nM)	Kirischuk et al., 1995e

[a] The full-size caffeine-induced $[Ca^{2+}]_i$ response requires charging of stores by releasable Ca^{2+}.
[b] The amplitude of caffeine-induced $[Ca^{2+}]_i$ transients is controlled by basal $[Ca^{2+}]_i$.

caffeine induced the elevation of $[Ca^{2+}]_i$ from the resting level to ~300-400 nM with the maximal rate of rise in the range of 150-200 nM/s. After reaching a peak, the $[Ca^{2+}]_i$ level started to decline in the presence of caffeine and within 80-100 s cytoplasmic calcium returned to the initial resting value. If the caffeine was washed out during this recovery phase $[Ca^{2+}]_i$ immediately dropped to the basal level. In the absence of extracellular calcium caffeine produced a similar rise in $[Ca^{2+}]_i$, indicating that caffeine released Ca^{2+} from the internal store. The amplitude of caffeine-triggered $[Ca^{2+}]_i$ transients in sensory neurones was reported to be modulated by basal $[Ca^{2+}]_i$ level (Mironov, 1994b): the maximal amplitudes of caffeine-induced $[Ca^{2+}]_i$ transients were observed at basal $[Ca^{2+}]_i$ close to 300-400 nM. At lower and higher $[Ca^{2+}]_i$ the amplitudes of calcium release became smaller, indicating presumably the bell-shaped regulation of the CICR channel by cytoplasmic Ca^{2+} concentration.

Concentration dependence

The action of methylxanthines on $[Ca^{2+}]_i$ is clearly intracellular and at millimolar drug concentrations $[Ca^{2+}]_i$ elevation develops rapidly, indicating that methylxanthines are approaching their intracellular targets quite fast. Fortunately, while measuring $[Ca^{2+}]_i$ with one of the ratiometric dyes, namely indo-1, it appeared possible simultaneously to monitor the intracellular caffeine concentration. Monitoring of the intracellular caffeine (as well as other methylxanthines) concentration was facilitated by the fact that methylxanthines bind to a Ca^{2+} indicator indo-1 (O'Neill *et al.*, 1990; Usachev and Verkhratsky, 1995) and quench its fluorescence in a wavelength-independent way. An important feature of methylxanthine-dependent quenching of indo-1 is its concentration dependence. Using the concentration-dependent quenching of indo-1 fluorescence by methylxanthines, it has been shown that methylxanthines indeed freely penetrate cellular membrane and the intracellular caffeine concentration equilibrates with the external concentration with a time constant of about $8s^{-1}$ (O'Neill *et al.*, 1990).

Caffeine and other methylxanthines released Ca^{2+} from the internal stores in nerve cells in a concentration-dependent manner. The threshold concentrations for caffeine are in the range of 0.5-1 mM and saturation is reached at about 5 mM (experiments on rat sensory neurones); IBMX and theophylline show similar concentration dependence (Usachev *et al.*, 1993; Usachev and Verkhratsky, 1995). Moreover, the submaximal caffeine concentrations could not fully discharge the calcium store. In experiments performed on cultured DRG neurones (Usachev *et al.*, 1993) we have found that these cells responded to application of 2 mM caffeine by transient $[Ca^{2+}]_i$ elevation with an average amplitude of 76 ± 31 nM. The successive challenge with 2 mM caffeine applied 30 s later failed to produce a $[Ca^{2+}]_i$ response; however, 10 mM caffeine induced $[Ca^{2+}]_i$ transients with an average amplitude of 232 ± 17 nM. This property matches the 'quantal' or 'incremental' calcium release from $InsP_3$- sensitive stores; similar 'quantal' caffeine-induced Ca^{2+} liberation was also observed in chromaffin cells (Cheeck *et al.*, 1993).

The concentration dependence presumably reflects the number of activated CICR channels, while 'quantal' release might indicate the existence of various ER compartments bearing different sensitivity to caffeine. In addition, such a property predicts a 'gradual', rather than an 'all-or-nothing' responsiveness of the CICR mechanism in nerve cells.

Depletion and refilling of calcium stores

Based on the general scheme of caffeine-induced calcium liberation (Fig. 3.4A) it is obvious that the kinetics of the caffeine-induced $[Ca^{2+}]_i$ transient is determined by the balance between Ca^{2+} release from the internal store, Ca^{2+} reuptake into the store, cytoplasmic Ca^{2+} buffering and Ca^{2+} extrusion to the extracellular space. Ca^{2+} release by itself is determined by the driving force for Ca^{2+} ions (assuming that ER Ca^{2+} channels are open throughout the caffeine application). After initiation of the release the driving force for Ca^{2+} ions falls because of (1) deprivation of the intraluminal free Ca^{2+} content and (2) increase of the cytoplasmic Ca^{2+} concentration. During release some Ca^{2+} ions are reloaded back into the store, and some are buffered and/or extruded outside. However, it seems that the most important mechanism responsible for the decay of the caffeine-induced $[Ca^{2+}]_i$ transients is associated with the depletion of ER-releasable Ca^{2+}.

The deprivation of internal stores by caffeine is clearly manifested by a decrease of the store responsiveness to caffeine upon subsequent application of the latter (Friel and Tsien, 1992a; Usachev *et al.*, 1993; Shmigol *et al.*, 1994a). An example of such depletion is shown in Fig. 3.5. It is quite evident that $[Ca^{2+}]_i$ responses to successive caffeine applications are smaller in amplitude. Extensive caffeine applications appear to be more effective for store depletion (Fig. 3.5B). The plasmalemmal Ca^{2+} extrusion obviously participates in the decay of caffeine-induced Ca^{2+} transients. Blockade of Ca^{2+} extrusion by La^{3+} decreased both the rate of Ca^{2+} store depletion and the velocity of the decay of the caffeine-induced $[Ca^{2+}]_i$ transients, reflecting an increased recirculation of Ca^{2+} between the ER and the cytoplasm (Usachev *et al.*, 1993). On the other hand, SERCA-driven Ca^{2+} uptake into ER stores also participates in the recovery of the stores responsiveness to caffeine, so finally the releasable Ca^{2+} content of the ER lumen is determined by competition between the activity of SERCA pumps (which are responsible for Ca^{2+} uptake by internal stores) and plasmalemmal calcium pumps (which underlie Ca^{2+} extrusion from a cell).

The major question is whether the refilling of internal stores could be fulfilled by calcium already existing in the cytoplasm, or whether it is necessary to initiate an additional calcium inflow from the external environment. A characteristic property of the peripheral neurones is the ability of caffeine-sensitive stores to restore their responsiveness to caffeine in steady-state conditions (Friel and Tsien, 1992a; Usachev *et al.*, 1993). Such a recovery of the amplitude of the caffeine-induced $[Ca^{2+}]_i$ transient (Fig. 3.5C) obviously reflects the complete replenishment of the calcium stores.

The deprivation of internal stores of releasable Ca^{2+} stimulates Ca^{2+} uptake into the ER. Quite often, following the washout of caffeine a subresting drop of $[Ca^{2+}]_i$ is observed (so-called 'post-caffeine undershoot') (Friel and Tsien, 1992a; Usachev *et al.*, 1993). This undershoot probably reflects the increased activity of SERCA pumps and is believed to be a sign of the activation of SERCA pumps following the depletion of internal stores. The speed of refilling of ER stores is greatly enhanced if additional Ca^{2+} has been injected into the cytoplasm: if the cell was depolarized after depletion of

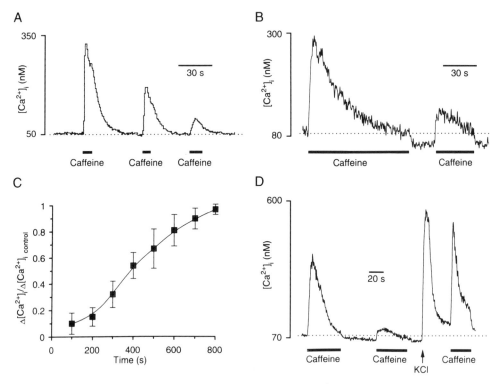

Figure 3.5. Depletion and refilling of caffeine-sensitive Ca^{2+} stores in rat DRG neurones (modified from Usachev *et al.*, 1993 with permission from Elsevier Science Ltd). (A, B) Examples of caffeine-induced $[Ca^{2+}]_i$ transients recorded in response to subsequent 20 mM caffeine administrations. (C) The time course of spontaneous refilling of the caffeine-sensitive Ca^{2+} stores. (D) Transmembrane calcium entry through voltage-activated calcium channels reloads the caffeine-sensitive internal calcium stores with releasable Ca^{2+}. The caffeine (20 mM) and high-potassium (50 mM K^+)-containing solutions were applied at times indicated below the $[Ca^{2+}]_i$ trace

stores by caffeine the succeeding application of caffeine induced a full-size $[Ca^{2+}]_i$ response (Fig. 3.5D). Moreover, quite often the amplitude of this $[Ca^{2+}]_i$ response (elicited immediately after the end of depolarization-triggered $[Ca^{2+}]_i$ transient) was significantly larger as compared with the initial caffeine-induced $[Ca^{2+}]_i$ elevation (Thayer *et al.*, 1988; Usachev *et al.*, 1993).

Thus Ca^{2+} entry via voltage-operated calcium channels may serve as an additional source of calcium ions which could be trapped by caffeine-sensitive stores. In addition, Ca^{2+} influx during the depolarization can overload these stores, indicating an involvement of the caffeine-sensitive calcium pools in sequestration of cytoplasmic calcium during depolarization-induced $[Ca^{2+}]_i$ transients.

Heterogeneous expression of the CICR mechanism in mammalian sensory neurones

Our investigations of caffeine-sensitive Ca^{2+} release in mammalian sensory neurones demonstrated that caffeine-triggered $[Ca^{2+}]_i$ transients can be elicited only in a certain

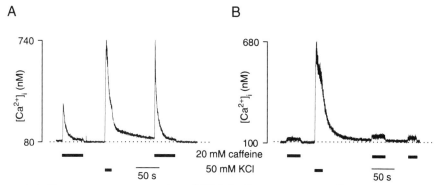

Figure 3.6. Heterogeneous expression of CICR/caffeine-sensitive Ca^{2+} stores in mouse sensory neurones (from Shmigol *et al.*, 1994b with permission from Rapid Communications of Oxford, Ltd). The $[Ca^{2+}]_i$ was recorded from large (A) and small (B) mouse DRG neurones by means of indo-1-based microfluorimetry. Caffeine was able to induce intracellular Ca^{2+} release only in large neurones

subpopulation of cells. Sensory neurones from both mice and rats appeared to be heterogeneous in respect to the expression of caffeine-releasable calcium stores: we have found that the diameter of DRG neurones strongly correlated with the appearance of caffeine-induced $[Ca^{2+}]_i$ transients.

It is widely accepted that the diameters of somata of sensory neurones in dorsal root ganglia correlate with the conduction velocity of their axons and sensory modalities: rapidly conducting Aα and Aβ axons which presumably transmit proprioceptive and tactile information belong to neurones with the largest cell bodies, whereas slow conducting Aδ and C-type axons which are believed to transmit pain and thermal information are attached to neurones with small somata (Harper and Lawson, 1985). In addition, DRG neurones of different size generate action potentials with characteristic features and express distinct patterns of voltage-gated Ca^{2+} channels (see chapter 2). We found that caffeine is able to elevate $[Ca^{2+}]_i$ only in large DRG neurones; in contrast to large DRG neurones, cells with small soma diameter displayed either no response to caffeine, or responded by low-amplitude steady-state $[Ca^{2+}]_i$ elevation. Moreover, depolarization-triggered $[Ca^{2+}]_i$ transients did not modulate the subsequent responses to caffeine (Fig. 3.6). This led us to suggest that caffeine-sensitive ER stores are almost absent in small-diameter DRG neurones. Similar to our observations, a subpopulation of chick DRG neurones was also found to be insensitive to caffeine, suggesting the absence of functioning CICR in these cells (Mironov *et al.*, 1993). Furthermore, CICR-related ER Ca^{2+} stores may be unevenly distributed within the same neurone: caffeine usually evoked higher $[Ca^{2+}]_i$ transients in the soma of cultured DRG neurones as compared with their processes (Thayer *et al.*, 1987); analysis of $[Ca^{2+}]_i$ signal in the isolated nerve endings of neurohypophyseal cells did not reveal the existence of CICR in this compartment at all (Stuenkel, 1994).

Caffeine-induced $[Ca^{2+}]_i$ elevation in central neurones

Investigation of the properties of caffeine-induced Ca^{2+} release in mammalian central neurones revealed some differences as compared to the peripheral ones. First of all,

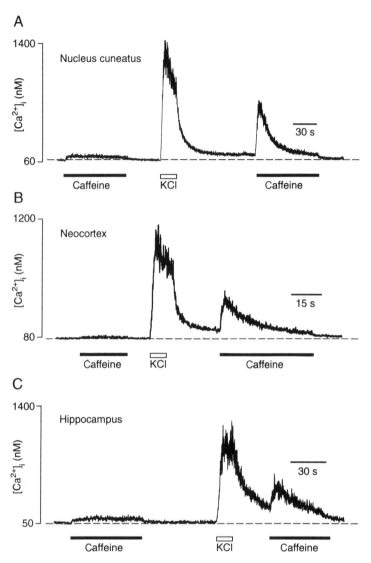

Figure 3.7. Filling of the caffeine-sensitive stores in cultured central neurones by voltage-induced Ca^{2+} entry (from Shmigol *et al.*, 1994a with permission from Springer-Verlag). $[Ca^{2+}]_i$ was recorded from indo-1/AM-loaded neurones. Caffeine (20 mM) and KCl (50 mM) were applied as shown on the graph

generally, the amplitudes of caffeine-induced $[Ca^{2+}]_i$ transients recorded at rest were substantially smaller in central neurones. However, in many cell types a depolarization-induced Ca^{2+} entry into these neurones markedly increased the amplitudes of consecutive caffeine-triggered $[Ca^{2+}]_i$ transient.

As an example Fig. 3.7 shows $[Ca^{2+}]_i$ recordings performed on cultured neurones obtained from three different brain regions: neocortex, nucleus cuneatus and hippocampus (Shmigol *et al.*, 1994a). The amplitudes of caffeine-induced $[Ca^{2+}]_i$

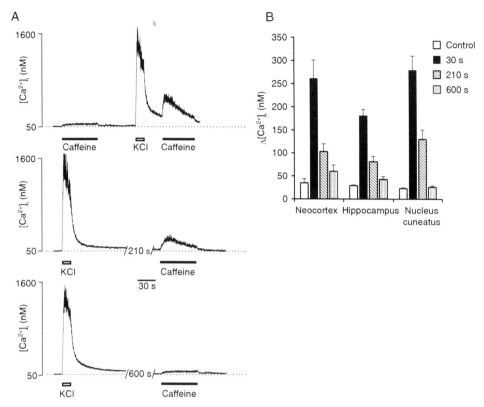

Figure 3.8. Spontaneous loss of releasable calcium from caffeine-sensitive pools in cultured central neurone (from Shmigol *et al.*, 1994a with permission from Springer-Verlag). (A) The $[Ca^{2+}]_i$ was recorded from indo-1/AM-loaded rat nucleus cuneatus neurone. The caffeine (20 mM)-induced $[Ca^{2+}]_i$ transients were recorded at different times (indicated on the graph) after the end of conditioning depolarization (50 mM KCl). The increase of the time gap between conditioning depolarization and caffeine challenge caused significant decrease of the amplitudes of caffeine-triggered $[Ca^{2+}]_i$ transients, reflecting spontaneous depletion of caffeine-sensitive calcium stores. (B) Mean (± s.e.m.) amplitudes of caffeine-mediated $[Ca^{2+}]_i$ transients recorded form various central neurones at different times (indicated on the graph) after conditioning depolarization

transients recorded 30 s after the end of neurone depolarization reached on average 745% as compared to control ones in neocortical, 624% in hippocampal and 1213% in nuclear cuneatus neurones, respectively. Surprisingly, the loading of caffeine-sensitive stores by Ca^{2+} entry through the plasma membrane was transient and within several minutes these stores spontaneously lost their releasable Ca^{2+} content; this could be studied by varying the time interval between charging depolarization and caffeine application. As an example of the spontaneous depletion of caffeine-sensitive depots Fig. 3.8 shows $[Ca^{2+}]_i$ recordings from a nucleus cuneatus neurone. It is evident that 10 min after loading the stores by depolarization they lost releasable Ca^{2+} ions. The same time dependence for the spontaneous depletion of caffeine-sensitive pools was also found in neocortical and hippocampal neurones.

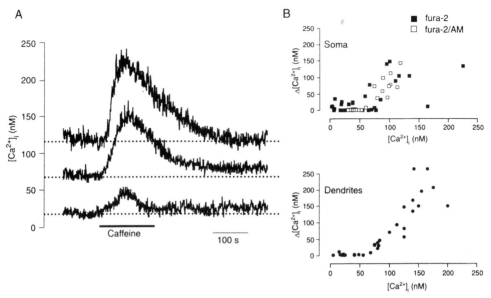

Fig 3.9. Caffeine-induced Ca^{2+} release in Purkinje cerebellar neurones is regulated by basal [Ca^{2+}]$_i$ (from Kano *et al.*, 1995; reproudced by permission of The Physiological Society). (A) Caffeine-induced [Ca^{2+}]$_i$ transients were recorded from fura-2-loaded voltage-clamped Purkinje neurone in rat cerebellar slice at different basal [Ca^{2+}]$_i$. (B) Amplitudes of caffeine-induced [Ca^{2+}]$_i$ transients measured separately from soma and dendrites of Purkinje neurones plotted versus basal [Ca^{2+}]$_i$

   Similarly to described results, the charging of calcium stores by depolarization-induced Ca^{2+} entry as a prerequisite for full-size caffeine-induced [Ca^{2+}]$_i$ response have been found in other types of central neurones, including cerebellar granule (Irving *et al.*, 1992a) and Purkinje neurones (Brorson *et al.*, 1991).

   The pharmacological properties of caffeine-triggered Ca^{2+} release in neurones from CNS did not differ substantially from those observed in cells from the peripheral nervous system (see Table 3.1). However, the sensitivity of at least one class of central neurones, namely cerebellar granule cells, to caffeine appeared to be somewhat lower as compared with peripheral neurones and other types of central neurones. In both cultured granule neurones (Irving *et al.*, 1992a) and the same neurones studied in acutely prepared cerebellar slices (Kirischuk *et al.*, 1995e) the threshold for caffeine was found to be in a range of 5 mM and the maximal [Ca^{2+}]$_i$ response was observed at caffeine concentrations of 30-50 mM. The reasons for such a decreased sensitivity remain unclear.

   In another class of central neurones, namely in cerebellar Purkinje neurones, the situation seems to be even more complicated. It appears that the amplitude of the caffeine-induced Ca^{2+} release is controlled by the resting [Ca^{2+}]$_i$ level, which precedes the caffeine application. In resting conditions application of 20 mM caffeine to Purkinje neurones sitting in a cerebellar slice had either no effect on [Ca^{2+}]$_i$ or induced a tiny [Ca^{2+}]$_i$ response. However, increasing the resting [Ca^{2+}]$_i$ led to an almost linear increase of the amplitude of caffeine-mediated [Ca^{2+}]$_i$ response (Kano *et al.*, 1995). This kind of positive regulation by basal [Ca^{2+}]$_i$ is demonstrated in Fig. 3.9. It seems that in

Purkinje neurones resting $[Ca^{2+}]_i$ controls both the filling state and the ability of the Ca^{2+}-gated Ca^{2+} release channel to be open in response to appropriate stimuli.

These results led us to the suggestion that, although having quite similar pharmacological properties, Ca^{2+} stores in peripheral and central neurones differ in Ca^{2+} ion handling. In peripheral sensory and sympathetic neurones under resting conditions the Ca^{2+} stores are continuously filled by releasable Ca^{2+}, and after discharging they spontaneously refill. In contrast, in central neurones caffeine-sensitive stores have a minute amount of releasable Ca^{2+} under resting conditions; nevertheless they can be rapidly but transiently charged by depolarization-triggered Ca^{2+} entry. The Ca^{2+} stores in central neurones, in contrast to peripheral ones, display a spontaneous depletion of releasable Ca^{2+}.

Pharmacological modulation of caffeine-induced $[Ca^{2+}]_i$ transients in nerve cells

Inhibitors of CICR channels

Various substances known to interact with Ca^{2+}-gated Ca^{2+} release channels (see chapter 3) effectively inhibit caffeine-induced $[Ca^{2+}]_i$ transients in peripheral and central neurones (Table 3.1). Fig. 3.10 presents several examples of pharmacological blockade of caffeine-triggered $[Ca^{2+}]_i$ responses measured in mammalian neurones. Among different blockers ryanodine demonstrated clear use dependence, while other substances inhibit caffeine-induced $[Ca^{2+}]_i$ transients in a concentration-dependent way.

Thapsigargin blocks caffeine-induced $[Ca^{2+}]_i$ release in nerve cells

As has been pointed in chapter 3, Ca^{2+} uptake into the ER stores is achieved via the activity of SERCA pumps, which can be selectively blocked by the tumour promoter thapsigargin (Thastrup *et al.*, 1990; Lytton *et al.*, 1991). Treatment of peripheral neurones by thapsigargin (20-50 nM) inhibited caffeine-induced $[Ca^{2+}]_i$ transients by preventing the reloading of ER calcium stores (Shmigol *et al.*, 1994b, 1995a). Thapsigargin effectively blocked both steady-state replenishment of calcium stores and the loading of them by depolarization-triggered Ca^{2+} entry (Fig. 3.11).

It has to be noted, however, that apart from the modification of SERCA pumps, thapsigargin possesses several side-effects. In micromolar concentrations it inhibits voltage-gated calcium currents in adrenal glomerulosa cells (Roussier *et al.*, 1993) and rat DRG neurones (Shmigol *et al.*, 1995a). Similarly, thapsigargin and another SERCA pump blocker, 2,5-*t*-butylhydroquinone (tBHQ), inhibited HVA calcium currents in GH_3 pituitary cells, whereas cyclopiazonic acid (which also demonstrates SERCA-inhibiting activity) did not (Nelson *et al.*, 1994). Thapsigargin was also reported to collapse the mitochondrial membrane potential and induce Ca^{2+} release from the mitochondrial pool (Vercesi *et al.*, 1993).

In numerous observations on various cells outside the nervous system the blockade of the SERCA pump by thapsigargin was found to be associated with a significant elevation in $[Ca^{2+}]_i$ (see Petersen *et al.*, 1994 for review). In contrast, in neurones resting $[Ca^{2+}]_i$ levels were not affected by thapsigargin application, or thapsigargin induced only a tiny elevation of $[Ca^{2+}]_i$. This was true not only for DRG neurones (Shmigol *et*

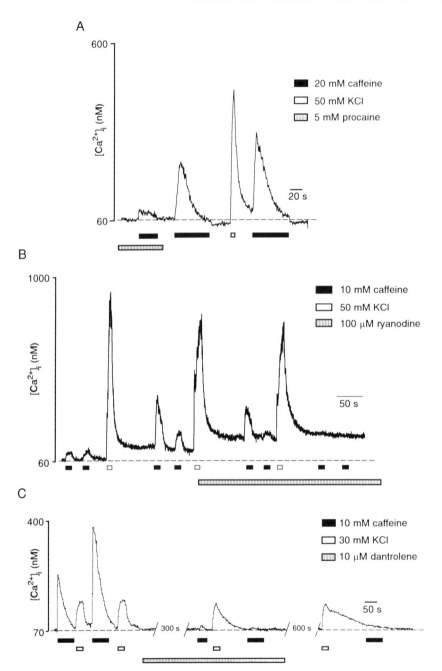

Figure 3.10. Pharmacological properties of caffeine-induced Ca^{2+} release in mammalian neurones. The examples of inhibitory action of procaine, ryanodine and dantrolene on caffeine-triggered Ca^{2+} release were taken from experiments on cultured rat DRG (A, C) and hippocampal (B) neurones (A, C: from Usachev *et al.*, 1993 with permission from Elsevier Science Ltd; B: from Kirischuk and Verkhratsky, own observations)

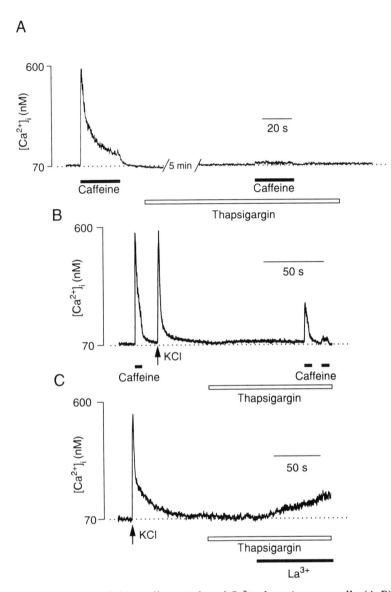

Figure 3.11. Thapsigargin inhibits caffeine-induced Ca^{2+} release in nerve cells. (A, B) Examples of caffeine-induced [Ca^{2+}]$_i$ transients recorded from indo-1-loaded mouse DRG neurones treated with thapsigargin. (C) Blockade of plasmalemmal Ca^{2+} extrusion unmasks thapsigargin-induced [Ca^{2+}]$_i$ elevation. Time for applications of caffeine (20 mM), KCl (50 mM), La^{3+} (3 mM) and thapsigargin (50 nM) are shown on the graph (A: from Shmigol *et al.*,1995b with permission of The Physiological Society; B, C: from own observations)

al., 1994b, 1995a) but also for spinal cord neurones (Salter and Hicks, 1994), septal neurones (Bleakman *et al.*, 1993) and cerebellar granule cells (cultured: Irving *et al.*, 1992a; cerebellar slices: Kirischuk *et al.*, 1995e). In the case of chicken sensory neurones, however, thapsigargin was reported to significantly elevate [Ca^{2+}]$_i$

(Mironov *et al.*, 1993), although in this paper the action of thapsigargin was shown to be reversible. Such a reversibility contradicts the commonly accepted view that thapsigargin covalently and irreversibly binds to SERCA pumps. The discrepancies of thapsigargin action on $[Ca^{2+}]_i$ presumably reflect the different relative importance of various components of $[Ca^{2+}]_i$ homeostasis in different cells. From the basic point of view, blockade of SERCA pumps may initiate $[Ca^{2+}]_i$ elevation only in cases when resting Ca^{2+} leakage from the stores overcomes the intrinsic buffer/extrusion capacity of the cell. The absence of thapsigargin-induced $[Ca^{2+}]_i$ rise in neurones makes it likely that the resting $[Ca^{2+}]_i$ level is strongly controlled by mechanisms other than SERCA pumping, such as highly efficient cytosolic Ca^{2+} buffer mechanisms, Ca^{2+} uptake into mitochondria or Ca^{2+} extrusion into the extracellular space. Indeed, the inhibition of plasmalemmal Ca^{2+} extrusion by La^{3+} reveals the slow rise of $[Ca^{2+}]_i$ in thapsigargin-treated mouse DRG neurones (Fig. 3.11C), which obviously reflects Ca^{2+} leakage from the stores.

ACTIVATION OF CICR IN NEURONES BY PLASMALEMMAL Ca^{2+} ENTRY

Experiments with methylxanthines unequivocally demonstrated that many nerve cells express functionally available CICR machinery. However, obviously the cell would never face millimolar concentrations of methylxanthines; thus it is important to understand whether CICR may be activated in physiological conditions. The question whether Ca^{2+} influx through plasmalemmal Ca^{2+} channels may activate CICR, which in turn would serve as an amplifier of depolarization-induced $[Ca^{2+}]_i$ signal was open until recently.

First indirect evidences concerning the involvement of the CICR mechanism in Ca^{2+} signal generation in neuronal cells came from the comparison of depolarization-induced $[Ca^{2+}]_i$ transients in normal conditions and upon pharmacological modulation of the state of calcium stores. These experiments were designed to find out whether pharmacological modification of internal stores (including depletion of stores by prolonged caffeine exposure or blockade of CICR by ryanodine) could change the amplitude and speed of rise of depolarization-activated $[Ca^{2+}]_i$ transients. From the conceptual point of view, it is possible to assume that if CICR is indeed involved in the amplification of depolarization-triggered $[Ca^{2+}]_i$ transients, the depletion of caffeine-sensitive stores would attenuate both amplitude and rate of rise of $[Ca^{2+}]_i$ elevation produced by membrane depolarization. Vice versa, the sensitization of CICR channels by, for example, low doses of caffeine would facilitate the development of depolarization-induced $[Ca^{2+}]_i$ transients. Indeed, in experiments on bullfrog sympathetic neurones (Friel and Tsien, 1992a) and rat DRG neurones (Usachev *et al.*, 1993) these theoretical assumptions were completely confirmed (see Fig. 3.12). Cells superfusion with 1 mM caffeine led to an increase in the rate of rise and the amplitude of depolarization-induced $[Ca^{2+}]_i$ transients, while store depletion by 20 mM of caffeine reduced both these parameters. Blockade of the CICR mechanism by ryanodine attenuated the amplitudes and rate of rise of depolarization-induced $[Ca^{2+}]_i$ transients (Friel and Tsien, 1992a; Usachev *et al.*, 1993). Similarly to the peripheral neurones, the sensitization of the CICR mechanism by caffeine in cerebellar Purkinje neurones significantly enhances the amplitude and duration of depolarization-

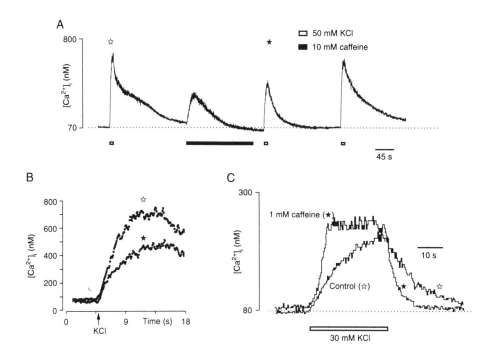

Figure 3.12. Manipulation with caffeine-sensitive stores affects depolarization-triggered $[Ca^{2+}]_i$ transients in rat indo-1/AM-loaded DRG neurones (from Usachev *et al.*, 1993 with permission from Elsevier Science Ltd). (A) Comparison of control response to 50 mM KCl, and $[Ca^{2+}]_i$ responses to 50 mM KCl taken after caffeine-induced depletion of the ER stores. Note a clear decrease of both the amplitude and the rate of rise of the depolarization-induced $[Ca^{2+}]_i$ transient after caffeine conditioning. (B) Control depolarization-induced $[Ca^{2+}]_i$ transient (marked by a white star in A) and the same transient after caffeine conditioning (marked by a black star) are superimposed in an expanded time scale. The amplitude and the rate of rise of depolarization-evoked $[Ca^{2+}]_i$ transients were 603 nM and 202 nM/s in control and 393 nM and 122 nM/s after caffeine-induced depletion of internal calcium stores. (C) Similarly, control $[Ca^{2+}]_i$ transients in response to 30 mM KCl exposure is superimposed with $[Ca^{2+}]_i$ transient recorded in the presence of 1 mM caffeine. In the presence of 1 mM caffeine $[Ca^{2+}]_i$ transients increased more rapidly and recovered more quickly. The maximal rate of rise was 30 nM/s in control and 72 nM/s in the presence of 1 mM caffeine; the time constant of the recovery was 12.4 s in control and it decreased to 2.5 s in the presence of 1 mM caffeine

triggered $[Ca^{2+}]_i$ transients (Fig. 3.13). In cultured embryonic spinal *Xenopus* neurones caffeine and ryanodine decreased the amplitude and affected the kinetics of the depolarization-triggered $[Ca^{2+}]_i$ transients (Barish, 1991b).

However, in order to prove directly the existence of CICR in neuronal cells in physiological conditions one has to compare the amount of Ca^{2+} ions entering the cytoplasm during depolarization through plasmalemmal Ca^{2+} channels with the actual increase in $[Ca^{2+}]_i$ evoked by this depolarization. Experiments performed recently on a number of neuronal preparations (including sympathetic, sensory and cerebellar Purkinje neurones) demonstrated a marked non-linearity between Ca^{2+} entry via voltage-operated channels and amplitude of the cytoplasmic calcium

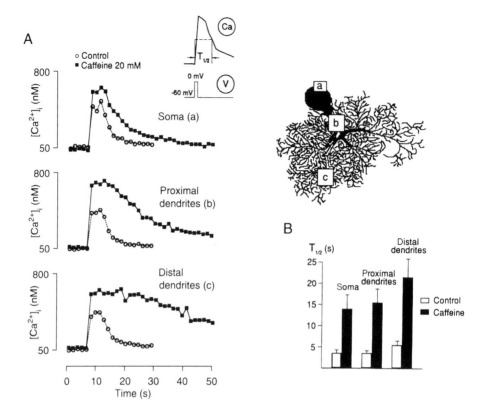

Figure 3.13. Caffeine enhances depolarization-triggered $[Ca^{2+}]_i$ transients in cerebellar Purkinje neurone (from Kano *et al.*, 1995; reproduced by permission of The Physiological Society). $[Ca^{2+}]_i$ was recorded from voltage-clamped fura-2-loaded Purkinje neurone in rat cerebellar slice by means of CCD-based video-imaging. The fluorescent-intensity picture of the Purkinje neurone together with regions from which the integral of the $[Ca^{2+}]_i$ transients were calculated (white boxes) are shown in the inset. (A) The application of 20 mM caffeine by itself did not elevate $[Ca^{2+}]_i$. However, in the presence of 20 mM caffeine the amplitude and duration of depolarization-induced (1 s voltage step from -60 to 0 mV) $[Ca^{2+}]_i$ transients were significantly enhanced. (B) The mean values (± s.e.m.) for the half-time of $[Ca^{2+}]_i$ transient recovery measured separately in soma and dendrites in control conditions and in the presence of caffeine

elevation. In order to compare Ca^{2+} entry with the cytoplasmic calcium elevation, these experiments were performed on voltage-clamped neurones with simultaneous recording of $[Ca^{2+}]_i$ and transmembrane Ca^{2+} current.

The amount of Ca^{2+} translocated through the plasma membrane can be estimated from the I_{Ca} integral (which reflects the net transmembrane charge movement). Than the amplitude of the corresponding $[Ca^{2+}]_i$ transient was divided on either charge or actual amount of transported Ca^{2+} ions, giving the so-called 'unit calcium transient' (Hua *et al.*, 1993). These unit calcium transients were then compared for Ca^{2+} currents of different duration or amplitudes. Assuming that transmembrane calcium current is only one source of Ca^{2+} ions, one should expect linear relations between amount of

Ca^{2+} entering the cell and $[Ca^{2+}]_i$ transients; thus the unit calcium transient should be constant regardless of the integral of calcium current. Supralinear relations between unit calcium transient and the amount of transmembrane calcium entry would reflect either appearance of CICR delivering additional Ca^{2+} ions, or saturation of cytoplasmic Ca^{2+} buffers and/or fast extrusion systems.

Fig. 3.14 demonstrates results of such an experiment performed on freshly isolated rat DRG neurones (Shmigol et al., 1995b). The amount of Ca^{2+} influx was varied either by applying depolarizing pulses with duration between 20 and 500 ms (Fig 3.14A,C) or by increasing the extracellular Ca^{2+} concentration from 2 mM to 8 mM (Fig 3.14B). In both cases the amplitudes of $[Ca^{2+}]_i$ transients increased to a higher level than expected from the amount of Ca^{2+} entry. While the unit calcium transient was almost constant with pulse durations up to 100 ms, pulses lasting 200 ms or longer gave a steep rise in the unit transient, indicating the occurrence of CICR. Similarly, upon elevation of extracellular Ca^{2+} concentration the amplitude of $[Ca^{2+}]_i$ transient rose to a much greater extent than the integral of I_{Ca}, increasing simultaneously the unit calcium transient. Depletion of internal stores by 20 mM caffeine abolished this supralinearity; in the presence of caffeine unit calcium transient became constant at all I_{Ca} durations. Sensitization of the CICR mechanism by 1 mM caffeine produced an opposite effect, significantly increasing the amplitude of $[Ca^{2+}]_i$ transients and unit calcium transient without changing the parameters of I_{Ca}.

Similar supralinear relations between the amplitude of $[Ca^{2+}]_i$ transient and net Ca^{2+} influx through voltage-gated plasmalemmal channels have been observed in bullfrog sympathetic ganglia (Hua et al., 1993) and in rat cerebellar Purkinje cells (Llano et al., 1994). For bullfrog sympathetic neurones (Hua et al., 1993) the additional evidence for CICR arose from double-pulse experiments: when the $[Ca^{2+}]_i$ transients were induced by two brief depolarizations, the second $[Ca^{2+}]_i$ transient was facilitated. This facilitation decreased while increasing the interpulse interval and could be blocked by dantrolene.

An additional piece of evidence favouring the physiological existence of CICR in nerve cells came from experiments with ryanodine (Shmigol et al., 1995b). Intracellular perfusion of DRG neurones with 10 μM ryanodine (Fig. 3.15) significantly modified the parameters of the I_{Ca}-induced $[Ca^{2+}]_i$ transient: the first transient became much larger and its recovery was considerably prolonged, while the second and following transients were markedly inhibited, without any apparent changes in Ca^{2+} current. In addition, caffeine, applied after the first depolarization failed to induce any $[Ca^{2+}]_i$ elevation. These data are well explained from the theory of ryanodine action: the first depolarization opens CICR channels, and ryanodine binds to them, locking ER channels in an open state; this explains the potentiation of the first depolarization-induced $[Ca^{2+}]_i$ transient. Afterwards, however, ER stores lose the ability to accumulate Ca^{2+} due to continuous leakage of intraluminal Ca^{2+}, and CICR become unavailable for both caffeine and I_{Ca} activation.

Certainly, a very interesting question is whether CICR may amplify the $[Ca^{2+}]_i$ signal occurring not under voltage-clamp conditions (which still remain somehow artificial) but during physiological electrical activity of the neurone. In order to resolve this problem, the DRG neurones were studied under current-clamp using a whole-cell recording configuration, and action potentials were evoked by just

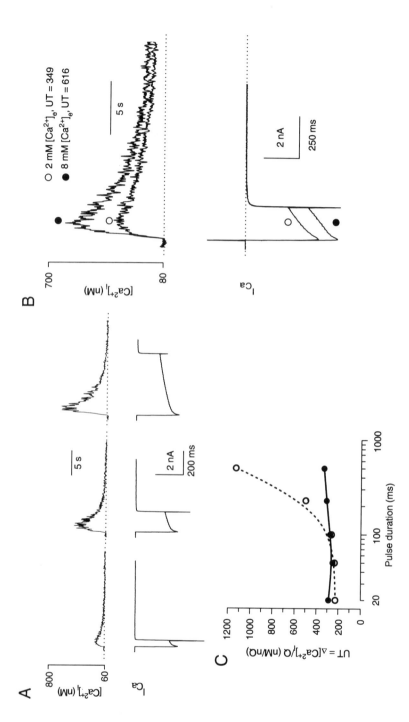

Figure 3.14. Contribution of CICR into voltage-triggered $[Ca^{2+}]_i$ transients in rat DRG neurones (from Shmigol *et al.*, 1995b; reproduced by permission of The Physiological Society). The Ca^{2+} entry was graded by increasing the duration of voltage steps (A) or by increasing the extracellular Ca^{2+} concentration (B). In both cases, the amplitude of $[Ca^{2+}]_i$ transients rose relatively higher as compared with the integral of I_{Ca}. The $\Delta[Ca^{2+}]_i/Q$ ratio ('unit calcium transient', see text for explanation) was higher at larger Ca^{2+} loads (C), indicating the occurrence of CICR

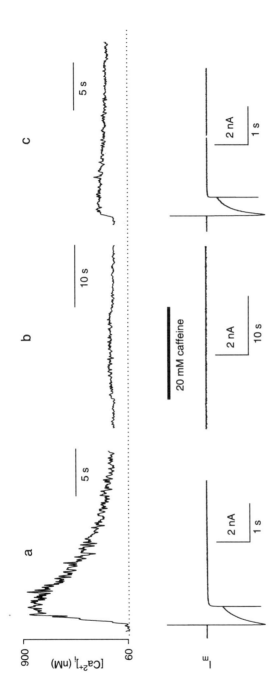

Figure 3.15. Ryanodine affects caffeine- and depolarization-induced $[Ca^{2+}]$ transient on rat DRG neurone (from Shmigol *et al.*, 1995b; reproduced by permission of The Physiological Society). The simultaneous recordings of $[Ca^{2+}]_c$ (top) and I_{Ca} (bottom) performed after 5 min cell dialysis with internal solution enriched with 10 μM ryanodine are shown: (a) first depolarization after 5 min cell dialysis; (b) 1 min after the first trace, application of 20 mM caffeine no longer induces $[Ca^{2+}]_i$ elevation; (c) second clamp pulse applied 1 min after washout of caffeine. While I_{Ca} is similar to that during the first trace $[Ca^{2+}]_i$ transient is reduced by 80%. Holding potential −60 mV; 500 ms clamp steps to 0 mV

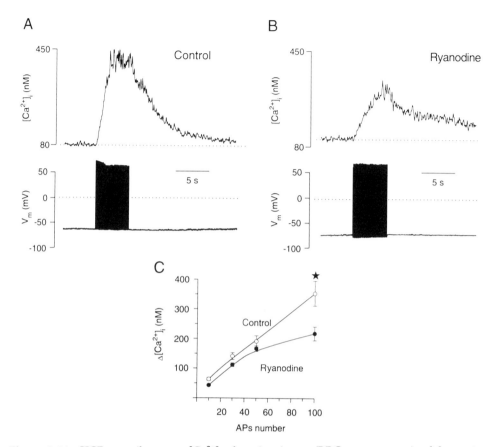

Figure 3.16. CICR contributes to [Ca^{2+}]$_i$ elevation in rat DRG neurone trained by action potentials (from Shmigol *et al.*, 1995b; reproduced by permission of The Physiological Society). (A, B) [Ca^{2+}]$_i$ transient evoked by 100 action potentials (20 Hz stimulation frequency) before (A) and after a 5 min exposure to 100 μM ryanodine (B) in the bath. (C) Means ± s.e.m. of Δ[Ca^{2+}]$_i$ evoked by action potentials as a function of the number of action potentials (frequency of stimulation 20 Hz) for control conditions and in ryanodine-treated neurones. Star marks the significant difference at 100 action potentials ($p < 0.05$)

suprathreshold current pulses. The amplitude of the [Ca^{2+}]$_i$ transient increased with increasing number of action potentials delivered to the cell with a fixed frequency. Extracellularly applied ryanodine (100 μM) reduced the amplitude of [Ca^{2+}]$_i$ responses (Fig. 3.16), suggesting that CICR can contribute to the changes in [Ca^{2+}]$_i$ provided the electrical activity of the neurone is high.

The major difference between different types of neurones studied so far is the amount of 'trigger' Ca^{2+} ions (resulting from their transmembrane influx) which are sufficient for inducing measurable CICR. The higher sensitivity of the CICR mechanism seems to be found in cerebellar Purkinje neurones where even short Ca^{2+} currents (60-100 ms in duration) were able to initiate CICR. Ca^{2+}-sensitive ER stores are more reluctant in sympathetic and sensory neurones where the duration of triggering I_{Ca} must be in the range of hundreds milliseconds. Moreover, compared with muscle preparation, the initiation of CICR in neurones obviously needs much more trigger Ca^{2+} entering the cell. In neurones short depolarization or single action potentials did not trigger CICR, while in cardiomyocytes pulses as short as 4 ms triggered maximal CICR (Han et al., 1994). Presumably, the difference can be connected to the function of CICR and the density of CICR channels. In neurones CICR amplifies Ca^{2+} influx depending on the electrical activity; cardiac CICR is specialized for secure coupling between excitation and contraction. This specialization of CICR in muscle preparations is based on a much higher density of CICR channels in muscle as compared to nerve cells: the specific activity for [^{3}H]ryanodine binding (which reflects the channel density) in the brain is only about 2-10% of that from muscle (Ogawa, 1994).

Furthermore, as density of transmembrane Ca^{2+} channel current in cardiomyocytes and neurones is comparable, the difference cannot be attributed to the amount of trigger Ca^{2+}. Instead, the amplification gain of CICR may differ due to a different Ca^{2+} load of the intracellular stores. Furthermore, the ultrastructure may be specialized for an effective CICR in cardiomyocytes but not in neurones. In cardiomyocytes, a single plasmalemmal calcium channel faces approximately eight CICR channels/RYRs of the sarcoplasmic reticulum across a 15 nm narrow 'junctional gap'. Ca^{2+} accumulation in the gap space facilitates the activation of multiple RYRs (Isenberg and Han, 1994). In neurones information about the co-localization of plasmalemmal Ca^{2+} channels and ER Ca^{2+} release channels/RYRs is absent, hence one can only speculate that a specialized ultrastructure here is less prominent than in cardiomyocytes. Since activation of CICR in neurones requires a relatively large Ca^{2+} influx (multiple action potentials, etc.) one could assume that Ca^{2+} ions have to diffuse from the plasmalemma to RYRs localized at the ER deeply in the cytosol. Over a distance of 50 nm or more, Ca^{2+} diffusion with binding dissipates the high local subplasmalemmal $[Ca^{2+}]$ (Yamada and Zucker, 1992). In this respect, the higher sensitivity of CICR to trigger Ca^{2+} in Purkinje neurones becomes understandable: these neurones express the highest density of RYRs in the brain, and the ER channels seem to be localized in close proximity to the plasma membrane.

In case of a long-lasting (or repetitive) Ca^{2+} influx, most of the Ca^{2+}-binding capacity may be exhausted; diffusion may be less hindered, and increases in the local $[Ca^{2+}]$ may be high enough for activation of CICR. Once CICR has started, the Ca^{2+} release flux may activate Ca^{2+}-gated Ca^{2+} release channels in the neighbourhood and CICR may continue for some time. This positive feedback explains why the depolarization-triggered $[Ca^{2+}]_i$ transient always continued to increase when Ca^{2+} influx was terminated.

cADPR AS A POTENTIAL REGULATOR OF CICR IN NEURONES

For quite a long time methylxanthines and ryanodine were the only one known modulators of Ca^{2+} release via Ca^{2+}-gated Ca^{2+}-release channels, and certainly it was important to find an endogenous substance able to modulate the state of these channels. Recently, such an endogenous substance which may function as a physiological modulator (or perhaps a second messenger) of Ca^{2+}-induced Ca^{2+} release has been found. The candidate for such a role is an NAD^+ metabolite, cyclic ADP ribose (cADPR; molecular weight 541), which derives from NAD^+ due to the activity of ADP ribosyl cyclase.

The ability of cADPR to liberate Ca^{2+} ions from the internal stores was discovered by Lee and his co-workers (Clapper et al., 1987). They found that NAD^+ was able to produce a huge Ca^{2+} release with a certain time lag after NAD^+ administration. Finally it appeared that NAD^+ itself does not have Ca^{2+}-releasing activity. However, it served as a substrate for ADP ribosyl cyclase; cADPR produced from NAD^+ activates Ca^{2+} release at a nanomolar concentration (Lee et al., 1989).

Turnover of cADPR

Synthesis of cADPR is controlled by two major subtypes of ADP ribosyl cyclase: one of them is a 29 kDa cytosolic protein, and the second appears to be a membrane-bound enzyme. Both types of cADP ribosyl cyclase have been detected in a number of tissues including nervous system (see Galione, 1993, 1994 for review). The membrane-associated isoform of cADP ribosyl cyclase possesses an extracellular enzymatic domain (which was shown at least for red blood cells; Lee et al., 1993), suggesting that cADPR may also be involved in intercellular signal transmission. The catabolism of cADPR is mediated via membrane-associated cADPR hydrolase, which degrades cADPR to ADP ribose. The cADPR hydrolase is usually co-localized with the cADP ribosyl cyclase.

Ca^{2+}-liberating activity of cADPR

Experiments on sea urchin eggs demonstrated that cADPR induces Ca^{2+} release from the internal stores at nanomolar concentrations (K_D ~18 nM), being thus the most potent Ca^{2+}-liberating agent described so far (Galione, 1993, 1994). The action of cADPR also required the presence of an accessory protein, most likely calmodulin (Lee et al., 1994). The cADPR-induced Ca^{2+} release can be antagonized by ryanodine, ruthenium red and procaine and potentiated by caffeine, suggesting that cADPR specifically activates the CICR mechanism (Galione, 1994). The binding sites for ryanodine and cADPR appeared to be different, but nevertheless they seem to be tightly coupled. The releasing activity of cADPR was shown to be confined only to cardiac and brain isoforms of the Ca^{2+}-gated Ca^{2+} channels (RYRs 2 and 3) (Meszaros et al., 1993; Galione, 1994); however, at micromolar concentrations cADPR induced Ca^{2+} release from rabbit skeletal muscle sarcoplasmic reticulum (Morrissette et al., 1993), although this observation remains unique.

At the molecular level cADPR was reported to bind to the putative ATP-binding site of the CICR channel/RYR molecule; moreover, it was found that cADPR (as well as ADP ribose and β-NAD^+) competes with ATP for this binding site (Sitsapesan et al., 1994). Assuming much higher concentrations of ATP, β-NAD^+ and other adenine nucleotides in the cell, it seems unlikely that cADPR may resume its ability to activate CICR under physiological conditions, although this suggestion has to be confirmed.

Recent investigations demonstrate that cADPR also stimulates Ca^{2+} release from caffeine/ryanodine-sensitive ER compartments in secretory cells (Thorn et al., 1994; Takesawa et al., 1994), brain (White et al., 1993) and heart microsomes (Meszaros et al., 1993). At 1 μM concentration cADPR was found to activate directly cardiac (Meszaros et al., 1993) but not skeletal (Galione et al., 1991; Meszaros et al., 1993) Ca^{2+}-gated Ca^{2+}

channels incorporated into the planar lipid membranes. The resting cADPR concentration in brain tissue was estimated to be close to 100-200 nM (Walseth et al., 1991), which is much higher than the K_D for Ca^{2+} release activation determined in sea urchin egg. This may indicate either a different sensitivity of ER Ca^{2+} release channels in mammalian tissue or, in fact, cADPR may serve as a regulator, rather than an activator of ER Ca^{2+} release channels in neurones. It is still a question whether cADPR may act as a distinct second messenger, or whether its action is confined to the sensitization of Ca^{2+} release channels to calcium, which would potentiate CICR in turn. It is also not clear what kind of signal-transducing pathway may control the production of cADPR. One of the possible ways suggested is the involvement of cGMP as an intermediate transmitter which activates cGMP-dependent protein kinase and the latter subsequently activates cADP ribosyl cyclase (Galione, 1994; Galione et al., 1993). The intracellular concentration of cGMP, in turn, may be regulated by plasmalemmal receptors, coupled with guanylate cyclase (GC) or by NO, which was also reported to activate GC. The latter mechanism was recently proposed for intestinal cells, in which NO induced cytoplasmic Ca^{2+} signals associated with Ca^{2+} release from ryanodine-sensitive internal stores (Publicover et al., 1993). In sea urchin eggs and rat pancreatic β cells evidence supportive of the second messenger role of cADPR also have been found. In sea urchin eggs the level of cADPR is controlled by cGMP (Galione, 1994), while in pancreatic β cells cADPR production (and subsequent calcium release) is directly stimulated by glucose (Takesawa et al., 1993; Galione, 1993).

Several attempts have been made to reveal the action of cADPR on $[Ca^{2+}]_i$ in neuronal cells. The first clue about the Ca^{2+}-regulating potency of cADPR in neural cells came from experiments on voltage-clamped DRG neurones (Currie et al., 1993). In this investigation Ca^{2+}-activated K^+ current was measured as an indicator of CICR occurrence. It appeared that cADPR may activate potassium currents, thus suggesting the occurrence of Ca^{2+} release. Later the action of cADPR on $[Ca^{2+}]_i$ was directly studied on voltage-clamped bullfrog sympathetic (Hua et al., 1994) and mouse DRG (Shmigol et al., 1995c) neurones. In both species intracellular administration of cADPR did not induce Ca^{2+} release but significantly potentiated CICR triggered by plasmalemmal Ca^{2+} entry. In cADPR-loaded neurones a significant increase of the unit Ca^{2+} transient was observed, suggesting enhancement of CICR evoked by Ca^{2+} entry (Fig. 3.17).

AGONIST-MEDIATED $[Ca^{2+}]_i$ ELEVATION IN NEURONES

The mechanism of neurotransmitter-evoked $[Ca^{2+}]_i$ signals is less straightforward as compared with depolarization-induced $[Ca^{2+}]_i$ elevation. The majority of neurotransmitters interact with several receptor subtypes, which may be co-localized in the same cell or in the same postsynaptic regions. Synaptic transmission is often associated with the generation of intracellular Ca^{2+} signals the characteristics of which are determined by a number of distinct mechanisms. The pathways for excitatory neurotransmitter-induced $[Ca^{2+}]_i$ elevation comprise the following: (1) binding to ionotropic receptors resulting in membrane depolarization, which causes activation

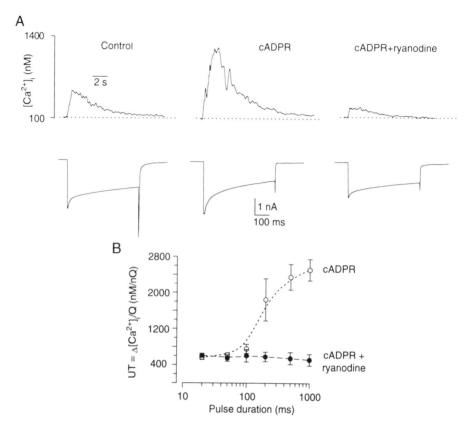

Figure 3.17. Cyclic ADP-ribose enhances CICR in mouse sensory neurones (Shmigol *et al*, 1995c; reproduced by permission). (A) $[Ca^{2+}]_i$ and I_{Ca} were recorded simultaneously in control conditions and after the intracellular administration of 1 μM of cADPR. (B) The dependence of 'unit calcium transient' from the duration of I_{Ca} recorded in the presence of cADPR and mixture of cADPR and ryanodine. Note that 'supralinear' increase in unit calcium transient starts at shorter I_{Ca} duration as compared with normal (see Figure 3.14) conditions

of voltage-dependent plasmalemmal calcium channels; (2) a number of subsets of ionotropic receptors possess significant Ca^{2+} permeability (see chapter 2) which also participate in Ca^{2+} delivery to the cytoplasm; (3) Ca^{2+} influx via both voltage- and ligand-operated channels may induce CICR, which will further amplify the signal; and (4) neurotransmitters activate several subclasses of metabotropic receptors, coupled with PI turnover and subsequent Ca^{2+} release from the $InsP_3$-sensitive calcium stores. All these pathways may act simultaneously, producing complicated cytoplasmic Ca^{2+} responses. Table 3.2 summarizes the relative importance of these mechanisms in various neurones challenged with different neurotransmitters.

In Fig. 3.18 an example of glutamate-evoked $[Ca^{2+}]_i$ response recorded from a granule cell in a cerebellar slice is shown. This response is determined by all three major pathways, characteristic for neurotransmitter-driven $[Ca^{2+}]_i$ transients. The dissection of these components may be achieved by step-by-step inhibition of the response components. First, inhibition of sodium current either by TTX or Na^+

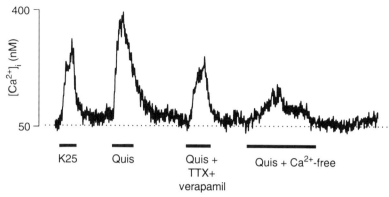

Figure 3.18. Separation of different pathways involved in glutamate-induced $[Ca^{2+}]_i$ signal generation in granule neurones from cerebellar slice (Kirischuk *et al*, 1995e; reproduced with permission). $[Ca^{2+}]_i$ was recorded from fura-2-loaded neurone in response to KCl, and glutamate agonist quisqualate (100 μM) as indicated on the graph. Quisquatate was applied in normal solution, after blockade of voltage-gated channels with TTX and Ca^{2+} antagonists and in Ca^{2+}-free extracellular solution

removal from the bath diminished Ca^{2+} entry via voltage-operated channels. The remaining component is presumably comprised of Ca^{2+} entry via ionotropic receptors and InsP$_3$-mediated Ca^{2+} release. Removal of Ca^{2+} ions from the bath revealed the IICR-associated component in a pure form. Similarly, different components interplay in agonist-induced $[Ca^{2+}]_i$ responses in other types of neuronal cells.

PLASMALEMMAL Ca^{2+} INFLUX FOLLOWING ACTIVATION OF VOLTAGE-GATED CHANNELS

The activation of plasmalemmal ligand-activated channels by neurotransmitters and neuroactive substances usually leads to the generation of inward depolarizing currents of variable (primarily cationic) nature. Depending on the density of the ligand-activated channels these inward currents might depolarize cellular membrane beyond the threshold for voltage-gated Ca^{2+} channels. Opening of the latter usually serves as a main route for Ca^{2+} influx.

Although both electrical stimulation (action potentials) and neurotransmitters activate the same pathway for Ca^{2+} entry (voltage-gated channels), the peculiarities of the resulting $[Ca^{2+}]_i$ signals may differ considerably. The depolarization induced by the action potential lasts for several milliseconds and induces a quite generalized cellular response with opening of voltage-gated channels over the whole cellular surface. In contrast, neurotransmitters may act for a notably longer period of time and their effects are highly localized, being often restricted to tiny postsynaptic regions.

Excitatory amino acids

The ability of excitatory amino acids (EAA: glutamate and its agonists kainate and AMPA) to induce $[Ca^{2+}]_i$ elevation has been demonstrated in many types of

Table 3.2. Agonist-mediated Ca^{2+} elevation

Preparation/cell type	Agonist	Mechanism of [Ca^{2+}]i rise			References
		VGCCs[a]	LGCCs[a]	Release from ER stores	
Culture/rat/DRG	Bradykinin	–	–	+++ (IICR)	Thayer et al. (1987)
Culture/rat/dorsal horn neurones	Glutamate	+++	++	–	Reichling and MacDermott (1993)
	NMDA	++	+++	–	
Cultural/rat/superior cervical ganglion neurones	Nicotinic cholinoreceptor agonists	–	+++	–	Trouslard et al. (1993)
Acutely isolated/chick/ciliary ganglion	ATP (10 µM)	++	++	–	Abe et al. (1995)
Acutely isolated/rat/thalamus, hippocampus	ATP (1–100 µM)	–	–	+++ (IICR)	Mironov (1994a)
Culture/rat/Hypothalamus	ATP	+++	–	–	Chen et al. (1994)
Culture/rat/dorsal spinal cord	ATP	+/–	+/–(?)	–	Salter and Hicks (1994)
Culture/rat/dorsal horn	GABA	+++			Reichling et al. (1994)
	Glycine	+++			
Culture/rat/septum	Glutamate, NMDA, AMPA, KA	+++	+(?) (NMDA component)		Bleakman et al. (1993)
Culture/mouse/striatum	Glutamate, NMDA	+++	++ (NMDA component)	–	Murphy et al. (1987)
Culture/rat/hippocampus	GABA	+++	(?)	–	Segal (1993)
Culture/rat/hippocampus	PAF	–		+++(IICR)	Bito et al. (1992)
Culture/rat/hippocampus	Quisqualate	+	–	+++ (IICR, CICR?)	Murphy and Miller (1989b), Furuya et al. (1989), Shirasaki et al. (1994)

Preparation	Agonist				Reference
Culture/rat/hippocampus	NMDA	+++	+++	++ (CICR)	Segal and Manor (1992)
Culture/rat/hippocampus; pyramidal neurones	Glutamate	+++	++ (NMDA component)	-	Glaum et al. (1990)
Cutlure/rat/cerebellar granule neurones	NMDA	++	++	++ (CICR)	Simpson et al. (1993)
Culture/rat/cerebellar granule neurones	Glutamate	++	+	++	Irving et al. (1992a, 1992b), Holopainen et al. (1989, 1990)
	trans-ACPD	-		+++	
	ACh	-		+++ (IICR)	
	CCh				
Culture /rat cerebellar Purkinje neurones	AMPA/KA	+++	+++	-	Brorson et al. (1994)
Slice/rat/neocortex	Glutamate	+	+++	-	Yuste and Katz (1991)
Slice/rat/hippocampus, CA1 neurones	Stimulation of native glutam-atergic synaptic input		++	+++ (CICR)	Alford et al. (1993)
Slice/rat/hippocampus, CA1 neurones	NMDA, trans-ACPD	-	-	++ (IICR)	
Slice/rat/cerebellar Purkinje neurones	Glutamate	++	(?)	+++	Llano et al. (1991)
	Quisqualate	-	-		
Slice/mouse/cerebellar granule neurones	Glutamate	+++	+	+	Kirischuk et al. (1995e)
	Quisqualate				
Slice/chicken/nucleus magnocellularis	Glutamate	+++	+ (?)	+	Zirpel et al. (1995)
	AMPA	+++	+	-	
	Kainate	++	+	-	
	NMDA	++	++	-	
	Quisqualate		-	++ (IICR)	
	trans-ACPD	-	-	+++ (IICR)	

[a]VGCC, voltage-gated calcium channels; LGCC, ligand-gated calcium channels.

mammalian neurones. They trigger $[Ca^{2+}]_i$ rise in spinal cord (MacDermott *et al.*, 1986), hippocampal (Segal and Manor, 1992) and cortical (McMillan *et al.*, 1990) neurones, etc.; the initial studies of EAA effects on $[Ca^{2+}]_i$ were comprehensively reviewed by Mayer and Westrbrook (1987a) and by Collingridge and Lester (1989). The action of EAA on $[Ca^{2+}]_i$ is quite complex and is determined by the wide variety of their receptors; the latter are responsible either for the generation of inward cationic currents (sometimes with significant Ca^{2+} component—see below) and the alteration of intracellular levels of second messengers ($InsP_3$ and cAMP) which also might activate intracellular Ca^{2+} release. Whatever the particular mechanisms of cellular excitation by EAA are, usually they depolarize the cell and trigger Ca^{2+} entry via voltage-gated channels. The relative involvement of different Ca^{2+}-gated channels subtypes in EAA-triggered $[Ca^{2+}]_i$ elevation remains to be elucidated.

Acetylcholine

Acetylcholine ionotropic responses in the nervous system are mediated by various subclasses of NChRs (see chapter 1). Activation of NChRs effectively depolarizes neurones with subsequent Ca^{2+} entry via voltage-gated channels. In addition, Ca^{2+} may permeate neuronal NChRs (see below). Unfortunately, however, there are only a few studies available concerning the mechanisms of NChR-mediated $[Ca^{2+}]_i$ signalling in nerve cells. (Decker and Dani, 1990; Feiber and Adams, 1991; Mulle *et al.*, 1992)

ATP: Ionotropic purinoreceptors

The existence of ATP-gated ionic currents in nerve tissue was first discovered in 1983 in rat sensory neurones (Krishtal *et al.*, 1983). Later, ATP-gated cation-selective ion channels (coupled with P_{2X} and P_{2Y} purinoreceptors) were found in various peripheral and central mammalian neurones (Bean, 1992; Edwards and Gibb, 1993; Edwards, 1994). The ATP-induced cation conductance effectively depolarized nerve cells and the ATP-triggered elevation of $[Ca^{2+}]_i$ mediated via activation of P_{2Y} purinoreceptors was observed in chick ciliary ganglion cells (Abe *et al.*, 1995), whereas in rat hypothalamic neurones ATP-driven $[Ca^{2+}]_i$ rise was mediated by P_{2X} purinoreceptors (Chen *et al.*, 1994).

GABA

GABA (γ-aminobutyric acid) is generally considered to be the most common inhibitory transmitter in the nervous system. GABA acts through the activation of two subtypes of ionotropic ($GABA_A$ and $GABA_C$) and one metabotropic ($GABA_B$) receptors. The functional properties of GABA receptors are determined by their subunit composition (Verdoorn *et al.*, 1990), and may vary considerably. Traditionally, both $GABA_A$ and $GABA_C$ receptors were thought to generate transmembrane flux of chloride ions (Bormann, 1988), which usually enter the cells down the electrochemical gradient (assuming an E_{Cl} of ~-70 mV and a resting membrane potential of ~-70 to -50 mV) thus causing neuronal hyperpolarization. Recently, however, the existence of a novel $GABA_A$ receptor subtype linked to the cationic (Na^+- and presumably

Ca^{2+}-permeable) channel which is responsible for depolarization in certain populations of nerve cells or in cells during early ontogenetic stages was suggested (Cherubini *et al.*, 1991; Lambert *et al.*, 1991). In addition, even acting through the conventional $GABA_A$ anion-permeable channel GABA might depolarize the cell if the latter creates the outward driving force for Cl^- ions. Possibly, both mechanisms are accounted for the generation of $[Ca^{2+}]_i$ transients recorded from several types of vertebrate neurones in response to GABA applications (early postnatal cerebellar granule cells—Connor *et al.*, 1987; postnatal neocortical neurones—Yuste and Katz, 1991; cultured hippocampal neurones—Segal, 1993; and dorsal horn neurones—Reichling *et al.*, 1994).

The activation of $GABA_A$ receptor-coupled cationic channels was suggested to produce depolarization with subsequent voltage-gated Ca^{2+} channel openings and $[Ca^{2+}]_i$ elevation in cultured hippocampal neurones (Segal, 1993). In dorsal horn neurones GABA also triggered $[Ca^{2+}]_i$ elevation; however, the mechanism of depolarization was completely different, being associated with Cl^--permeable channels (Reichling *et al.*, 1994). These neurones seem to maintain unusually high intracellular Cl^- concentrations (>22 mM) which allows Cl^- efflux (and, therefore, generation of depolarizing current) at resting membrane potential. This Cl^- current-associated depolarization was high enough in order to activate voltage-gated Ca^{2+} channels. Pharmacological analysis of GABA-triggered $[Ca^{2+}]_i$ transients with Ca^{2+} channel agonists revealed that both L- (nimodipine-sensitive) and N- (ω-conotoxin-sensitive) Ca^{2+} channels were involved in the generation of Ca^{2+} fluxes.

Glycine

Similarly to GABA, glycine receptors are permeable to Cl^- ions. Glycine was reported to generate $[Ca^{2+}]_i$ elevation in dorsal horn neurones due to Cl^--dependent depolarization and subsequent opening of voltage-gated Ca^{2+} channels (Reichling *et al.*, 1994).

Ca^{2+} INFLUX VIA LIGAND-GATED CHANNELS

The second major route for Ca^{2+} entry induced by neurotransmitters is associated with direct Ca^{2+} inflow through ligand-gated channels. For quite a long time it was believed that activation of neuronal ligand-gated channels may induce Ca^{2+} influx only indirectly, due to the generation of Na^+ depolarizing currents with subsequent opening of voltage-gated Ca^{2+} channels. This paradigm was first broken after the discovery of high calcium permeability of one of the subclasses of neuronal glutamate-gated channels—the NMDA receptors (Mayer and Westbrook, 1987a,b; see chapter 2). The activation of NMDA ionotropic receptors with subsequent Ca^{2+} entry via both NMDA-gated and voltage-gated Ca^{2+} channels was found to be responsible for Ca^{2+} signal generation in many types of central neurones (Table 3.2).

Subsequently appreciable calcium permeability was discovered for other subtypes of glutamate receptors. The evidence concerning calcium permeability of non-NMDA receptors came from experiments utilizing either recordings of glutamate-induced $[Ca^{2+}]_i$ transients in Na^+-free solutions, in solutions containing high concentrations of voltage-gated calcium channels blockers, or using quenching of fura-2 by Co^{2+} which is thought to permeate AMPA/KA channels but not voltage-gated Ca^{2+} channels. The

Table 3.3. Fractional Ca^{2+} permeability of ionotropic receptors

Preparation	Fractional Ca^{2+} current (%)	References
Recombinant GluR channels		Burnashev et al. (1995)
NMDA	8 (NR1–NR2C)–11 (NR1–NR2A)	
AMPA	0.5 (GluR-A/B)–3.9 (GluR-D)	
KA	0.2 (GluR-6 edited)–1.5 (GluR-6 unedited)	
Slices/rat/medical septum neurones/GluR channels		Schneggenburger et al. (1993)
NMDA	6.8	
AMPA/KA	1.4	
Slices/mouse/cerebellar Bergmann glial cells/GluR		Kirischuk and Verkhratsky (1994)
Neonatal (P6)	< 0.2	
Adult (P20)	2.5–3	
Culture/rat, bovine/adrenal chromaffin cells		Vernino et al. (1994)
Neuronal NChR type	4	
Muscle NChR type	2	
Culture/adrenal chromaffin cells/NChR	2.5	Zhou and Neher (1993a)

indication for Ca^{2+}-permeable AMPA/KA receptors was found for many types of cultured central neurones (e.g. striatal neurones—Murphy and Miller, 1989a; hippocampal neurones—Iino et al., 1990; Ogura et al., 1990; Segal and Manor, 1992; cerebellar granule neurones—Holopainen et al., 1989; cerebellar Purkinje neurones—Brorson et al., 1994).

Recently direct measurements of the fractional Ca^{2+} current (i.e. the part of the total transmembrane current carried by Ca^{2+} ions) recorded upon activation of glutamate receptors in physiological conditions have been performed on both cloned GluR channels and GluR channels *in situ* (the available data on fractional Ca^{2+} permeability of different types of ligand-operated channels are summarized in Table 3.3). This fractional calcium current was quite variable, fluctuating between <0.2% for homomeric GluR-B AMPA receptor and 8-11% for NMDA receptors. The fractional Ca^{2+} current determined for medial septum neurones *in situ* varied between 1.4% for AMPA/KA receptors and 6.8% for NMDA receptors, suggesting that Ca^{2+} entry via non-NMDA channels is only four times less compared with NMDA channels.

Almost simultaneously with the discovery of Ca^{2+} influx through GluR channels, a relatively high calcium permeability was found for nicotinic cholinoreceptors, expressed in the central nervous system. As compared to the muscle subtype, neuronal NChRs have higher Ca^{2+} permeability and additionally current through neuronal NChRs is modulated by extracellular Ca^{2+} concentration (Vernino et al.,

1992). The fractional permeability of neuronal NChR determined for bovine and rat chromaffin cells varied between 2.5% (Vernino et al., 1994) and 4.1% (Vernino et al., 1992) in physiological solutions ($[Ca^{2+}]_o$ 2-2.5 mM). The BTX-sensitive ChR also possesses Ca^{2+} permeability, which is mainly determined by the α_7-subunit: homomeric α_7 receptors expressed in Xenopus oocytes showed Ca^{2+} permeability comparable with those for NMDA receptors (Seguela et al., 1993). In certain regions of the nervous system the α_7 subunits dominate (e.g. ciliary ganglia—Corriveau and Berg, 1993) which may be important for the $[Ca^{2+}]_i$ signal arising from NChR activation.

Calcium permeability was also suggested for some other ligand-gated channels, including P_1 and P_2 purinoreceptors; $GABA_A$ receptors (cation-permeable), etc. For neuronal ATP-gated channels (P_2 receptors) the relative Ca^{2+}/Na^+ permeability ratio varied between 2 : 1 for isolated nucleus tractus solitarii neurones (Ueno et al., 1992) and 1 : 3 in sensory neurones (Bean et al., 1990). The fractional Ca^{2+} contribution to the ionic currents induced by all these ligands has to be elucidated.

INSP₃-INDUCED Ca²⁺ RELEASE IN NERVE CELLS

Although $InsP_3$ turnover and $InsP_3$-induced Ca^{2+} release have been studied in a wide variety of cells, and IICR has been suggested to play an important role in development of a number of important brain functions (like neuronal integrative function, long-term potentiation, learning and memory) there are still a very limited number of experimental data describing IICR peculiarities in nerve cells. The direct action of intracellular administration of $InsP_3$ on $[Ca^{2+}]_i$ has been examined so far only in molluscan neurones and in chick sensory neurones. Pressure injections of $InsP_3$ (which gave an estimated intracellular concentration of ~1 μM) into non-identified snail neurones induced $[Ca^{2+}]_i$ transients with average amplitudes 500-600 nM. These transients persisted in Ca^{2+}-free external solutions and, interestingly, in snail neurones $InsP_3$-sensitive and caffeine-sensitive stores showed clear functional and spatial distribution. Caffeine-sensitive stores seemed to be preferentially localized close to the cellular membrane, while $InsP_3$-induced responses were recorded from the centre of the neurone (Kostyuk and Kirischuk, 1993).

Similarly, pressure injection of 1 μM of $InsP_3$ into chick DRG neurones evoked large $[Ca^{2+}]_i$ transients (amplitude range 200-300 nM) in almost 80% of cells tested (Mironov, 1994b). The $InsP_3$ effects were mimicked by the non-hydrolysed GTP analogue $GTP\gamma S$, indicating the involvement of G proteins as an intermediate step in the activation of PLC and subsequent $InsP_3$ formation.

Under physiological conditions the activation of the phospholipase C family, which underlie the synthesis of $InsP_3$, is controlled by a number of metabotropic receptors widely expressed in the nervous system. These receptors share many structural and functional properties; in particular, all of them are composed of seven membrane-spanning domains and are coupled to phospholipase C via various subsets of G proteins. The metabotropic receptor family is responsible for the effects of numerous neurotransmitters and neuromodulators—glutamate, acetylcholine, ATP, noradrenaline, 5-hydroxytryptamine (serotonin), etc.

Glutamate metabotropic receptors

Molecular studies (reviewed by Nakanishi, 1992; Hollman and Heihemann, 1994) revealed that metabotropic glutamate receptors (mGluRs) belong to a broad gene family. At least six types of mGluRs (mGluR1-6; Table 3.4) with distinct pharmacological properties have been discovered and molecularly characterized so far (with exception of mGluR6, which has not been fully characterized yet). Similarly to other G protein-linked receptors mGluRs comprise seven transmembrane domains; however, their amino acid structure differs significantly from the other representatives of the G protein-coupled receptor family. The six isoforms of mGluRs represent two groups which are distinguished by their intracellular effects. Only two mGluRs, namely mGluR1 and mGluR5, are coupled with β-1 phospholipase C (PLCβ-1), thus participating in InsP$_3$ formation; four other isoforms (mGluR2, 3, 4 and 6) are linked to the inhibitory shoulder of the cAMP messenger system (see Nakanishi, 1992; Hollman and Heihemann, 1994 for review). The mGluR-controlled activation of PLC is mediated via an ample family of G proteins (Sternweis and Smrcka, 1992). Based on pharmacological studies the existence of an additional mGluR coupled with InsP$_3$ formation was postulated, although it has not yet been purified (Hollman and Heihemann, 1994). Apart from stimulation of InsP$_3$ production, mGluR1 is coupled with cAMP production and arachidonic acid release presumably via different subsets of G proteins (Aramori and Nakanishi, 1992); mGluR5 solely interferes with InsP$_3$ turnover. The successful expression of mGluR1 and mGluR5 in a transfected cell line demonstrated that both of them stimulate cleavage of PIP$_2$, InsP$_3$ production and subsequent Ca^{2+} mobilization from the internal stores.

Both mGluR1 and mGluR5 are expressed throughout the brain (see Table 3.4; Hollman and Heihemann, 1994; Tanabe et al., 1993), with some regions of preferential expression of one of the subtypes. mGluR1 is preferentially expressed in cerebellum, substantia nigra, olfactory bulb and superior colliculus, whereas mGluR5 dominates in cerebral cortex, CA1 region of hippocampus and nucleus accumbens. Interestingly, in cerebellum mGluR5 appears only for a short period during development; adult cerebellar cells completely lack it. A high concentration of mGluR5 was also found in nociceptive dorsal horn neurones of the rat (Vidnynszky et al., 1995).

Glutamate-induced [Ca^{2+}]$_i$ release

Glutamate-initiated increase of InsP$_3$ formation was initially described for cultured striatal neurones (Sladeczek et al., 1985); subsequently such an effect was also discovered in various brain regions, e.g. in hippocampal (Nicoletti et al., 1986a) and cerebellar (Nicoletti et al., 1986b; Blackstone et al., 1989) neurones. The ability of glutamate to trigger Ca^{2+} release from internal stores was first discovered in rat cultured hippocampal neurones stimulated with different GluR agonists (Murphy and Miller, 1989b; Furuya et al., 1989). In these experiments glutamate and quisqualate were shown to evoke a biphasic [Ca^{2+}]$_i$ response comprised of Ca^{2+} mobilization from the internal stores and transmembrane Ca^{2+} influx. The existence of glutamate-induced IICR-mediated via mGluR5 receptors was recently confirmed in rat pyramidal CA1 hippocampal neurones (Shirasaki et al., 1994). In the latter experiments voltage access

Table 3.4. General properties of metabotropic glutamate receptors

Receptor subtype	Molecular weight, kDa (number of amino acid residues)	Preferential agonists	Mechanisms of action	Preferential expression in the brain
mGluR1	133 (1179)	Quis > Glu > trans-ACPD	InsP$_3$/Ca^{2+} release	Cerebellar Purkinje neurones, hippocampal CA2–CA4 pyramidal neurones, thalamus
mGluR2	96 (854)	trans-ACPD > Glu > Quis	cAMP turnover	Gentate gyrus, cerebral cortex, olfactory bulb
mGluR3	99 (857)	trans-ACPD > Glu > Quis	cAMP turnover	Cerebral cortex, thalamus, glia
mGluR4	102 (880)	L-AP4 > Glu	cAMP turnover	Cerebellar granule neurones
mGluR5	128 (1151)	Quis > Glu > transACPD	InsP$_3$/Ca^{2+} release	Striatum, cerebral cortex, hippocampus (CA1–CA4); dorsal horn of the spinal cord
mGluR6	?	trans-ACPD?	cAMP turnover?	?

Glu, glutamate; Quis, quisqualate; trans-ACPD, L-AP4, L-2-amino-4-phosphonobutyrate.

was achieved using a 'perforated' patch-clamp technique; breaking through and intracellular dialysis rapidly abolished IICR, thus suggesting the existence of as yet unknown cytoplasmic factors which control IICR availability. Similarly to caffeine-releasable ER stores in central neurones, quisqualate-sensitive pool demonstrated the fast spontaneous depletion of releasable Ca^{2+} content; in order to evoke quisqualate-triggered Ca^{2+} release hippocampal neurones must be trained with depolarization providing the refilling of the ER stores.

Later mGluR-driven $[Ca^{2+}]_i$ elevation was described in cultured cerebellar granule cells treated with either glutamate or the metabotropic agonist trans-ACPD (Irving et al., 1992a, 1992b). Recently, Ca^{2+} mobilization from the internal stores triggered by metabotropic glutamate receptors was found in neurones in situ in acutely prepared cerebellar and hippocampal slices. First, Llano et al. (1991) demonstrated quisqualate-induced Ca^{2+} release in dendrites of cerebellar Purkinje cells in acutely prepared slices; subsequently, utilizing a similar preparation, quisqualate-triggered IICR was found in cerebellar granule cells (Kirischuk et al., 1995e). In both cases trans-ACPD was much less effective as compared with quisqualate, thus supporting the idea of preferential expression of mGluR1 in cerebellar Purkinje neurones. The involvement of mGluR1 was also suggested in the generation of glutamate-triggered IICR in nucleus magnocellularis neurones studied in chicken brain slices (Zirpel et al., 1995). The involvement of mGluR-driven IICR (as revealed by the specific mGluR antagonist MCPG) in the $[Ca^{2+}]_i$ response evoked in situ by the stimulation of native glutamatergic synaptic inputs was observed in a subpopulation of hippocampal CA1 neurones (Frenguelli et al., 1993). In experiments on hippocampal slices, Jaffe and Brown (1994) found that trans-ACPD induces local $[Ca^{2+}]_i$ rises in dendrites (presumably due to IICR) which may afterwards propagate to the soma through the dendritic tree. The replenishment of the InsP$_3$-sensitive stores in this preparation also required voltage-triggered Ca^{2+} entry.

Muscarinic cholinoreceptors

The metabotropic effect of acetylcholine is mediated via the family of muscarinic receptors (M_1 to M_5), which are typical G protein-coupled metabotropic receptors. Among them the M_3 subtype is coupled with PLC and InsP$_3$ production. The activation of M_3 MChRs increases cytosolic level of InsP$_3$ (Whitham et al., 1991) and mobilizes Ca^{2+} via the generation of IICR in phaeochromocytoma PC12 cells and cultured cerebellar granule neurones (Irving et al., 1992a, 1992b). In the latter, activation of MChRs releases Ca^{2+} from the same pool as glutamate, although the MChR-sensitive pathway was insensitive to pertussis toxin, suggesting the probable involvement of Gq/G11 proteins (Irving et al., 1992b).

ATP: Metabotropic purinoreceptors

Metabotropic purinorepectors have been recently characterized at the molecular level and cDNAs for both P_{2Y} and P_{2U} receptors have been cloned (Lustig et al., 1993; Webb et al., 1993). Structurally, $P_{2Y/U}$ receptors are similar to other G protein-coupled receptors and demonstrate a seven-transmembrane domain structure. P_{2Y} receptors are thought to activate PLCβ-1 in a pertussis toxin-sensitive manner, which suggests the involvement of G proteins, while P_{2U} receptors interact with PLC in pertussis toxin-sensitive and -insensitive pathways. These pathways involve the newly identified G_q/G_{11} class of heterotrimeric G proteins, which do not show pertussis toxin-mediated ADP ribosylation (Strathmann and Simon, 1990; Dubyak and El-Moatassim, 1993). Increase in InsP$_3$ production following $P_{2Y/U}$ receptor stimulation was observed in various tissues, including neuronal preparations (Allsup and Boarder, 1990).

So far the ATP-induced Ca^{2+} release from internal stores has been characterized for hippocampal and thalamic neurones kept in short-term culture (Mironov, 1994a). In these neurones ATP clearly evoked intracellular Ca^{2+} release mediated through P_{2Y} purinoreceptors. Such ATP-triggered Ca^{2+} transients were not associated with generation of membrane current and persisted in Ca^{2+}-free extracellular media. The ATP-triggered IICR was antagonized by the SERCA blockers thapsigargin and 2,5-di(tertbutyl)1,4-benzohydroquinone (t-BHQ); surprisingly it was also effectively blocked by ryanodine in micromolar concentrations.

INTERACTIONS BETWEEN CICR AND IICR IN NERVE CELLS

One of the most intriguing questions in investigations of the properties of intracellular calcium release is the interaction between IICR and CICR and understanding whether the cell possesses a single ER compartment bearing both InsP$_3$-receptors and RYRs/CICR channels, or whether IICR and CICR develop from separate Ca^{2+} pools.

The data concerning functional continuity versus functional segregation of InsP$_3$ and Ca^{2+}/caffeine/ryanodine-sensitive pools are still quite limited and controversial. Experiments performed on whole-brain microsomes and synaptosomes revealed that they are sensitive to both caffeine and InsP$_3$, suggesting co-localization of both types of release in at least some central neurones (Gandhi and Ross, 1987; Martinez-Serrano and Satrustegui, 1989; Palade et al., 1989). For cultured hippocampal neurones, for example, Murphy and Miller (1989b) found that the discharging of the Ca^{2+}-sensitive pool by caffeine did not affect the IICR activated by quisqualate, thus suggesting the existence of separate Ca^{2+} pools. However, later experiments performed on the same neurones demonstrated the IICR never could be activated after caffeine application, indicating tight coupling between IICR and CICR pools (Shirasaki et al., 1994). In snail neurones no interaction between either release mechanism has been observed, as can be seen from examples presented in Fig. 3.19. Moreover, in these cells the localization of InsP$_3$- and Ca^{2+}/caffeine-sensitive pools is also distinct: caffeine-induced release occurs near the plasma membrane, whereas InsP$_3$-mediated Ca^{2+} liberation occurs in the deeper cellular areas. Similarly, in cultured DRG neurones bradykinin (stimulator of InsP$_3$ production) releases Ca^{2+} in both soma and processes, while caffeine induces much larger $[Ca^{2+}]_i$ responses in the soma (Thayer et al., 1987). Conversely, data favouring the existence of a single Ca^{2+} store involved in both CICR and IICR were obtained in cultured cerebellar granule neurones (Irving et al., 1992a). The interactions between stores might be even more complicated: for instance, challenging of dorsal horn neurones by substance P (InsP$_3$-generating agent) depletes caffeine-sensitive stores, but caffeine does not affect the response to substance P (Henzi and MacDermott, 1992), which may suggest that InsP$_3$-stimulated release could activate CICR.

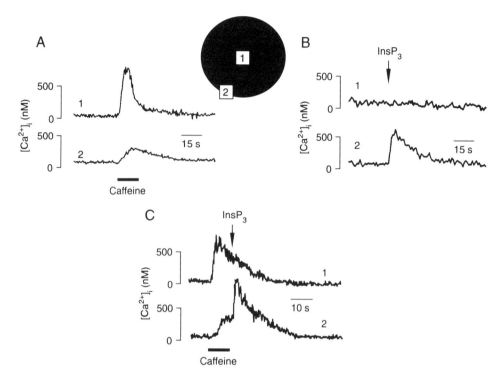

Figure 3.19. Spatial and functional separation of Ca^{2+}/caffeine- and InsP$_3$-sensitive Ca^{2+} release in snail neurone (from Kostyuk and Kirischuk, 1993 with permission). (A) $[Ca^{2+}]_i$ was recorded separately from two regions (one close to the membrane, the second in the centre) of the neurone as shown in the inset. Caffeine evoked a large $[Ca^{2+}]_i$ transient near the membrane, while in the centre of the neurone $[Ca^{2+}]_i$ elevation was much smaller. (B) Similarly, $[Ca^{2+}]_i$ was recorded upon the intracellular injection of InsP$_3$ (denoted by an arrow); the InsP$_3$-induced $[Ca^{2+}]_i$ transient was larger in the centre of the cell. (C) Caffeine and InsP$_3$ act on separate Ca^{2+} pools. The experiment was performed as described in A and B. InsP$_3$ injected immediately after caffeine application evoked an additional $[Ca^{2+}]_i$ rise in the centre of the neurone

Thus, the existence of functionally segregated or co-localized release mechanisms seems to vary considerably between various neuronal types, which may be an important determinant of $[Ca^{2+}]_i$ signalling in different areas of the nervous system.

Another phenomenon which may involve interplay between intracellular Ca^{2+} pools is the oscillations in $[Ca^{2+}]_i$. Regular fluctuations of cytoplasmic calcium occurring in response to certain biologically active substances play an important role in physiological activity of various eukaryotic cells. The $[Ca^{2+}]_i$ oscillations were observed in many types of cells outside the nervous system (see Miyazaki, 1993; Amundsen and Clapham, 1993; Petersen *et al.*, 1994 for review). In nerve cells the oscillations of $[Ca^{2+}]_i$ were observed in snail neurones (Kostyuk *et al.*, 1989), in bullfrog sympathetic neurones (Nohmi *et al.*, 1992a; Friel and Tsieu, 1992b) and in a certain population of hippocampal neurones (Murphy and Miller, 1989b). In both cases, oscillations were induced by caffeine exposure and required activation of continuous

Ca^{2+} entry. The mechanisms of the $[Ca^{2+}]_i$ oscillations presumably comprise interactions between Ca^{2+} release, refilling of internal stores and $[Ca^{2+}]_i$ modulation of the availability of the ER Ca^{2+} release channels, although the mechanism of this kind of $[Ca^{2+}]_i$ signalling in nervous tissue obviously has to be investigated in more detail.

SPATIAL ASPECTS OF INTRACELLULAR CALCIUM SIGNALLING

All results we have discussed previously concern changes in $[Ca^{2+}]_i$ all over the cell. However, in reality the distribution of cytoplasmic free calcium is not homogeneous, and a number of steep intracellular Ca^{2+} gradients may occur accompanying physiological cellular reactions. This intracellular heterogeneity of $[Ca^{2+}]_i$ signals are especially important for neurones endowed with striking specialization of various subcellular compartments. There are at least two manifestations of spatial organization of intracellular calcium signals: one which can be seen at a 'macrocellular' level (represented by $[Ca^{2+}]_i$ waves or local $[Ca^{2+}]_i$ spikes due to a peculiar concentration of Ca^{2+} channels or receptors involved in calcium signalling), and the second represented by appearance of 'microdomains' of elevated calcium.

Surprisingly, there are not many data concerning the spatial organization of 'macro' calcium signal within nerve cells. Good examples are specific generation of glutamate-induced IICR in dendrites of cerebellar Purkinje neurones (Llano et al., 1991) or appearance of radial $[Ca^{2+}]_i$ gradients in the soma of voltage-clamped sympathetic neurones (Hernandez-Cruz et al., 1990). Obviously, progress in video-imaging techniques will considerably increase our understanding of spatial organization of neuronal $[Ca^{2+}]_i$ signalling in the near future.

The problem of 'micro' calcium signals seems to be even more intriguing. Initially the idea about local organization of $[Ca^{2+}]_i$ signals came from theoretical assumptions which simulate the diffusion of Ca^{2+} ions in the cytoplasm after their entry via membrane channels (see review by Augustine and Neher, 1992b). These assumptions predict that $[Ca^{2+}]_i$ may rise to hundreds of micromoles in tiny compartments, and the microdomains with high Ca^{2+} concentration may survive for several milliseconds. Unfortunately the currently available techniques for recording spatial development of $[Ca^{2+}]_i$ signals are far from the detection of micromolar Ca^{2+} transients in a time range of several milliseconds, which has made the problem of local $[Ca^{2+}]_i$ signalling one of the most challenging questions in the whole calcium field. However, in recent years evidence (mostly indirect) supporting the idea of local $[Ca^{2+}]_i$ signals has appeared.

First, Llinas et al. (1992) using synthetic n-aequorin-J (which has a Ca^{2+} sensitivity of the order of 100 μM—Shimomura et al., 1989)-based Ca^{2+} recordings demonstrated that synaptically activated Ca^{2+} entry via plasmalemmal channels can indeed elevate $[Ca^{2+}]$ to levels > 100 μM in a tiny compartment (~1 μm in diameter) in close proximity with postsynaptic active zones. The duration of these high-Ca^{2+} microdomains did not exceed several milliseconds. Using mitochondria-targeted aequorin Rizzutto et al. (1993) demonstrated that Ca^{2+} fluxes through InsP$_3$-gated channels may also generate micromolar local Ca^{2+} gradients which are sensed by neighbouring mitochondria.

Second, a number of studies have revealed that neuronal dendritic spines form a very specialized compartment, which are relatively isolated from the rest of the neurone, and the spines might be a very good place for generating the local Ca^{2+} signals. Initially the isolation of dendritic spines in respect to $[Ca^{2+}]_i$ signals was shown by Müller and Connor (1991; see also Connor et al., 1994), who found that synaptic activation produced a $[Ca^{2+}]_i$ rise in individual spines, leaving dendrites unaffected. Similarly, purely dendritic $[Ca^{2+}]_i$ transients were not transmitted to the spines (Guthrie et al., 1991), thus indicating their unique segregation. Keeping in mind that dendritic spines play an important role in synaptic transmission in the central nervous system, local $[Ca^{2+}]_i$ signals in spines might be highly important for neuronal integrative functions. Similarly, local $[Ca^{2+}]_i$ signals arising near the ER Ca^{2+} release channels may serve as a signal targeting specifically localized enzymes.

TERMINATION OF CALCIUM SIGNALS

Being always under high pressure from intracellularly aimed Ca^{2+} gradients, eukaryotic cells have developed a sophisticated system for elimination of Ca^{2+} from the cytoplasm. This system includes (1) Ca^{2+} extrusion into the extracellular space by an ATP-driven plasmalemmal Ca^{2+} pump and an Na^+/Ca^{2+} exchanger mechanism and (2) calcium uptake by ER stores and intracellular organelles. The overlapping activity of these transporters and their competition with calcium buffers for Ca^{2+} entering into the cytoplasm actually terminate the $[Ca^{2+}]_i$ signal and determine the recovery kinetics of $[Ca^{2+}]_i$ transients.

ROLE OF THE PLASMALEMMAL Ca^{2+} PUMP

The plasmalemmal calcium pump (PMCA) serves as a low-affinity system which is able to operate at low $[Ca^{2+}]_i$, thus effectively participating in maintaining $[Ca^{2+}]_i$ at physiological concentrations. The plasmalemmal Ca^{2+} pump which ejects Ca^{2+} ions from the cytoplasm into the extracellular space was discovered by Schatzmann in 1966. Similarly to SERCA pumps, PMCA belongs to the family of P-type ion motif ATPases. PMCA exists in several isoforms encoded by a multigene family (Table 3.5); additional diversity comes from an alternative splicing. All isoforms of PMCA are relatively large proteins (~1200 amino acid residues; molecular weight ~130-135 kDa) with a similar functional architecture. The most common model proposes 10 transmembrane domains and a large region protruding into the cytoplasm (see Carafoli, 1992 for review).

The activity of PMCA is controlled by cytoplasmic Ca^{2+} and by a number of biologically active substances. The most important among them are Ca^{2+} ions themselves and calmodulin. Increase in cytoplasmic calcium activates the pump and calmodulin increases the affinity of the calcium pump and its maximal transport rate. The most commonly used blockers of the Ca^{2+} pump are vanadate and lantanides.

Methods for measurement of Ca^{2+} extrusion from cells are much less developed compared to measurement of intracellular Ca^{2+} levels. Usually radioisotope techniques and multicellular preparations are used for this purpose, and they estimate only slow extrusion processes. In our group a technique has been developed which allows

Table 3.5   Molecular diversity of plasmalemmal Ca^{2+} pumps (from Carafoli, 1992)

PMCA1	PMCA2	PMCA3	PMCA4
1a, 1b, 1c, 1d, 1e[a]	2b, 2f[a]	3a	4a, 4b, 4g[a]
1176–1258[b]	1099–1198[b]	1159[b]	1169–1205[b]

[a] Isoforms arising from alternative slicing.
[b] Number of amino acids; some isoform sequences are incomplete.

measurement of the extrusion of Ca^{2+} ions in parallel with the changes of their level in the cytosol, and it has provided the first direct data about the kinetics and intensity of this process (Tepikin et al., 1991, 1994). The technique is based on the formation of a microchamber around the isolated cell with a volume of extracellular solution of 4-7 nl (approximately 10 times greater than that of the cell). The microchamber was in fact a drop of extracellular solution covered with a layer of non-fluorescent oil to avoid evaporation. An isolated cell loaded with fluorescent indicator (fura-2) was placed in the centre of the drop, which contains another Ca^{2+} indicator (antipyrylazo III) working at different wavelengths. This allows parallel measurement of Ca^{2+} level changes both inside and outside the cell. A disadvantage of this technique is the fact that the presence of the indicator (a strong Ca^{2+} buffer) in the extracellular solution decreases the free Ca^{2+} concentration here well below the physiological level; therefore no Ca^{2+} transients can be induced by opening of plasmalemmal channels; however, they can be modelled by direct injection of Ca^{2+} through an intracellular microelectrode or release from intracellular stores.

Measurements have shown that Ca^{2+} ion extrusion from the cell starts in parallel with the rise of the intracellular Ca^{2+} signal (Fig. 3.20). During increase of $[Ca^{2+}]_i$ to 0.2-0.5 μM, the velocity of Ca^{2+} extrusion from a snail neurone varied between 0.3 and 4.6 $\mu M/s$ per cell volume. During caffeine-induced Ca^{2+} transients a stimulation of calcium extrusion took place, reaching a velocity of 5.0 $\mu M/s$ per cell volume. An approximate comparison indicates that at least 30% of Ca^{2+} injected into the cytosol is immediately extruded into the extracellular solution. This value may be somewhat overestimated because of the low free Ca^{2+} level in the drop, which may facilitate Ca^{2+} extrusion. The data obtained seem to be of a general significance, as similar measurements on secretory cells (the only difference being in using fluo-3 as the extracellular indicator) gave a mean value of $39\% \pm 12\%$ Ca^{2+} loss during a cystokinin-evoked Ca^{2+} spike (Tepikin et al., 1992).

The importance of plasmalemmal Ca^{2+} pumping in the formation of $[Ca^{2+}]_i$ signal was also confirmed in experiments on sensory neurones, where inhibition of PMCA by extracellularly applied La^{3+} significantly prolonged the recovery of depolarization-triggered $[Ca^{2+}]_i$ transients (Usachev et al., 1993, see also Fig. 3.21). The simultaneous blockade of both ER calcium pumps and PMCA pumps almost completely blocked the recovery of $[Ca^{2+}]_i$ signal, indicating the leading role of ATP-driven Ca^{2+} pumping in the termination of $[Ca^{2+}]_i$ signal in nerve cells.

The results obtained confirm the suggestion that Ca^{2+} extrusion is in fact a rapid process with kinetics comparable to those of cytosolic Ca^{2+} transients (in the range of seconds) and can substantially influence the amplitude and time course of the latter. The mechanisms directly responsible for such extrusion are still not well analysed. It

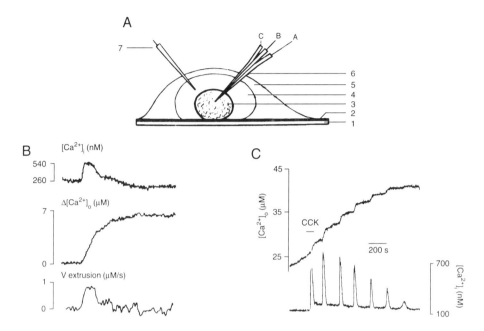

Figure 3.20. Extrusion of Ca^{2+} from a single cell measured by the microdroplet technique (from Tepikin *et al.*, 1991, 1992 with permission of Springer-Verlag). (A) Scheme of the microdroplet: (1) glass plate; (2) silicon layer; (3) isolated cell; (4) extracellular solution; (5) non-fluorescent oil; (6) three-barrel microelectrode with barrels A and B filled with 2.5 M KCl for voltage-clamp and barrel C with 0.2 M $CaCl_2$ for Ca^{2+} injection; (7) micropipette for drug application. (B) Short injection of Ca^{2+} into a snail neurone inducing a Ca^{2+} transient (top record) and parallel changes in extracellular Ca^{2+} level (middle record); rate of Ca^{2+} extrusion is shown in the bottom record. (C) Rhythmic Ca^{2+} transients triggered in a pancreatic islet cell by short application of cholecystokinin (CCK) (lower record) and changes in extracellular Ca^{2+} level induced by immediate Ca^{2+} extrusion

is most probable, at least in nerve cells, that the leading role in this process is played by plasmalemmal and ER Ca-ATPases (cf. Kostyuk *et al.*, 1989).

ROLE OF SODIUM/CALCIUM EXCHANGE

The fundamental property of the Na^+/Ca^{2+} exchange mechanism is its ability to translocate Ca^{2+} ions from the cytoplasm to the extracellular space, i.e. against a high electrochemical gradient by utilizing the electrochemical gradient of sodium ions. This mechanism has been found and extensively characterized in various excitable and non-excitable cells (reviewed by Blaustein *et al.*, 1991). In nervous cells the involvement of the Na^+/Ca^{2+} exchanger in $[Ca^{2+}]_i$ regulation was initially observed in experiments on invertebrate axons and isolated neurones.

In mammalian neurones the question of the relative importance of Na^+/Ca^{2+} exchanges in maintaining the resting $[Ca^{2+}]_i$ and in Ca^{2+} extrusion after neuronal excitation was addressed in a limited number of studies. However, the data available show a clear difference between peripheral and central neurones. In peripheral

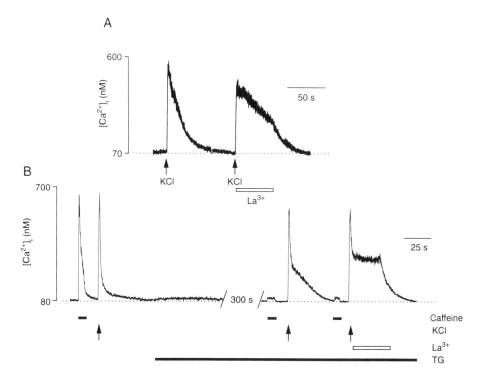

Figure 3.21. Major determinants of $[Ca^{2+}]_i$ signal recovery in mouse DRG neurone (own observations). (A) Blockade of plasmalemmal Ca^{2+} extrusion by La^{3+} (3 mM) significantly slows down the recovery of KCl (50 mM)-induced $[Ca^{2+}]_i$ transient. (B) Simultaneous inhibition of ER calcium uptake (thapsigargin TG 50 nM) and plasmalemmal Ca^{2+} extrusion (La^{3+} 3 mM) almost completely inhibited the recovery of depolarization-triggered $[Ca^{2+}]_i$ transient

neurones (rat DRG cells) Na^+ removal from the extracellular solution did not change appreciably either basal $[Ca^{2+}]_i$ or recovery kinetics of $[Ca^{2+}]_i$ transients (Thayer and Miller, 1990; Benham *et al.*, 1992; Duchen *et al.*, 1990; Shmigol *et al.*, 1995b). In contrast, in central neurones (rat brain synaptosomes—Taglialatela *et al.*, 1990; cultured hippocampal neurones—Segal and Manor, 1992; Koch and Barish, 1994; cultured cerebellar granule neurones—Kiedrowski *et al.*, 1994; acutely dissociated neurones from nucleus basalis—Tatsumi and Katayama, 1993) the Na^+/Ca^{2+} exchanger was shown to affect significantly the recovery phase of $[Ca^{2+}]_i$ transients and (sometimes) alter resting $[Ca^{2+}]_i$. The importance of Na^+/Ca^{2+} homeostasis in $[Ca^{2+}]_i$ handling in central neurones is also supported by the finding that blockade of the exchanger potentiates glutamate neurotoxicity (Mattson *et al.*, 1989; Andreeva *et al.*, 1991). Furthermore, Ca^{2+} entry via the Na^+/Ca^{2+} exchanger mechanism functioning in reverse mode was reported to enhance and prolong the glutamate-triggered $[Ca^{2+}]_i$ transient in cerebellar granule neurones. The simultaneous recording of $[Ca^{2+}]_i$ and $[Na^+]_i$ in these neurones demonstrated that cytoplasmic sodium concentration, upon glutamate exposure, may rise to 60 mM, thus reversing the exchanger and provoking additional Ca^{2+} entry through this mechanism (Kiedrowski *et al.*, 1994).

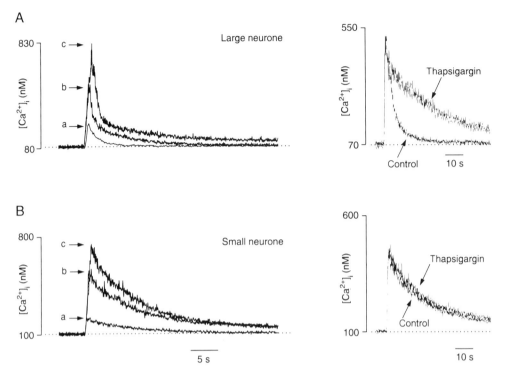

Figure 3.22. The role of SERCA-driven Ca^{2+} uptake by intracellular stores in Ca^{2+} signal termination in mouse sensory neurones (from Shmigol *et al.*, 1994b with permission from Rapid Communications of Oxford, Ltd). (A) Depolarization-induced $[Ca^{2+}]_i$ transients in DRG neurones with small and large cell bodies. Superimposed $[Ca^{2+}]_i$ transients in response to 300 ms (a), 500 ms (b) and 1 s (c) applications of 50 mM KCl solutions recorded in large and small neurones. The RP was −62 mV for the neurone shown in A and -67 mV for the neurone shown in B. The application of 50 mM KCl-containing solution depolarized the cells to -15 mV in large and −17 mV in small neurone respectively. Note the clear difference in recovery kinetics of $[Ca^{2+}]_i$ transients. (B) Superimposed records of $[Ca^{2+}]_i$ transients evoked by 2 s application of 50 mM KCl external solution measured from large and small DRG neurones in control conditions and after 5 min cell incubation with 50 nM thapsigargin. Thapsigargin clearly affects $[Ca^{2+}]_i$ transient recovery only in a large cell

ROLE OF UPTAKE BY ER STORES

Although it is quite clear that nerve cells are endowed with SERCA pumps, which allows Ca^{2+} accumulation in the ER stores, our knowledge concerning the relative importance of ER Ca^{2+} uptake in the termination of cytoplasmic Ca^{2+} signal is very limited. Emptying of the caffeine-sensitive ER stores (which would presumably enhance the rate of Ca^{2+} reuptake) was found to accelerate the rate of decay of the subsequent depolarization-triggered $[Ca^{2+}]_i$ transient (Friel and Tsien, 1992; Usachev *et al.*, 1993); however, other authors have reported insignificance of ER Ca^{2+} accumulation in recovery of $[Ca^{2+}]_i$ transients (Benham *et al.*, 1992).

The influence of direct blockade of SERCA-driven pumping on the kinetics of depolarization-induced $[Ca^{2+}]_i$ elevation was characterized on acutely isolated mouse

DRG neurones (Shmigol *et al.*, 1994b). As was pointed above, a subpopulation of these neurones (namely nociceptive sensory neurones with small somata) does not express caffeine-sensitive ER stores, presumably lacking a Ca^{2+} accumulation in this particular store. Analysis of the recovery kinetics of the depolarization-triggered $[Ca^{2+}]_i$ transient in mouse DRG neurones revealed that it was significantly faster in large versus small neurones (Fig. 3.22). In order to account for these differences in functional activity of SERCA pumps, these neurones were treated with thapsigargin, and it appeared that inhibition of ER Ca^{2+} uptake markedly slowed the recovery of depolarization-triggered $[Ca^{2+}]_i$ transients only in large DRG neurones, and left it unaffected in small ones (Fig. 3.22B). These results suggest that SERCA-mediated Ca^{2+} uptake into the ER stores may significantly determine the $[Ca^{2+}]_i$ signal kinetics only in certain neuronal subpopulations.

OTHER INTRACELLULAR SYSTEMS INVOLVED IN $[Ca^{2+}]_i$ HOMEOSTASIS

Mitochondria

Historically, mitochondria were the first intracellular organelles found to be associated with the regulation of $[Ca^{2+}]_i$: for quite a long time it was generally accepted that Ca^{2+} sequestration by mitochondria was the main mechanism of $[Ca^{2+}]_i$ homeostasis in eukaryotic cells (see Carafoli and Crompton, 1976 for review). Later, however, the point of view on mitochondrial Ca^{2+} sequestration changed towards the idea that it might be important only at high $[Ca^{2+}]_i$ (> 500 nM).

The accumulation of Ca^{2+} ions by mitochondria is achieved via an electrogenic uniporter; that is, the high proton electrochemical gradient, which provides the driving force for Ca^{2+} flow into the mitochondrial matrix. The H^+ gradient, created by mitochondrial proton transport systems, makes the inner mitochondrial membrane potential highly negative (up to −200 mV). The mitochondrial membrane appears almost impermeable to Na^+ and K^+ but it displays a highly active Ca^{2+} electrogenic transporter, which allows massive Ca^{2+} influx down the electrochemical gradient, so that the intramitochondrial Ca^{2+} concentration may reach levels of hundreds of micromoles. The nature of this transporter remains unclear, although it was hypothesized that it might be a highly mitochondria-specific calcium channel (Bragadin *et al.*, 1979). Simultaneously, the mitochondrial membrane contains electrically neutral H^+/Ca^{2+} and Na^+/Ca^{2+} exchangers which prevent mitochondria from Ca^{2+} overload.

Collapsing of the mitochondrial membrane potential (by uncouplers of oxidative phosphorylation or blockers of electron transport) causes release of Ca^{2+} ions. This release is mediated by several pathways (see recent review by Pozzan *et al.*, 1994), including passive Ca^{2+} outflow, persistent activity of electroneutral exchanger and activation of a 'mega' cationic channel with enormously high conductance (~1 nS) (Bernardi *et al.*, 1992).

The role of mitochondrial accumulation in $[Ca^{2+}]_i$ homeostasis in nerve cells and its involvement in the clearing of Ca^{2+} ions from the cytoplasm after periods of neuronal activity remains a challenging question. Usually for probing mitochondrial $[Ca^{2+}]_i$ homeostatic functions mitochondrial uncoupling agents—protonophores (*m*-chloro-phenyl-hydrazone, CCCP; and *p*-trifluoromethoxyphenylhydrazone, FCCP)—are the tools of choice (Thayer and Miller, 1990; Friel and Tsien, 1994), although they were reported to release Ca^{2+} from non-mitochondrial stores in *Helisoma* neurones (Jensen and Rehder, 1991). The common idea which emerged from experiments concerning the influence of mitochondrial uncouplers on $[Ca^{2+}]_i$ and $[Ca^{2+}]_i$ transients is that mitochondria may be an important Ca^{2+} buffer in conditions of moderate and high Ca^{2+} load of nerve cells (Thayer and Miller, 1990; Duchen *et al.*, 1990; Friel and Tsien, 1994). The common assumption is that mitochondria start to sequester Ca^{2+} when the $[Ca^{2+}]_i$ rises above a certain 'set-point', which for neurones may lie in the range of 300-600 nM (Thayer and Miller, 1990). Mitochondrial Ca^{2+} uptake may limit the peak of cytosolic $[Ca^{2+}]_i$ elevation, thus serving as a neuroprotector factor. In addition, mitochondria may represent a dynamic system which is not only responsible for fast Ca^{2+} accumulation, but may also release Ca^{2+} when $[Ca^{2+}]_i$ is below the 'set-point', thus leading to the prolongation of $[Ca^{2+}]_i$ signal recovery. Such a prolongation was indeed found in sensory (Thayer and Miller, 1990) and sympathetic (Friel and Tsien, 1994) neurones, and it might be important for temporal amplification of the calcium signal. In addition, Ca^{2+} ions accumulated by mitochondria could provide Ca^{2+} signal to metabolic processes. Another important role of mitochondrial Ca^{2+} uptake might be determined by their preferential intracellular localization in the neighbourhood of Ca^{2+} entry sites (e.g. near plasma membrane) where local Ca^{2+} concentration could be exceptionally high (>1-10 μM). In particular, mitochondria were suggested to be preferentially localized near the sites of InsP$_3$ release, where they can face micromolar calcium concentrations produced by IICR in a small microdomain (Rizzuto *et al.*, 1993). In this case mitochondria may be involved in regulation of $[Ca^{2+}]$ in such a microcompartment.

Nucleus

It is still very unclear whether the nucleus can act as a functionally distinct $[Ca^{2+}]_i$-handling subcompartment. Initial studies of the permeability of nuclear membrane revealed that many hydrophilic compounds with a molecular weight as high as 20 kDa can freely penetrate the nuclear envelope (Peters, 1986). Recently, however, video-imaging and especially high-resolution confocal microscopy recordings of intracellular Ca^{2+} distribution have demonstrated the existence of Ca^{2+} concentration gradients between nucleus and cytosol. Several groups have reported that calcium concentration in the nerve cell nucleus increased faster and reached higher levels than cytosolic Ca^{2+} after depolarization-induced Ca^{2+} entry (sympathetic, sensory and hippocampal neurones—Segal and Manor, 1992; Hernandez-Cruz *et al.*, 1990; Hernandez-Cruz *et al.*, 1991; Przywara *et al.*, 1991; Birch *et al.*, 1992). Such a heterogeneity of nuclear Ca^{2+} signal presumes the existence of a specialized amplification system, located in the neuronal envelope. The generation of an intranuclear Ca^{2+} signal might be of special importance taking into account that gene expression and other intranuclear reactions are strongly influenced by calcium ions. Indeed, there are several clues indicating the possible association of neuronal development and nuclear Ca^{2+} signals. Nuclear Ca^{2+} transients were reported to be coupled to neurite outgrowth in DRG neurones (Birch *et al.*, 1992). Furthermore, nuclear Ca^{2+} signals undergo developmental changes: prominent nuclear Ca^{2+} signals were observed in embryonic DRG neurones, whereas they became much smaller in postnatal neurones (Utzschneider et al., 1994).

Unfortunately, some caution is needed when analysing the results of Ca^{2+} indicator imaging studies; artefacts can arise from a number of conditions, including differences in viscosity in the cytoplasm and intranuclear medium, dye distribution, etc. Simultaneously with experimental evidence favouring the idea of intranuclear Ca^{2+} gradients, a number of authors have failed to observe differences in $[Ca^{2+}]$ between nucleus and cytoplasm (Marrion and Adams, 1992; Nohmi et al., 1992b; Neher and Augustine, 1992). Recently, O'Malley (1994) made a very careful examination of Ca^{2+} permeability in the nuclear envelope of sympathetic bullfrog neurones using fluo-3 confocal microscopy and intracellular perfusion with Ca^{2+} buffers. His experiments suggest that Ca^{2+} freely penetrates the nuclear envelope, and there is no evidence supporting the existence of Ca^{2+} gradients between nucleus and cytoplasm. Generally, based on currently available knowledge, it is impossible to confirm unequivocally or rule out the importance of the nucleus as a separate component of $[Ca^{2+}]_i$ homeostasis.

CONCLUSIONS

The injection of Ca^{2+} ions into the cell through the highly coordinated activity of plasmalemmal and intracellular calcium-permeable channels is the main source of temporary elevation of free Ca^{2+} level in the cytosol (the 'calcium signal') during cellular activity. However, this signal is substantially modified by several cellular mechanisms functioning on different time scales. The most rapid one is the buffering of injected ions by cytosolic buffers, mainly by Ca^{2+}-binding proteins, which occurs in a time range of milliseconds. Despite this speed, substantial spatial gradients of free Ca^{2+} still occur inside the cell, reaching millimolar concentrations near the injection sites; this might be important for triggering further cellular reactions having comparatively low sensitivity to Ca^{2+}. Altogether, not more than 1% of the injected ions remain free for exerting their physicochemical activity inside the cell.

Two other mechanisms—extrusion of Ca^{2+} ions back into the extracellular space and their uptake or release by intracellular stores, both depending on the activity of membrane ATPases—function on a time scale of seconds; nevertheless they can substantially modify the amplitude and kinetics of the calcium signal. Obviously, the relative role of these mechanisms might be substantially different depending on the type of cell, the stage of its development, as well as on possible pathological conditions. However, data on the individual features of the Ca^{2+}-handling mechanisms in nerve cells are still quite scarce, and this problem should be extensively studied.

4   Calcium Signalling in Glial Cells

Traditionally glial cells were regarded as a passive non-excitable element of the nervous system which mainly serve as structural and nutritional units. The first attempts to investigate the electrogenesis of glial cells were made in the early 1960s by Kuffler and his colleagues (Kuffler and Potter, 1964; Orkand *et al.*, 1966). The initial studies seemed to confirm the conservative paradigm, demonstrating the absence of voltage-gated ionic conductances in glial cells (Ransom and Goldring, 1973). However, an extensive investigation of glial cell electrophysiology, started at the beginning of 1980s after the introduction of the patch-clamp technique, finally demonstrated that glia expresses the same complex variety of ionic channels and neurotransmitter receptors as neurones do; moreover, the expression of these signalling molecules is highly labile and undergoes substantial changes during ontogenesis. The physiology of membrane ion channels and receptors in glial cells have been extensively reviewed recently (Barres *et al.*, 1988, 1990a; Bevan, 1990; Ritchie J.M., 1992; Sontheimer, 1994; Kettenmann *et al.*, 1993), so only a few introductory remarks will be made here.

The predominant membrane conductance in glial cells is associated with potassium channels, although glia expresses a number of voltage-gated channels, selective for Na^+, Ca^{2+} and anions. These channels (which were always regarded as an attribute of excitable cells) have been detected in various types of isolated glial cells as well as in glia *in situ*. In addition to voltage-gated channels, glial cells express a wide pattern of membrane receptors, both ionotropic and metabotropic (see Blankenfeld and Kettenmann, 1992 for review).

The investigation of Ca^{2+} handling in glial cells started in the late 1980s, and clearly demonstrated that glia possesses the ability to generate quite complex and organized $[Ca^{2+}]_i$ signals. These $[Ca^{2+}]_i$ signals together with electrical membrane responses might be an important determinant for glial-to-neuronal interactions, allowing a two-directional information exchange. In this chapter we will review the current knowledge of the mechanisms of $[Ca^{2+}]_i$ homeostasis and $[Ca^{2+}]_i$ signalling in glial cells.

Ca^{2+} DISTRIBUTION IN GLIAL CELLS

The application of microfluorometric techniques using Ca^{2+} indicators allowed precise measurements of free intracellular Ca^{2+} concentration in glial cells. Table 4.1 summarizes some of these data. An interesting feature of resting $[Ca^{2+}]_i$ in glial cells is its prominent variability not only between different subtypes of glia, but also within the same population of cells. Resting calcium in many different types of glial cells

Table 4.1 Resting [Ca²⁺]i in glial cells

Preparation/cell type	Method of [Ca²⁺]i recording	Resting [Ca²⁺]i	References
Glial cell lines			
Glioma C6	fura-2	75–200	Lin *et al.* (1992)
Glioma C6BU-1	quin-2	10–100	Ogura *et al.* (1986)
Oligodendrocytes			
Culture/brainstem	fura-2	70	Moorman and Hume (1994)
Culture/cerebrum	indo-1	5–120	Dyer and Benjamins (1990)
Astrocytes			
Culture/rat/cortex	fura-2	34 ± 4	Jensen and Chui (1990)
Culture/rat/hippocampus	fura-2	150	Ogata *et al.* (1994)
Acutely isolated/rat/ hippocampus	indo-1	5–400	Duffy and MacVicar (1994)
Culture/rat/cortex	fura-2	85–220	Goldman *et al.* (1994)
Culture/cortex	fura-2	50–160	Gabellini *et al.* (1991)
Slice/mouse/cerebellar Bergmann glial cells	fura-2	30–200	Kirischuk and Verkhratsky (1994)

varies between 30-40 and 200-400 nM. Certainly, this variability may reflect method-induced artefacts; however, it may also indicate the high lability of $[Ca^{2+}]_i$ homeostasis in glial cells which allows resting $[Ca^{2+}]_i$ to fluctuate over a wide range. The majority of experiments with $[Ca^{2+}]_i$ recordings in glial cells have been done using membrane-permeable forms of calcium indicators; thus all the problems associated with such methods (uncertain calibration, dye compartmentalization, dye photo-bleaching, etc.) has to be considered. This may, of course, influence the significance of the quantification of resting $[Ca^{2+}]_i$ in glial cells. Nevertheless, even in experiments performed on Bergmann glial cells in cerebellar slices (Kirischuk and Verkhratsky, 1995) with careful intracellular calibration procedures the $[Ca^{2+}]_i$ scattered between 30 and 200 nM. This did not reflect cell damage, because in all cases the resting potential determined by whole-cell recordings was sufficiently high (-75 to -60 mV); so we might suggest that such a high variability in resting $[Ca^{2+}]_i$ has a certain physiological meaning, reflecting for example the participation of glial cells in regulation of interstitial calcium.

As is the case with other eukaryotic cells, free cytoplasmic Ca^{2+} represents the minor part of total calcium in glial cells. The bulk Ca^{2+} is associated with endoplasmic reticulum (ER) Ca^{2+} stores, which seems to be quite elaborated in glial cells, mitochondria and Golgi apparatus (see Finkbeiner, 1993 for review). Interestingly, *Aplysia* glial cells were found to have an unusual analogue of Ca^{2+} stores—so-called 'gliagrana' (Keicher *et al.*, 1991)—which may retain an enormously high (up to 50-100 mM) Ca^{2+} concentration. The density of these gliagrana varied with fluctuation in extracellular Ca^{2+} (Keicher *et al.*, 1992), once more suggesting the possible involvement of glia in regulation of interstitial calcium concentration.

$[Ca^{2+}]_i$ MOBILIZATION IN GLIAL CELLS: AN OVERVIEW

Although many subtypes of glial cells express voltage-gated plasmalemmal channels, including those which generate inward depolarizing currents (Na^+ and Ca^{2+}), glia still remains unexcitable from the formally physiological point of view: glial cells are unable to generate action potentials. Therefore, the primary events which underlie generation of calcium fluxes are coupled with reception of chemical changes in the glial environment. In contrast to neurones, where electrical excitation plays a key role in $[Ca^{2+}]_i$ signal generation, in glial cells this function is achieved mainly by plasmalemmal receptors. Glial cells express a wide selection of both ionotropic and metabotropic receptors, the activation of which brings to the game a number of different mechanisms, finally altering $[Ca^{2+}]_i$. One important consideration also has to be mentioned here: glial cells are facing not only biologically active chemical substances released from neurones during their activity, but they are also forced to sense changes to the ionic microenvironment in the interstitium. These changes might be quite remarkable: for example, interstitial potassium ion concentration may rise to 10-15 mM under normal conditions (Sykova, 1992) and may be as high as 80 mM during brain failure (e.g. anoxia—Blank and Kirschner, 1977; hypoglycaemia—Astrup and Norberg, 1976; and spreading depression—Nicholson *et al.*, 1978). That is, KCl depolarization, which quite often is regarded as unphysiological, appears to be a natural stimulus for glia.

Table 4.2 summarizes the involvement of different mechanisms in $[Ca^{2+}]_i$ signal generation in glial cells in response to various neurotransmitters and neuroactive substances. The basic features of these mechanisms are discussed in the following sections.

VOLTAGE-GATED Ca^{2+} CHANNELS AND $[Ca^{2+}]_i$ SIGNALLING

SCHWANN CELLS

So far the only one group (Amedee *et al.*, 1991) has reported the existence of voltage-gated Ca^{2+} currents in Schwann cells from the organotypic culture of mouse dorsal root ganglia. In these experiments both T and L types of whole-cell Ca^{2+} currents were detected pharmacologically and kinetically. The expression of Ca^{2+} channels in Schwann cells ultimately required the presence of DRG neurones in the culture system, suggesting its regulation by unknown neurone-derived factors. We do not know yet how these channels may be involved in the generation of $[Ca^{2+}]_i$ signals in Schwann cells.

ASTROCYTES

MacVicar (1984) first demonstrated that electrical stimulation of cultured cerebral astrocytes superfused with 10 mM Ba^{2+}-containing solutions evokes spike-like responses. These spikes were considered as a sign of the expression of voltage-gated Ca^{2+} channels. Later, voltage-clamp experiments revealed voltage-triggered Ca^{2+} currents in salamander retinal Müller cells (Newman, 1985), cultured astrocytes from rat optic nerve (Barres *et al.*, 1988, 1990b), human retinal astrocytes (Puro and Mano, 1991) and rat cerebrum (Barres *et al.*, 1989). Interestingly, the ultimate prerequisite for expression of calcium channels was the addition into the culture medium of certain factors, namely cAMP, noradrenaline (MacVicar and Tse, 1988; Barres *et al.*, 1989), serum factors (Barres *et al.*, 1989), or co-cultivation of astrocytes with neurones (Corvalan *et al.*, 1990). This means that the expression of calcium channels in astrocytes is presumably also controlled by the neuronal environment, which may be an important clue for studying neurone-glial interactions.

Astrocytes have been shown to express at least two subsets of calcium channels: at the whole-cell level both low- and high-voltage activated Ca^{2+} currents were detected. The LVA current was very similar to the T current observed in neuronal preparations, while the HVA current appeared to be sensitive to dihydropyridines, thus reflecting the activity of L-type calcium channels. However, it has to be noted that so far Ca^{2+} currents have been observed only in cultured astrocytes; experiments *in situ* (Walz and MacVicar, 1988) did not reveal voltage-gated Ca^{2+} permeability, although there have not been many such attempts.

Ca^{2+} influx via voltage-gated Ca^{2+} channels was high enough to increase substantially $[Ca^{2+}]_i$ in cultured hippocampal, cortical and suprachiasmatic nucleus astrocytes (Finkbeiner, 1993; Fatatis and Russel, 1992; MacVicar *et al.*, 1991) and in freshly isolated hippocampal astrocytes (Duffy and MacVicar, 1994). The amplitude of 50 mM K^+ depolarization-induced $[Ca^{2+}]_i$ transients measured with microfluorometric

Table 4.2. Stimulus-evoked [Ca²⁺]$_i$ elevation in glial cells

Preparation/cell type	Stimulus	Mechanism of [Ca²⁺]$_i$ rise			References
		VGCCs[a]	LGCCs[a]	Release from internal stores	
Schwann cells					
Frog neuromuscular junction preparation	ATP ACh	- -	- -	+++ +++	Jahromi et al. (1992, Reist and Smith (1992)
Culture/rat/sciatic nerve	ACh, histamine, glutamate	-(?)	++(?)	+++	Yoder et al. (1992), Lyons et al. (1992)
Oligodendrocytes					
Culture/mouse cortex, rabbit retina	Depolarization (KCl)	+++	-	-	Kirischuk et al. (1995d), Borges et al. (1994)
Culture/rat/optic nerve	PDGF (2 ng/ml)	-	-	+++	Hart et al. (1989)
Culture/rat/cortex Culture/mouse/oligodendrocyte precursors	Myelin extract GABA (1–100 µM)	- +++	- -	+++ +++	Moorman and Hume (1994) Kirchhoff and Kettenmann (1992)
Culture/mouse/oligodendrocyte precursors	Kainate (100 µM)	+++	-(?)	-	Borges et al. (1994)
Culture/mouse cortex	ATP (1–100µM)	-	-	+++	Kirischuk et al. (1995c)
Slice/mouse/corpus callosum					
Culture/mouse cortex Culture/rabbit retina	FCCP (10 µM)	-	-	+++ (mitochondrial pool)	Kirischuk et al. (1995b)
Culture/mouse/cerebrum	Antibodies to galactocerebroside	-	-	+++	Dyer and Benjamins (1990)
Culture/mouse/cortex	NGF	-	-	+++	Engel et al. (1994)
Astrocytes					
Human astrocytoma (1321N1, UC-11NG)	Histamine ACh (MChR)	-	-	+++	Yanai et al. (1992), Lucherini and Gruenstein (1992), Noronha-Blob et al. (1987)
Culture/rat/spinal cord	Glutamate (100 µM)	++	-(?)	+++	Ahmed et al. (1990)
Culture/rat/hippocampus, cortex, mouse/cortex Acutely isolated/rat/hippocampus	Depolarization (KCl)	+++	-	-	Fatatis and Russel (1992), MacVicar et al. (1991), Finkbeiner (1993)

Preparation	Agonist/stimulus			References
Culture/neonatal rat brain	Bradikinine (0.01–10 μM)	–	+++	Duffy and MacVicar (1994), Gimpl et al. (1992)
Culture/neonatal rat brain	Neuropeptide Y	+++	–	Gimpl et al. (1993)
Culture/rat/cerebrum	α-Adrenoagonists	+(?)	+++	Enkvist et al. (1989a, McCarthy and Salm (1991); Shao and McCarthy (1993, 1994)
Culture/rat/cerebrum (astrocyte types 1,2)	Histamine	–	+++	McCarthy and Salm (1991), Inagaki and Wada (1994)
Culture/rat/cerebrum (astrocyte type 1)	ATP (10 μM) Noradrenaline (100 μM) Histamine (1 mM) Carbachol (1 mM)	–	+++	Salm and McCarthy (1990), Shao and McCarthy (1993)
Culture/rat/cerebrum (astrocyte type 1)	Prostaglandin $F_{2\alpha}$		+++	Ito et al. (1992), Inagaki and Wada (1994)
Culture/mouse/striatum	Adenosine	++	++(?)	Delumenau et al. (1991a, 1991b)
	Tachykinin NK-1	+(?)	–	
Culture/rat/neurohypophysis	Vasopressin	+	+++	Hatton et al. (1992)
	Oxytocin		+++	
Mixture culture/neonatal rat brain (primarily astrocytic)	Mechanical stimulation Thapsigargin	+/–	–	Charles et al. (1993)
Culture/rat/dorsal spinal cord	ATP	–	+++	Salter and Hicks (1994)
Culture/rat/cortex	Glutamate (100 μM)	++	++	Jensen and Chui (1990)
	Quisqualate (10 μM)	+	+++	Holzwarth et al. (1994)
	Kainate (10 μM)	–		
Culture/rat/hippocampus	GABA	+++	–	Fraser et al. (1994)
Culture/rat/cortex	GABA$_A$ agonists	+	+(?)	Nilsson et al. (1993)
	GABA$_B$ agonists	–	++(?)	
Culture/rat/hippocampus	Adenosine (1 μM) + trans-ACPD (10 μM)	–	+++	Ogata et al. (1994)
Culture/rat/suprachiasmatic nucleus	Glutamate (100 μM) 5-HT	++	+	Van den Pol et al. (1992)
Acutely isolated/rat/hippocampus	Endothelin 3	+	+++	Suppatapone et al. (1989)
Culture/rat/cerebellum/Optic nerve/ rat/ astrocyte type 1(?)	Electrical stimulation of axon; glutamate	–	+++	Kriegler and Chiu (1993)
Slice/mouse/cerebellar Bergmann glial cells	ATP (100 μM)	–	+++	Kirischuk et al. (1995a)
Microglial cells				
Culture/mouse brain	ATP	+++	–(?)	Waltz et al. (1993)

[a]VGCC, voltage-gated calcium channels; LGCC, ligand-gated calcium channels.

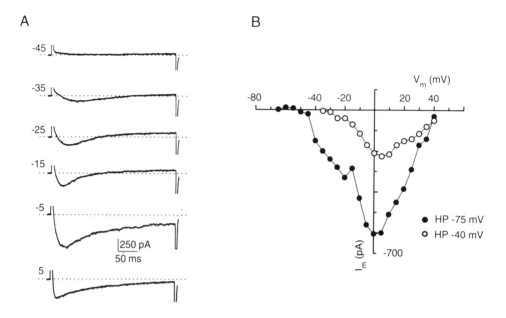

Figure 4.1. Voltage-gated calcium currents in mouse oligodendrocytes (from Blankenfeld *et al.*, 1992 with permission from Oxford University Press). (A) Examples of whole-cell Ca^{2+} currents measured from mature oligodendrocyte. For current measurements Ba^{2+} ions were used as the main permeable cation in the extracellular solution. (B) I–V curves of Ca^{2+} currents measured from mature oligodendrocyte precursors and mature oligodendrocytes. The I–V curve measured from holding potential –70 mV shows a clear hump, suggesting the existence of LVA and HVA current components. Shift of the holding potential to –40 mV eliminated the LVA Ca^{2+} current component due to steady-state inactivation

fura-2 and indo-1-based techniques reached 400-800 nM (Fatatis and Russel, 1992; MacVicar *et al.*, 1991). The high K^+-induced $[Ca^{2+}]_i$ elevation measured from astrocytes was clearly associated with Ca^{2+} entry via plasmalemmal voltage-gated channels: these $[Ca^{2+}]_i$ transients were blocked by Ca^{2+} removal from the bath, and substantially inhibited by organic (verapamil) and inorganic (Cd^{2+}, Co^{2+}) calcium antagonists (Duffy and MacVicar, 1994). In addition to voltage-gated plasmalemmal calcium channels Ca^{2+} ions may enter the astrocytes via stretch-activated (Puro, 1991a) and Ca^{2+}-activated Ca^{2+}-permeable channels (Puro, 1991b) found in human retinal Müller cells.

OLIGODENDROCYTES

Probably the first calcium currents were recorded from oligodendrocytes in 1987 by Grantyn and Kettenmann (personal communication). Later on voltage-gated calcium currents were characterized in cultured mouse oligodendrocytic precursors (Verkhratsky *et al.*, 1990). The density of these channels was found to be very low, and whole-cell calcium currents were detected only in conditions when high concentrations of Ba^{2+} ions were used as current carrier. Oligodendrocytic precursors demonstrated both

LVA (presumably T) and HVA Ca^{2+} currents. Later both these currents were found in mature oligodendrocytes (Fig. 4.1), and, moreover, it appeared that the expression of Ca^{2+} channels underwent substantial changes during oligodendrocyte development (Blankenfeld *et al.*, 1992). The investigation of the developmental changes of ionic channel expression in the oligodendrocyte lineage was facilitated by the discovery of a number of developmental stage-specific antibodies (so-called O series antibodies) which unequivocally distinguish between early glial precursors (O-negative), immature (O4-positive) and mature (O10-positive) oligodendrocytes (Sommer and Schachner, 1981, 1982). Ca^{2+} channels are present in early glial precursor cells; they are not detected in immature oligodendrocytes, but they reappear in more mature oligodendrocytes (Blankenfeld *et al.*, 1992).

The expression of Ca^{2+} channels in oligodendrocytic precursors was subsequently confirmed *in situ* in patch-clamp experiments performed on slices from mouse corpus callosum (Berger *et al.*, 1991). The question concerning expression of Ca^{2+} channels in mature oligodendrocytes *in vivo* still remains open.

Detailed investigation of depolarization-induced $[Ca^{2+}]_i$ transients was performed on cultured oligodendrocytes from mouse cortex and rabbit retina using high-resolution laser scanning confocal microscopy (Kirischuk *et al.*, 1995d). Depolarization of oligodendrocytes with application of 50 mM K^+ extracellular solutions led to the development of $[Ca^{2+}]_i$ transients as revealed by fluo-3-based measurements. These $[Ca^{2+}]_i$ transients disappeared after Ca^{2+} removal from the bath, were blocked by Ca^{2+} antagonists (Cd^{2+} and verapamil), and potentiated by Ca^{2+} agonist BAY K 8644, suggesting major involvement of voltage-gated Ca^{2+} channels (Kirischuk *et al.*, 1995d). Line-scan high temporal resolution recordings additionally demonstrated that depolarization triggered a fast increase in $[Ca^{2+}]_i$ beneath the membrane with subsequent spreading of Ca^{2+} ions towards the centre of the cell (Fig. 4.2).

Depolarization-induced $[Ca^{2+}]_i$ transients in addition demonstrated a distinct spatial heterogeneity, being more pronounced in oligodendrocytic processes. As shown in Fig. 4.3A, a moderate depolarization of the oligodendrocyte precursor by 20 mM K^+ led to an increase of fluo-3 fluorescence in the processes only, while $[Ca^{2+}]_i$ levels in the soma remained unaffected. An increase in $[K^+]_o$ (and thus an increase in the degree of cellular depolarization) resulted in a progressive fall in the amplitude of $[Ca^{2+}]_i$ elevation in processes, while in the soma $[Ca^{2+}]_i$ transients became larger (Kirischuk *et al.*, 1995d). Furthermore, $[Ca^{2+}]_i$ signals in processes and in somata of oligodendrocytic precursors can be dissected pharmacologically: Ni^{2+} (antagonist of low-voltage-activated Ca^{2+} channels) inhibited depolarization-induced $[Ca^{2+}]_i$ transients only in the processes (Fig. 4.3B), while dihydropyridines affected somatic depolarization-triggered $[Ca^{2+}]_i$ responses.

An uneven distribution of Ca^{2+} channels was also observed in mature oligodendrocytes (Fig. 4.4); depolarization-induced $[Ca^{2+}]_i$ increase was mainly confined to the processes whereas $[Ca^{2+}]_i$ levels in the soma increased to a much smaller extent. In mature oligodendrocytes $[Ca^{2+}]_i$ signal in processes is mediated by both LVA and HVA Ca^{2+} channels.

Interestingly, 10 mM of extracellular K^+—the concentration which was observed in the extracellular space during neuronal activity in white matter (see above)—also caused a clearly detectable increase in $[Ca^{2+}]_i$ (Fig. 4.4C). Therefore, activation of

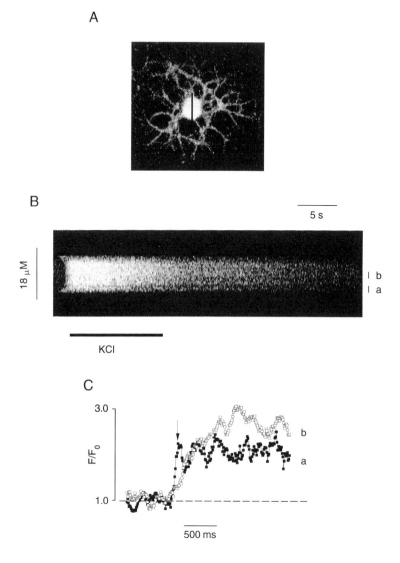

Fig 4.2. Activation of Ca²⁺ channels causes fast Ca²⁺ entry into oligodendrocytes (from Kirischuk *et al.*, 1995d with permission from Wiley-Liss, a division of John Wiley & Sons, Inc). To resolve the Ca²⁺ dynamics close to the plasma membrane Ca²⁺ distribution was measured by laser confocal microfluorimetry using the line scan mode. (A) Experimental protocol: the line was positioned through the centre of the cell soma and transient changes in Ca²⁺ were resolved with a time resolution of 10 ms per line scan. (B) Sequence of scans along the selected line: brighter regions correspond to higher [Ca²⁺]ᵢ levels. (C) At two locations in the cell, marked as a and b in B, the fluo-3 fluorescence change was resolved with a high time resolution during the onset of high-K⁺ application. It is evident that close to the membrane (a) the Ca²⁺ increase occurred much faster

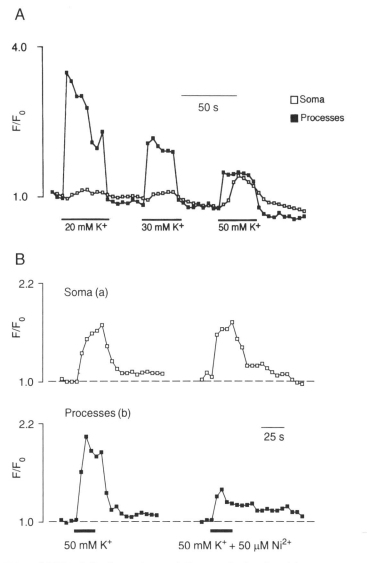

Figure 4.3. LVA and HVA Ca^{2+} channels are differentially localized between processes and soma of oligodendrocytic precursor (from Kirischuk *et al.*, 1995d with permission from Wiley-Liss, a division of John Wiley & Sons, Inc). (A) Fluorescence ratio (F/F_0) as a measure of $[Ca^{2+}]_i$ was recorded separately from processes and soma; $[K^+]_o$ was increased as indicated by bars. (B) Ni^{2+} ions suppressed depolarization-triggered $[Ca^{2+}]_i$ response only in processes of the oligodendrocyte precursors. $[Ca^{2+}]_i$ was separately recorded from the processes and soma by means of fluo-3 fluorescence

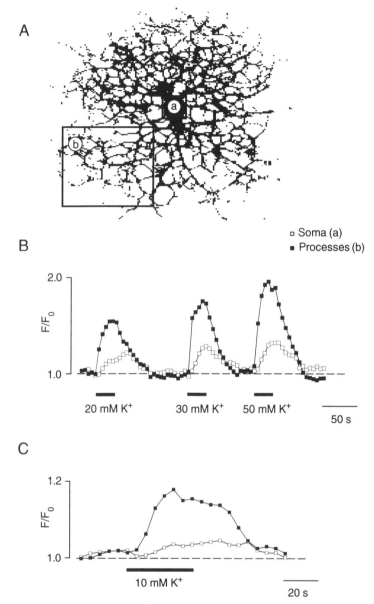

Figure 4.4. Depolarization-induced $[Ca^{2+}]_i$ transients in mature oligodendrocytes (from Kirischuk *et al.*, 1995d with permission from Wiley-Liss, a division of John Wiley & Sons, Inc). (A) The image of fluo-3-loaded mature oligodendrocyte. (B, C) $[Ca^{2+}]_i$ recordings (measured as a fluo-3 fluorescence ratio, F/F_o) from the soma and processes of the cell shown in A. $[K^+]_o$ was increased as indicated by bars

voltage-gated Ca^{2+} channels in oligodendrocytes may be significant (in respect to $[Ca^{2+}]_i$ signal generation) under physiological conditions.

MICROGLIAL CELLS

Microglial cells are probably the only representatives of glia which seem not to express voltage-gated Ca^{2+} channels. Neither electrophysiological (Bruner and Murphy, 1993) nor microfluorometric experiments revealed depolarization-triggered Ca^{2+} influx in microglia.

CALCIUM STORES AND Ca^{2+} RELEASE

As was mentioned at the beginning of this chapter, glial cells have an ER which can serve as a morphological substrate for rapidly exchanging Ca^{2+} stores. Unfortunately, we are still lacking information about the expression of different components of the Ca^{2+} release mechanism (Ca^{2+} release channels, SERCA pumps, Ca^{2+}-binding proteins, etc.) in glial cells. However, the available physiological data demonstrate one striking difference between neurones and glia in respect to the mechanisms of ER calcium release: it seems that glial cells lack CICR. Many trials for CICR discovery in glial cells (see, for example, Charles et al., 1993; Duffy and MacVicar, 1994; Kirischuk et al., 1995d; Peuchen et al., 1995) using caffeine and ryanodine failed; although this question is still open. Sometimes (e.g. Wood et al., 1993; Duffy and MacVicar, 1994) caffeine was observed to produce a small (< 50 nM) elevation in $[Ca^{2+}]_i$ in both oligocytes and astrocytes. However, in these experiments indo-1 was used as a $[Ca^{2+}]_i$ indicator, and the observed caffeine-induced $[Ca^{2+}]_i$ elevation may simply reflect artefacts coupled with caffeine-dependent quenching of indo-1. Certainly, some additional and more precisely aimed experiments are needed in order to confirm or refute CICR expression in glia. Very recently the indications for functional CICR were found in Schwann cells (Lev-Ram and Ellisman, 1995). In contrast, IICR is very elaborated in glia, and it seems to be involved in the majority of neurotransmitter effects in glial cells. Glial cells express a wide variety of metabotropic receptors coupled with $InsP_3$ production; increase in cytosolic concentration of $InsP_3$ in glial cells was observed in response to glutamate (Milani et al., 1989; Pearce et al., 1985), acetylcholine (Masters et al., 1984), ATP (Kastritsis et al., 1992; Kirischuk et al., 1995a, c), histamine (Arbones et al., 1988), endothelin (Lin et al., 1992), prostaglandins (Inagaki and Wada, 1994), noradrenaline (Pearce et al., 1985), angiotensin II (Tallant et al., 1991), arginine vasopressin (Hatton et al., 1992), substance P (Marriot et al., 1991), protein S-100 (Barger and Van Edlick, 1992), thrombin (Tas and Koshel, 1990), and many other neuroligands.

AGONIST-INDUCED CALCIUM SIGNALLING IN GLIAL CELLS

GLUTAMATE

Glutamate ionotropic receptors

Glutamate-induced calcium signalling is widely distributed among various types of glial cells. Glutamate-driven $[Ca^{2+}]_i$ transients have been shown for a variety of oligocytic and astrocytic cellular preparations (Table 4.2). In particular, ionotropic glutamate receptors which can induce $[Ca^{2+}]_i$ rise via different routes have been detected in cultured cells and in brain slices. Contrary to neurones, where glutamate-driven $[Ca^{2+}]_i$ signalling is associated mainly with NMDA receptors, in glial cells the leading role is linked to AMPA/kainate(KA) receptors. So far, only one group have reported NMDA-induced $[Ca^{2+}]_i$ rise in a minor subpopulation of cultured spinal cord astrocytes (Ahmed et al., 1990).

The molecular composition of AMPA/KA glutamate receptors has been detected for several subtypes of glial cells, and for certain populations of glial cells an appreciable Ca^{2+} permeability of glutamate-gated channels was demonstrated. In both corpus callosum astrocytes (Matute and Miledi, 1993) and in glial cells from the optic nerve (Jensen and Chiu, 1993) GluR-A and GluR-C are preferentially expressed, thus providing an expectation for reasonable Ca^{2+} permeability of these ionotropic receptors. The expression of mRNA from corpus callosum (Matute and Miledi, 1993) in oocytes revealed KA responses with prominent inward rectification, which is a characteristic property of Ca^{2+}-permeable GluR composition.

In cultured primary oligodendrocytes and oligodendrocytic precursors from rat cerebral cortex, as well as in the oligodendrocytic cell line CG-4 and type 2 astrocytes, Northern blot analysis revealed high expression of AMPA-related GluR-B, -C and -D as well as KA receptor-related GluR-6 and KA-2 subunits (Gallo et al., 1994). Polymerase chain reaction (PCR) performed on cultured cortical type 1 astrocytes and multipotential oligo/astrocyte progenitors demonstrated the expression of GluR-A, -B, -C, -D as well as GluR-6 (Holzwarth et al., 1994).

High expression of the GluR-B subunit, which determines Ca^{2+} impermeability of the glutamate receptor, suggests that the major route for glutamate-driven $[Ca^{2+}]_i$ elevation in glial cells must be coupled with membrane depolarization with subsequent opening of voltage-gated Ca^{2+} channels. Electrophysiological identification of glutamate-triggered cationic currents was performed on oligodendrocyte precursors (Wyllie et al., 1991; Patneau et al., 1994) and in mature oligodendrocytes (Patneau et al., 1994). This cationic conductance generated due to the activation of AMPA/KA receptors caused subsequent Ca^{2+} entry via voltage-gated plasmalemmal channels and $[Ca^{2+}]_i$ elevation, as was found in immunologically identified murine oligodendrocyte precursors and immature oligodendrocytes (Borges et al.,1994); blockade of voltage-gated Ca^{2+} channels abolished $[Ca^{2+}]_i$ rise in glutamate, AMPA or KA challenged unclamped cells, but did not affect significantly parameters of whole-cell currents through AMPA/KA receptors. In type 1 astrocytes and astrocytic precursors, however, microfluorometric investigations of glutamate (or KA)-triggered $[Ca^{2+}]_i$ transients revealed a large increase in $[Ca^{2+}]_i$ (up to 400-500 nM) even in Na^+-deficient extracellular solutions, which limited the ability of glutamate agonists to depolarize the cell (Enkvist et al., 1989b; Holzwarth et al., 1994). Moreover, Co^{2+} ions, which cannot permeate through voltage-gated Ca^{2+} channels, were shown to enter the glial cell upon KA application (as determined by fura-2 quenching—Holzwarth et al., 1994). This result suggests that AMPA/KA ionotropic receptors in glial cells exert Ca^{2+} permeability high enough to produce large-amplitude $[Ca^{2+}]_i$ transients. Glutamate-triggered $[Ca^{2+}]_i$ elevation was also observed in astrocytes in organotypic cultures, where glutamate was released from neighbouring neurones (Dani et al.,

1992), indicating the physiological significance of glutamate-induced $[Ca^{2+}]_i$ signalling in glial cells. How can glutamate-induced Ca^{2+} entry be related to high expression of GluR-B subunit which is thought to inhibit Ca^{2+} permeability in heteromeric glutamate receptors? The simplest explanation is that cortical glial cells may express a mixture of Ca^{2+}-permeable and -impermeable receptors, or that GluR-B subunit may appear in glial cells in unedited (Ca^{2+}-permeable) form. Another possibility may be coupled with the relatively low buffer capacity of glial cells, which will cause a large $[Ca^{2+}]_i$ elevation in response to a small Ca^{2+} influx. In this case even a low (but existing) Ca^{2+} influx via GluR-B-containing receptors might be sufficient to produce an appreciable $[Ca^{2+}]_i$ transient.

A different situation was found in cerebellar Bergmann glial cells. These cells completely lack voltage-gated plasmalemmal Ca^{2+} channels, and the only pathway for Ca^{2+} influx described so far is Ca^{2+} entry via KA ionotropic receptors. *In situ* hybridization analysis of cerebellar Bergmann glia showed high levels of GluR-A, -C, and -D mRNAs, but no expression of GluR-B (Burnashev *et al.*, 1992; Müller T. *et al.*, 1992). Consistent with this peculiar expression, Bergmann glial cells studied in cerebellar slices develop $[Ca^{2+}]_i$ transients linked to Ca^{2+} influx through AMPA/KA glutamate receptors (Müller T. *et al.*, 1992). The fractional Ca^{2+} permeability of these receptors was in the range of 2.5-3% (Kirischuk and Verkhratsky, 1994). Interestingly, cerebellar Bergmann cells *in situ* are also shown to express NMDA receptors, which, however, appear to be Ca^{2+}-impermeable (Müller T. *et al.*, 1993).

The Ca^{2+} permeability of AMPA/KA receptors in cerebellar Bergmann glial cells is also regulated during development: it was found recently (Kirischuk and Verkhratsky, 1995) that in young cerebellum slices (mice, between postnatal days 1 and 6) application of KA induced an inward current which was not associated with $[Ca^{2+}]_i$ rise. The Ca^{2+}-permeable receptors become significantly expressed only from postnatal day 16.

Glutamate metabotropic receptors

In situ hybridization (Tanabe *et al.*, 1993) revealed the expression of only mGluR-3 (preferential) and mGluR-4 in glial cells throughout the brain (with the exception of the rat optic nerve, where the expression of PLC coupled mGluRs (mGluR-1-?) was reported by Jensen and Chiu, 1993). These receptors are not linked to the activation of phospholipase C, being thereby non-effective in InsP$_3$ formation and triggering the IICR. However, numerous studies clearly demonstrated that a significant component of glutamate-induced $[Ca^{2+}]_i$ elevation in glial cells is associated with Ca^{2+} release from InsP$_3$-sensitive ER stores (cultured astrocytes—Ahmed *et al.*, 1990; Finkbeiner, 1993; Holzwarth *et al.*, 1994; oligodendrocytes—Kastritsis and McCarthy, 1993). Moreover, in many cases *trans*-ACPD, which is believed not to be the preferential agonist of mGluR-1 and -5 linked to PIP$_2$ hydrolysis, was very effective in inducing intracellular Ca^{2+} release in cultured astrocytes (Finkbeiner, 1993; Kim *et al.*, 1994). Therefore, we may assume that glial cells express members of the metabotropic GluRs family which are not entirely similar to those described so far in nervous tissue.

PURINORECEPTORS

ATP seems to be the most abundant and reliable $[Ca^{2+}]_i$ mobilizer in glial cells. ATP induces $[Ca^{2+}]_i$ elevation in all types of brain macroglia, in peripheral Schwann cells and in microglial cells.

Ionotropic ATP receptors

ATP-gated cationic channels have been found in cultured astrocytes (Shao and McCarthy, 1994; Walz et al., 1995) and microglial cells (Walz et al., 1993). In both preparations ATP activates cationic conductance via P_{2Y} purinoreceptors; however, the mechanism for $[Ca^{2+}]_i$ elevation was somewhat different. In cultured astrocytes Ca^{2+} entered the cytoplasm via both ATP-gated channels and voltage-gated Ca^{2+} channels, while in microglia Ca^{2+} entry through ATP-gated channels was the exclusive route for $[Ca^{2+}]_i$ elevation.

Metabotropic ATP receptors

The ATP driven formation of InsP$_3$ (through activation of $P_{2Y/U}$ receptors) is another mechanism for $[Ca^{2+}]_i$ elevation, widely expressed in glial cells. This mechanism may coexist with ionotropic Ca^{2+} elevation in astrocytes (Kastritsis et al., 1992) and microglial cells (Kirischuk and Verkhratsky, own observations) and it plays an important role in $[Ca^{2+}]_i$ mobilization in oligodendrocytes.

For the oligodendrocytic cell lineage the existence of ATP-mediated calcium signalling was discovered for both cultured cells from various CNS regions (Kastritsis and McCarthy, 1993; Kirischuk et al., 1995c) and in oligodendrocytes in situ in corpus callosum slices (Kirischuk et al., 1995c). Examples of ATP-triggered $[Ca^{2+}]_i$ transients measured with fluo-3-based laser confocal scanning microscopy from cultured oligodendrocytes are shown in Fig. 4.5. Oligodendrocytes acquired sensitivity to ATP during their development: ATP evoked $[Ca^{2+}]_i$ elevation only in late precursors and oligodendrocytes but not in early glial precursor cells. Similarly, while recording from corpus callosum slices ATP responses were measured only starting from postnatal day 12, when maturation of the majority of oligodendrocytes in the corpus callosum was completed. In contrast, at postnatal days 1-6, when glial elements of the corpus callosum are represented by precursor cells, ATP was ineffective. ATP-mediated $[Ca^{2+}]_i$ responses were not accompanied by generation of transmembrane current and it remained basically unchanged after 2-3 min incubation with Ca^{2+}-free solution, suggesting that ATP-mediated elevation of $[Ca^{2+}]_i$ is due to Ca^{2+} liberation from intracellular stores.

The characteristic pharmacology of ATP-induced $[Ca^{2+}]_i$ responses in oligodendrocytes is shown in Fig 4.6. The rank order of potency for the purine and pyrimidine nucleotides was: UTP $\geq$ ATP > ADP $\gg$ AMP = adenosine = α,β-methylene-ATP for retinal oligodendrocytes, and ADP $\geq$ ATP $\gg$ UTP = AMP = adenosine = α,β-methylene-ATP for cortical oligodendrocytes. In addition, sensitivity to ATP, ADP and UTP sometimes varied even among cells from the same culture, and slightly changed during oligodendrocyte development from late precursors to mature cells (Kirischuk

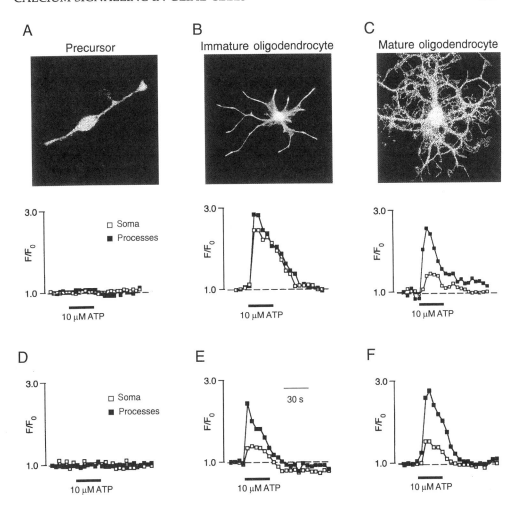

Figure 4.5. ATP-induced calcium signals in cultured oligodendrocytes at different developmental stages (from Kirischuk *et al.*, 1995c; reproduced by permission of The Physiological Society). (A–C) Upper panel shows images of mouse cortical oligodendrocyte precursor, mature and immature oligodendrocytes; lower panel shows [Ca^{2+}]$_i$ responses (recorded by fluo-3 fluorescence) measured from these cells. (D–F) Similar [Ca^{2+}]$_i$ responses in retinal oligodendrocyte precursor, immature and mature oligodendrocyte respectively

et al., 1995c). Such variability presumably indicates that oligodendrocytes may co-express P$_{2Y}$ and P$_{2U}$ purinoreceptors, both coupled with phospholipase C and InsP$_3$ turnover. ATP responses were also blocked by P$_2$ receptors agonist suramin, but at relatively high concentration (100 μM of suramin blocked the response by 85-90%).

ATP applications were shown to deplete the ER stores of releasable calcium, which was observed as a progressive decrease of the [Ca^{2+}]$_i$ transient amplitude in response to successive ATP challenges (Fig. 4.7.). The refilling of the internal stores was provided by the uptake of cytoplasmic Ca^{2+} due to the activity of SERCA pumps:

126

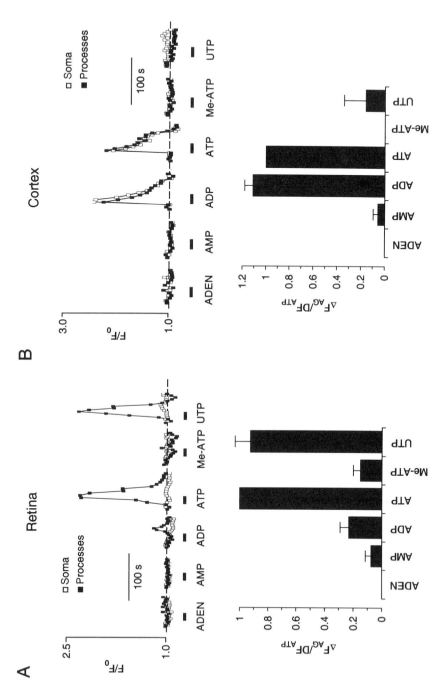

Figure 4.6. Agonist specificity of P₂ purinoreceptors involved in calcium signalling in oligodendrocytes (from Kirischuk *et al.*, 1995c; reproduced by permission of The Physiological Society). (A, B) The mean amplitudes of [Ca²⁺]ᵢ transients measured from cortical and retinal oligodendrocytes in response to various agonists of P₂ purinoreceptors. Representative [Ca²⁺]ᵢ traces are shown above

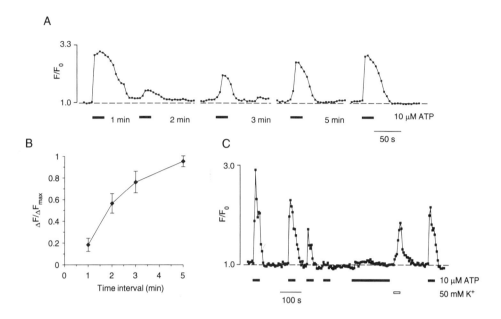

Figure 4.7. Depletion and refilling of ATP-sensitive Ca^{2+} stores in cortical oligodendrocyte (from Kirischuk *et al.*, 1995c; reproduced by permission of The Physiological Society). (A) ATP was applied with increasing time interval between the applications (time denoted at bottom). The $[Ca^{2+}]_i$ response (recorded as the fluo-3 fluorescence ratio) recovered to control conditions within an interval of 5 min. (B) The recovery time determined in experiments similar to those shown in A. Time between two ATP applications is indicated on the abscissa; the decrease of the response in relation to the control response is shown on the ordinate. Responses are normalized with respect to the control. (C) Depolarization-induced Ca^{2+} influx reloads internal stores. ATP (10 μM) and high $[K^+]_o$ (50 mM) were applied as indicated. Successive ATP applications led to a significant rundown of the response. The response could be restored by an exposure of the cell to an increase in $[K^+]_o$

depolarization-triggered injection of Ca^{2+} into the cytoplasm enhanced store replenishment, while SERCA inhibition by thapsigargin prevented Ca^{2+} uptake by the ER (Kirischuk *et al.*, 1995c). Interestingly, the rate of store refilling differed significantly between oligodendrocytes obtained from various brain structures: it was much faster in retinal versus cortical oligodendrocytes. The refilling of ER stores in oligodendrocytes ultimately required the presence of extracellular Ca^{2+}, suggesting the possible involvement of additional Ca^{2+} entry, activated probably by emptying of the stores (CRAC channels), although we failed to obtain direct evidence favouring this hypothesis.

ATP-triggered $[Ca^{2+}]_i$ responses did not develop evenly throughout the oligodendrocyte: usually the amplitudes of $[Ca^{2+}]_i$ elevations were significantly higher in dendrites as compared with the soma (cf. Fig. 4.5). This may indicate differential distribution of either P_2 purinoreceptors or ER calcium stores. The activation of $P_{2Y/U}$ purinoreceptors in oligodendrocytes was unequivocally demonstrated to trigger Ca^{2+} release via activation of $InsP_3$-gated intracellular channels: internal dialysis of oligodendrocytes with 1 μM of heparin abolished the $[Ca^{2+}]_i$ response (Fig. 4.8).

In cultured (Bruner and Murphy, 1993; Shao and McCarthy, 1995) astrocytes

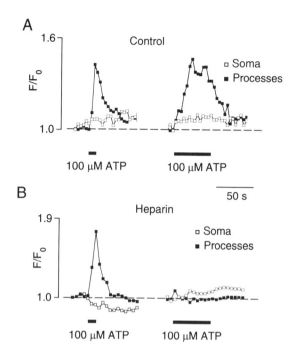

Figure 4.8. Heparin blocks ATP-mediated calcium signal in a retinal oligodendrocyte (modified from Kirischuk *et al.*, 1995c; reproduced by permission of The Physiological Society). (A) Mature oligodendrocytes were loaded with fluo-3/AM and the effect of ATP on $[Ca^{2+}]_i$ was recorded from the soma and processes (left trace). Subsequently the cell was approached with a patch pipette to form the whole-cell recording configuration. Thereby the cell was dialysed with the pipette solution containing fluo-3 pentapotassium salt. ATP induced a similar increase in $[Ca^{2+}]_i$ as prior to the dialysis (right trace). (B) In a similar recording paradigm as described in A an O10-positive oligodendrocyte was dialysed with a pipette solution additionally containing heparin (1 µM). The ATP response was blocked 5 min after the whole-cell recording configuration was established (right trace) as compared to the control prior to dialysis (left trace)

ATP-driven InsP$_3$ formation and $[Ca^{2+}]_i$ mobilization also went through P$_{2U}$ purinoreceptors. The IICR induced by ATP was blocked by thapsigargin and mimicked by flash-photolysis of intracellularly loaded caged-INsP$_3$ (Shao and McCarthy, 1995).

Very similar ATP-driven $[Ca^{2+}]_i$ responses were found in Bergmann glial cells (which represent the astrocytic branch of brain macroglia) in acutely prepared cerebellar slices (Kirischuk and Verkhratsky, 1995; Kirischuk *et al.*, 1995a). In Bergmann cells $[Ca^{2+}]_i$ mobilization was the result of P$_{2Y}$ purinoreceptor activation and was not associated with changes in plasmalemmal ionic conductance. Fig. 4.9 summarizes some basic properties of ATP-triggered calcium signals in Bergmann glial cells: the ATP-induced $[Ca^{2+}]_i$ transients persisted in Ca^{2+}-free external solution, and were inhibited by thapsigargin and intracellular administration of heparin. A very interesting feature of the ATP-triggered $[Ca^{2+}]_i$ mobilization in Bergmann glial cells is its strong modulation by background $[Ca^{2+}]_i$: the amplitude of ATP-responses was maximal at low resting $[Ca^{2+}]_i$ (30-50 nM), progressively decreased at higher

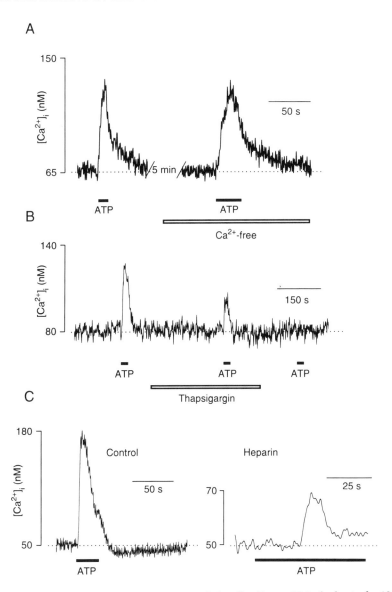

Figure 4.9. ATP induces IICR in Bergmann glial cells (from Kirischuk *et al.*, 1995a with permission). (A) ATP (100 μM) induces [Ca^{2+}]$_i$ elevation in control conditions and after 5 min slice superfusion with Ca^{2+}-free, EGTA-containing extracellular solution. (B) Thapsigargin (500 nM) inhibits ATP-induced [Ca^{2+}]$_i$ transients. (C) Intracellularly applied heparin (1 μM) blocks ATP-induced [Ca^{2+}]$_i$ signals. The control [Ca^{2+}]$_i$ transient was recorded from the fura-2/AM bulk loaded cell; the cell was then dialysed with heparin-containing pipette solution and 5 min later the second record (shown in the right panel) was taken

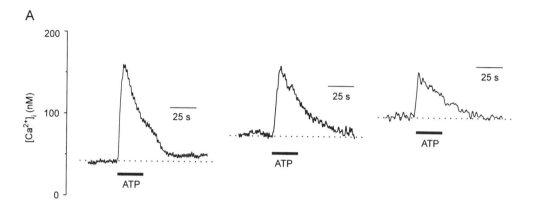

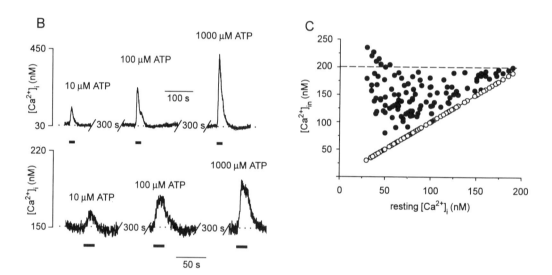

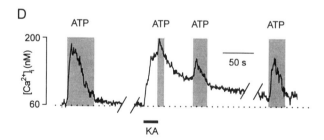

$[Ca^{2+}]_i$ and completely disappeared when $[Ca^{2+}]_i$ exceeded 200 nM (Fig. 4.10). The intimate mechanisms of this Ca^{2+}-dependent regulation remain unclear; it might be associated either with direct influence of cytoplasmic Ca^{2+} ions on $InsP_3$-gated ER channels, or $[Ca^{2+}]_i$ may affect other components of the $InsP_3$-sensitive pool. The availability of IICR in cerebellar Bergmann glial cells was also influenced by certain metabolic cytoplasmic factors, presumably due to the action on refilling properties of the ER stores: intracellular dialysis inhibited the replenishment of the $InsP_3$-releasable pool.

Similarly to ATP-induced calcium signalling in oligodendrocytes, confocal microscopy revealed the spatial heterogeneity of the ATP-triggered $[Ca^{2+}]_i$ signal in cerebellar Bergmann glial cells: $[Ca^{2+}]_i$ mobilization was always higher in cell processes as compared with the somatic region.

GABA

In contrast to neurones, where γ-aminobutyric acid (GABA) acts primarily as an inhibitory neurotransmitter, in glial cells application of GABA caused their depolarization. Such effects were found in both cultured (astrocytes—Kettenmann and Schachner, 1985; Kettenmann et al., 1987; oligodendrocytes—Blankenfeld et al., 1991) and slice (astrocytes—MacVicar et al., 1989; Sontheimer and Waxman, 1993; oligodendrocytes—Berger et al., 1992) preparations. These depolarizing GABA effects can be antagonized by the classic $GABA_A$ receptor antagonist bicuculine and the Cl⁻ channel blocker picrotoxin, and can be mimicked by the $GABA_A$ agonist muscimol. At the molecular level (experiments utilizing PCR technique) astrocytes were shown to express mRNA of $\alpha1$, $\alpha2$, $\beta1$, $\beta3$ and $\gamma1$ subunits of GABA receptors, which form homomeric or heteromeric Cl⁻-selective channels (Bovolin et al., 1992). Analysis of GABA-evoked currents supported the hypothesis of their Cl⁻ nature and showed that the Cl⁻ reversal potential in glial cells is very positive (namely about -35 mV), which determines the development of prominent Cl⁻ efflux with subsequent depolarization upon activation of $GABA_A$ receptors (see Blankenfeld and Kettenmann, 1992; Fraser et al., 1994 for review). The $GABA_A$-driven depolarization of glial cells activates voltage-gated plasmalemmal Ca^{2+} channels; Ca^{2+} influx through the latter produces $[Ca^{2+}]_i$ transients in astro- (Fraser et al., 1994) and oligodendroglia (Kirchhoff and Kettenmann, 1992). In both cases $[Ca^{2+}]_i$ responses were blocked by the Cl⁻ channel inhibitor picrotoxin and by the Ca^{2+} channel blocker verapamil. In cortical astrocytes,

---

Figure 4.10. ATP-induced Ca^{2+} elevation in Bergmann glial cells is controlled by resting $[Ca^{2+}]_i$ (from Kirischuk et al., 1995a with permission). (A) Examples of ATP-mediated $[Ca^{2+}]_i$ transients recorded from three fura-2/AM bulk loaded Bergmann glial cells. ATP (100 μM) was applied as indicated by bars. (B) $[Ca^{2+}]_i$ transients in response to increasing concentrations of ATP measured from two different Bergmann glial cells with different levels of basal $[Ca^{2+}]_i$ concentration. (C) Peak values of ATP-induced $[Ca^{2+}]_i$ transients measured from 112 Bergmann glial cells (solid circles) and resting $[Ca^{2+}]_i$ (open circles) are plotted against the corresponding resting $[Ca^{2+}]_i$ level. (D) ATP-induced $[Ca^{2+}]_i$ responses evoked upon experimental manipulation with $[Ca^{2+}]_i$. $[Ca^{2+}]_i$ transients evoked by ATP (100 μM) were recorded in control conditions and during the recovery phase of a kainate (100 μM)-triggered $[Ca^{2+}]_i$ elevation. Recordings were separated by 3 min intervals as indicated on the graph

however, Nilsson *et al.* (1993) found that $[Ca^{2+}]_i$ elevation produced by the $GABA_A$ agonist muscimol persisted in Ca^{2+}-free extracellular solution in a small subpopulation of type 1 cultured astrocytes, which may indicate yet unknown coupling of $GABA_A$ receptors with intracellular Ca^{2+} release. In addition to the $GABA_A$-mediated calcium signalling Nilsson *et al.* suggested an alternative pathway for Ca^{2+} entry associated with activation of $GABA_B$ receptor-coupled cationic channels with appreciable Ca^{2+} permeability. Other authors (Pearce and Murphy, 1988) demonstrated that glial $GABA_B$ receptors may inhibit formation of $InsP_3$, thus attenuating IICR induced by other neurotransmitters.

HISTAMINE

Glial cells were reported to express H1 histamine receptors coupled to the $InsP_3$/DAG intracellular signalling system and H2 receptors linked to adenylate cyclase (Inagaki and Wada, 1994). In respect to calcium signalling H1 receptors are of particular interest because of their potential link to IICR. The stimulation of H1 receptors in cultured astrocytes increased the turnover of $InsP_3$ (Arbones *et al.*, 1988) and generated $[Ca^{2+}]_i$ elevation due to IICR in astrocytoma lines (McDonough *et al.*, 1988; Yanai *et al.*, 1992; Lucherini and Gruenstein, 1992) and cultured astrocytes (Inagaki and Wada, 1994). Interestingly, histamine-induced $InsP_3$ formation was found only in type 2 cultured astrocytes (Kondou *et al.*, 1991). In accordance with this finding, microfluorometric experiments revealed that type 1 and type 2 astrocytes have a different sensitivity to histamine: while the majority of type 2 astrocytes responded to histamine with $[Ca^{2+}]_i$ elevation (Inagaki *et al.*, 1991a; Dave *et al.*, 1991), only a small subpopulation of type 1 astrocytes generated $[Ca^{2+}]_i$ transients upon histamine treatment (McCarthy and Salm, 1991).

As described above for ATP-induced calcium signalling, histamine induced $[Ca^{2+}]_i$ elevation preferentially in astrocyte processes (Inagaki *et al.*, 1991b; Inagaki and Wada, 1994). At submaximal histamine concentrations (0.1-1 μM) $[Ca^{2+}]_i$ rise was observed only at processes, while higher histamine concentrations (10-100 μM) induced an intracellular $[Ca^{2+}]_i$ wave, initiating in processes and spreading thereafter into the soma.

Similarly to astrocytes, histamine induced phosphoinositide hydrolysis and $InsP_3$ production in oligodendrocytes (Post and Dawson, 1992). This pathway underlies $[Ca^{2+}]_i$ elevation observed in immature and mature oligodendrocytes treated with histamine (Kastritsis and McCarthy, 1993).

OTHER LIGANDS RELATED TO CALCIUM SIGNALLING IN GLIAL CELLS

Development of the calcium signal in glial cells is initiated by numerous biologically active substances (see Table 4.2, and Finkbeiner, 1993 for review). In the majority of cases they act via activation of IICR from internal stores. Quite an important pathway in IICR generation in astrocytes is controlled by $\alpha 1$-adrenoreceptors (Shao and McCarthy, 1994). Similarly, the activation of muscarinic cholinoreceptors was also reported to produce $InsP_3$-mediated $[Ca^{2+}]_i$ responses in cultured astrocytes (Shao and McCarthy, 1993, 1994). However, it is still unclear whether MChRs are expressed in glial cells *in vivo*: a number of immunohistochemical studies did not reveal expression of MChRs in brain astroglia (e.g. Levey *et al.*, 1991). Generation of IICR-related $[Ca^{2+}]_i$ elevation in response to prostaglandin $F_{2\alpha}$ was found in cultured type 1 astrocytes (Inagaki and Wada, 1994). In contrast to histamine, which induced $[Ca^{2+}]_i$ elevation preferentially in type 2 astrocytes, prostaglandins mainly act on type 1 astrocytes (Ito *et al.*, 1992). In oligodendrocytes $[Ca^{2+}]_i$ mobilization (once more due to IICR) was observed in response to nerve growth factor (Engel *et al.*, 1994).

It is still unclear whether emptying of InsP$_3$-sensitive ER stores in glial cells is coupled with the generation of additional Ca^{2+} influx via CRAC channels. Although glial calcium stores show rapid depletion while incubated in Ca^{2+}-free media, and extracellular Ca^{2+} is ultimately required for their refilling (Peuchen *et al.*, 1995; Kirischuk *et al.*, 1995c), a direct demonstration of CRAC channel-mediated Ca^{2+} influx has not yet been achieved.

The IICR also participates in calcium signalling evoked by mechanical stimulation of astrocytic cultures (Charles *et al.*, 1991); it was blocked by heparin, which clearly shows the involvement of InsP$_3$-sensitive stores (Boitano *et al.*, 1992). $[Ca^{2+}]_i$ elevations were also observed in glial cells exposed to experimentally designed pathological conditions. Oligodendrocytes, for example, generate $[Ca^{2+}]_i$ oscillation originating from the intracellular stores in response to serum complement (Wood *et al.*, 1993), which is involved in cell damage and, particularly, in the initiation of the demyelinization of CNS structures. Calcium signalling also appeared in astrocytes which underwent swelling in response to hypotonic media (e.g. O'Connor and Kimelberg, 1993); the $[Ca^{2+}]_i$ elevation in this case was determined by both Ca^{2+} entry via voltage-gated channels and intracellular calcium release.

TERMINATION OF CALCIUM SIGNAL IN GLIAL CELLS

CALCIUM BUFFERING

Unfortunately, we have practically no information concerning the buffer properties of glial cell cytoplasm; this remains one of the most important questions in glial calcium homeostasis which has to be elucidated in the near future. Taking into account small densities of transmembrane ionic currents in glial cells which are often accompanied by large-amplitude (>1 μM) $[Ca^{2+}]_i$ transients, one may assume that the buffer capacity in glial cells may be substantially smaller as compared with neurones.

SODIUM/CALCIUM EXCHANGER

Several studies have demonstrated that $[Ca^{2+}]_i$ in glial cells is influenced by sodium transmembrane electrochemical gradient, suggesting the involvement of an Na^+/Ca^{2+} exchanger mechanism in astrocytic $[Ca^{2+}]_i$ homeostasis. Initial evidence concerning the existence of functional Na^+/Ca^{2+} exchange in glial cells came from radiotracer experiments demonstrating that fluxes of ^{45}Ca in glial cells are controlled by extracellular sodium concentration (Lazarewitch *et al.*, 1977). Alteration of transmembrane Na^+ gradient was reported to alter, in addition, the kinetic characteristics of the stimulus-evoked $[Ca^{2+}]_i$ transients in astrocytes (Finkbeiner, 1993). However, the relative importance of this mechanism in determination of resting $[Ca^{2+}]_i$ and in Ca^{2+} extrusion remains controversial (cf. Jensen and Chui, 1990; Duffy and MacVicar, 1994; versus Goldman *et al.*, 1994). A recent comprehensive study of the peculiarities of the Na^+/Ca^{2+} exchange mechanism in cultured cortical astrocytes clearly demonstrated (1) the existence of relatively high levels of mRNA encoding the heart isoform of the exchanger and (2) the prominent increase in $[Ca^{2+}]_i$ in ouabain-treated astrocytes after lowering the extracellular Na^+ concentration (Goldman *et al.*, 1994). Interestingly, the increase of $[Na^+]_i$ (by ouabain-induced blockade of the sodium pump) was the ultimate prerequisite for detection of $[Ca^{2+}]_i$ rise in sodium-deficient external solutions; simple manipulations with $[Na^+]_o$ were ineffective. Such a finding may explain the absence of dramatic $[Ca^{2+}]_i$ changes in previous experiments. In addition, it means that in order to induce Ca^{2+} influx into astrocytes via the Na^+/Ca^{2+} exchanger the transmembrane sodium gradient must be altered quite substantially.

Recently an ouabain-like compound functioning as a vertebrate adrenocortical hormone has been found (Hamlyn *et al.*, 1991); one may speculate that alteration of intracellular sodium concentration and subsequent activation of Ca^{2+} influx via the exchanger mechanism could represent the physiological pathway for ouabain action.

PLASMALEMMAL Ca^{2+} PUMP

Plasmalemmal Ca^{2+} pumps have been localized histochemically in Schwann cells and in cortical astrocytes and oligodendrocytes. The importance of Ca^{2+} extrusion via plasmalemmal Ca^{2+}-ATPases for termination of calcium signal was demonstrated in cultured cortical and retinal oligodendrocytes (Kirischuk *et al.*, 1995d). In these cells blockade of PMCA pumps by La^{3+} markedly slowed down the termination of depolarization-triggered $[Ca^{2+}]_i$ transients.

MITOCHONDRIA

The functional meaning of mitochondrial calcium accumulation with respect to $[Ca^{2+}]_i$ handling in glial cells practically has not yet been studied. Recently we investigated the possible role of mitochondria in $[Ca^{2+}]_i$ handling in oligodendrocytes. In contrast to neurones, treatment of oligodendrocytes by the mitochondrial uncoupler FCCP induced elevation of $[Ca^{2+}]_i$ for 200-400 nM above resting level (Kirischuk *et al.*, 1995b, 1995d). These data indicate that even in resting conditions mitochondria in oligodendrocytes contain appreciable amounts of releasable Ca^{2+}. However, FCCP exposure did not influence kinetic parameters of the depolarization-triggered $[Ca^{2+}]_i$ transients (Kirischuk *et al.*, 1995d), which means that mitochondrial Ca^{2+} accumulation does not play an important role in calcium signal termination in oligodendroglia (at least for moderate Ca^{2+} loads).

While studying FCCP-induced Ca^{2+} release in oligodendrocytes at different developmental stages we found pronounced spatial heterogeneity in mitochondrial-associated Ca^{2+} elevation in glial precursor cells. In these precursors FCCP-induced Ca^{2+} release was almost exclusively restricted to the cellular processes (Kirischuk *et al.*, 1995b). Similarly, the concentration of active mitochondria was revealed by the mitochondria-specific dye rhodamine 123 in the processes of glial precursors. This peculiar distribution disappeared at later stages of oligodendroglial development. Presumably, the preferential localization of active mitochondria in the processes of glial precursors might be important for energy supply for protein synthesis during cellular growth, and it could also be important for $[Ca^{2+}]_i$ handling in this subcellular compartment.

PLASTICITY OF $[Ca^{2+}]_i$ SIGNALLING IN GLIAL CELLS

Following the development of glial research, which expanded in recent years, we started to realize that glia is not only the major cellular element of the brain (up to 90% of the total number of cells in the CNS) but it possesses unique functional diversity and plasticity capabilities. Glial cells participate in many important processes in the brain, from leading the neurite outgrowth to formation of brain immunological reactions. Still the number of glial cell subtypes remains very limited, which basically means they are endowed with high plasticity potential, rapidly changing their properties in response to environmental demands.

This plasticity indeed exists, and it can be seen even *in vitro* at the single-cell level either in a form of morphological plasticity or in variation in the expression of various molecules involved in intercellular and intracellular signalling, including calcium signalling.

The ontogenetic plasticity of oligodendrocytes has been extensively studied during recent years. The development of oligodendroglia from their precursors to mature myelin-producing cells is associated with dramatic changes in the expression of ionic channels and neurotransmitter receptors. With respect to calcium signalling these changes comprise disappearance of numerous molecules which can induce depolarization-triggered calcium entry, and development of mechanisms responsible for Ca^{2+} release from internal sources. Indeed, the transition from oligodendrocyte precursor to the mature oligodendrocyte (Fig. 4.11) is accompanied by disappearance of fast Na^+ currents, voltage-dependent K^+ currents (Sontheimer *et al.*, 1989), glutamate (Borges *et al.*, 1994) and GABA (Blankenfeld *et al.*, 1991) receptors. Instead, oligodendrocytes acquire pathways for $InsP_3$-mediated Ca^{2+} release from internal stores (Kirischuk *et al.*, 1995c; Kastritsis and McCarthy, 1993). Expression of voltage-gated Ca^{2+} channels is transiently downregulated during the intermediate developmental stage (Blankenfeld *et al.*, 1992); later in mature oligodendrocytes they reappear and migrate to processes. These distinct developmental changes were initially observed *in vitro* in a culture system; subsequently they were confirmed in experiments *in situ* (Berger *et al.*, 1991, 1992).

This very distinct developmental scenario may presumably reflect the changes in functional specialization of oligodendrocytes. Oligodendrocytic precursors are forced to migrate extensively, searching for neurites, which they finally cover with myelin sheath. At that time they presumably need various plasmalemmal signalling molecules, which will sense neuronal activity and lead oligodendrocytic precursors to their targets. After establishing myelinization, oligodendrocytes lose the system of fast

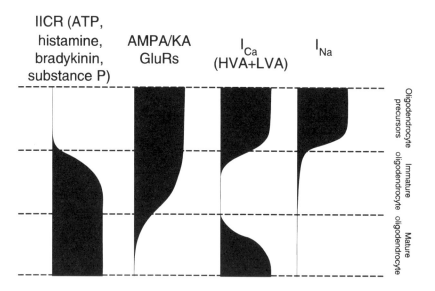

Figure 4.11. Developmental changes in calcium signalling-related neuroligand receptors expression in oligodendrocyte lineage

signalling (channels and ionotropic receptors) but they acquire receptors coupled with intracellular calcium release, which is presumably important for long-term neuronal-glial interactions.

The sensitivity of astrocytes to various neuroligands may vary in accordance with their origination from different brain regions. For instance, histamine and prostaglandin $F_{2\alpha}$ receptors coupled with InsP$_3$ turnover are highly expressed in cortical and hippocampal astrocytes, whereas they are almost absent in cerebellar astroglia (Hosli and Hosli, 1993). In addition, even astrocytes isolated from the same brain regions show remarkable variability in their sensitivity to different neuroligands. This variability seems to be an intrinsic property of astrocytes, rather than the result of the existence of genetically determined cellular subpopulations with different receptor phenotypes. This was clearly demonstrated in a series of elegant experiments performed by Shao and McCarthy (1993, 1994). They studied the heterogeneity of cultured astrocytes in respect to their sensitivity to various $[Ca^{2+}]_i$-mobilizing agents. In order to clarify whether different sensitivity to neuroligands is associated with the existence of several stable phenotypic clones, or whether it reflects an intrinsic potential of the astrocyte to vary the expression of different receptors, Shao and McCarthy cloned astrocytes isolated from the neonatal brain. They clearly showed that the divergence of astrocytic Ca^{2+}-mobilizing receptors occurs within a single clone, and moreover, the different sensitivity to neuroligands may appear between sister cells immediately after division. These results strongly support the existence of a high plasticity potential in astroglia.

SPATIOTEMPORAL ORGANIZATION OF CALCIUM SIGNAL IN GLIAL CELLS

In many cases, glial calcium signalling shows a very peculiar spatiotemporal organization. Quite often the $[Ca^{2+}]_i$ response of glial cells starts in a particular region of the cell and then travels to other areas, producing intracellular Ca^{2+} waves. Furthermore, many agonists evoke a complicated $[Ca^{2+}]_i$ response, which may last for many seconds in the form of $[Ca^{2+}]_i$ oscillations. The temporal organization of $[Ca^{2+}]_i$ responses has been comprehensively characterized in cultured astrocytes, yielding a detailed classification of the components of the calcium signal (Finkbeiner, 1993; Cornell-Bell and Finkbeiner, 1991; Kim *et al.*, 1994; Cornell-Bell *et al.*, 1990). The agonist-triggered $[Ca^{2+}]_i$ astrocytic responses are composed of an initial Ca^{2+} spike, which is believed to reflect Ca^{2+} release from internal stores, a sustained plateau and/or $[Ca^{2+}]_i$ oscillations. Both plateau and oscillations demonstrated a clear dependence of extracellular Ca^{2+}. The removal of extracellular Ca^{2+} eliminated or substantially reduced the plateau/oscillation phase of the agonist-triggered $[Ca^{2+}]_i$ response in astrocytes. This kind of temporal organization of the calcium signal was found in astrocytes challenged with numerous agonists, including glutamate and quisqualate (Cornell-Bell *et al.*, 1990; Jensen and Chui, 1990), histamine (Fukui *et al.*, 1991); noradrenaline (Salm and McCarthy, 1990); endothelin (Goldman *et al.*, 1991), ATP (Kastritsis *et al.*, 1992), etc. Interestingly, quite often the generation of a full $[Ca^{2+}]_i$ response (composed of initial spike and late plateau/oscillation phase) was concentration-dependent. Low agonist concentrations evoked only a monophasic spike-like $[Ca^{2+}]_i$ response, whereas at higher agonist concentrations it acquired the plateau or oscillation phase. The parameters of $[Ca^{2+}]_i$ response may vary in a wide range; even neighbouring cells in the same culture exhibited a quite different pattern of $[Ca^{2+}]_i$ responses (Finkbeiner, 1993).

While there are practically no doubts about the intracellular origin of the initial $[Ca^{2+}]_i$ spike, the precise mechanism responsible for the plateau/oscillation phase is still unclear. As was mentioned above, maintaining this phase requires extracellular Ca^{2+}; however, the nature of the transmembrane transporter mechanism is unclear. Although there was one report that inorganic Ca^{2+} antagonists inhibit the plateau phase of the agonist-triggered $[Ca^{2+}]_i$ response (see Finkbeiner, 1993), the involvement of voltage-gated plasmalemmal Ca^{2+} channels remains questionable. Another possible pathway for Ca^{2+} entry may be via CRAC channels, although their existence in glial cells has not yet been directly proved. Probably, $[Ca^{2+}]_i$ oscillations also involve $[Ca^{2+}]_i$ redistribution between the cytoplasm and ER stores and maintaining Ca^{2+} release, regulated by $[Ca^{2+}]_i$.

Simultaneously with distinct temporal organization, calcium signals in glial cells often demonstrate prominent spatial inhomogeneity. Usually $[Ca^{2+}]_i$ elevation starts in a certain cell region, and then propagates to other cell regions; moreover in astrocytic cultures, intracellular Ca^{2+} waves are able to cross intercellular borders, thus forming a Ca^{2+} wave which propagates through astrocytic networks. This intercellular Ca^{2+} wave may travel for long distances involving hundreds of cells within the network (Kim *et al.*, 1994). The velocity of Ca^{2+} wave propagation may fluctuate in a wide range between 10-20 and 40 $\mu m/s$ (Finkbeiner, 1993). This intercellular Ca^{2+} wave propagation is mediated via gap junctions, since uncoupling of the astrocytic network using gap junction blockers (halothane, octanol, protein kinase C or cytoplasmic acidification) inhibits intercellular Ca^{2+} waves without affecting Ca^{2+} signal generation in single cells (Finkbeiner, 1992; Enkvist and McCarthy, 1992).

Recent experiments utilizing high-resolution video-imaging techniques for investigation of $[Ca^{2+}]_i$ distribution demonstrate a very peculiar role of glial processes in calcium signal initiation. As already mentioned, exposure of cultured oligodendrocytes and astrocytes to various ligands (e.g. ATP, histamine; see above) evokes $[Ca^{2+}]_i$ elevation in processes, which can afterwards propagate towards the soma. The most peculiar situation was observed in cultured oligodendrocytes. In these cells, and especially in mature oligodendrocytes, both transmembrane Ca^{2+} influx and internal Ca^{2+} release are preferentially localized in the processes. Similarly, cultured astrocytes challenged by histamine also start to generate calcium signals in processes which then spread through the whole cell. These data may initiate the speculation that glial processes are the major signalling input which allows glial cells to communicate with neighbouring neurones.

CONCLUSIONS

Glial cells are equipped with an elaborated system which allows the generation of complex calcium signals. These signals are generated in response to various agonists and involve both transmembrane Ca^{2+} influx and intracellular Ca^{2+} release, predominantly from InsP$_3$-sensitive ER calcium stores. The calcium signal in many types of glial cells is initiated in their processes and then spreads inside the cell, generating intracellular Ca^{2+} waves. In glial cell networks Ca^{2+} waves may travel between cells over long distances. Glial cells also demonstrate high plasticity of calcium signalling pathways, which determine their functional diversity. The development of glia is associated with prominent changes in the mechanisms of calcium signalling. However, the experimental investigations of glial calcium signalling up to now were mainly descriptive, and we are still lacking the information about general mechanisms of $[Ca^{2+}]_i$ homeostasis in glial cells. In addition, the majority of the information concerning $[Ca^{2+}]_i$ handling in glial cells came from experiments on culture systems, raising the obvious question: how does the situation observed in cultured cells reflect the state of calcium signalling *in vivo*? Finally, the following questions are still unclear: what is the physiological meaning of calcium signalling in glia, and what are the intracellular targets and the natural stimuli which initiate glial $[Ca^{2+}]_i$ responses?

Summarizing the presented data, it would be important to clarify not only the general functional meaning of calcium signalling in neuronal cells, but also the specific role of different mechanisms participating in the formation of these signals. We shall start with the role of specific Ca^{2+} channels in triggering cell functions related to calcium signalling.

FUNCTIONAL ROLE OF LOW-VOLTAGE-ACTIVATED Ca^{2+} CHANNELS

The peculiar potential-dependent characteristics of LVA calcium channels (activation already at resting membrane potential level and rapid potential-dependent inactivation) imply their participation in the generation of membrane potential oscillations and, as a result, in bursts of action potentials. On one hand, this suggestion has been supported by the observation that a high density of LVA channels is encountered only in neurones inclined to produce such activity (thalamic neurones—Coulter et al., 1989; White et al., 1989; Dossi et al., 1992; neurones of substantia nigra—Kang and Kitai, 1993; medullary respiratory neurones—Richter et al., 1993; medium-sized sensory neurones in DRG—Scroggs and Fox, 1992b; Shmigol et al., 1995a). On the other hand, experiments on a neuronal computer model with variable densities of different voltage-dependent ion currents have also shown an extreme inclination to generate bursting activity in cases of elevated density of LVA Ca^{2+} channels (Veselovsky and Fedulova, unpublished data). From these findings it follows that selective suppression of LVA Ca^{2+} channels might be helpful in the treatment of epileptic seizures originating in brain neurones with such properties. In fact, this is the case with treatment of sensory seizures by ethosuximide, effectively depressing LVA I_{Ca} in thalamocortical relay neurones (Coulter et al., 1990) and DRG sensory neurones (Kostyuk et al., 1992a). In acutely isolated human neocortical neurones LVA currents could be depressed also by another antiepileptic substance—phenytoin—in concentrations within its therapeutic range (Sayer et al., 1993).

At the same time it is likely that the functional meaning of LVA Ca^{2+} channels is not limited only to electrical membrane phenomena. Despite the short mean open time of these channels, they can still produce a substantial intracellular Ca^{2+} transient, differing from the transients generated by other Ca^{2+} channels by its very fast time course. This suggestion has been verified in experiments on DRG neurones clamped by digitally constructed waveforms that simulate natural action potentials, with photometric determination of induced Ca^{2+} transients (McCobb and Beam, 1991). The measurements have shown that Ca^{2+} entry through LVA channels forms a disproportionately large fraction of the total Ca^{2+} entry (40–50%) during brief action potentials. The entry through HVA Ca^{2+} channels has increased more essentially as spike duration increased. Similar conclusions can be derived from our measurements of Ca^{2+} transients in DRG neurones of aged animals, in which LVA Ca^{2+} channels are practically absent. The depolarization-induced increase of $[Ca^{2+}]_i$ in old neurones was significantly lower in comparison with the cells isolated from adult rats, and the speed of its rise was considerably decreased (Kirischuk et al., 1992). These data suggest that LVA Ca^{2+} channels may be responsible for the fast injection of Ca^{2+} ions during neuronal activity, important for triggering of some specific cellular functions. Of special meaning in this respect could be observations that LVA channels in brain neurones are mostly expressed in terminal dendritic branches; in hippocampal neurones they were completely lost after surgical cut-off of dendritic branches, and in cultured hypothalamic neurones they were absent before dendrites originated during culturing (Müller T.H. et al., 1992; Karst et al., 1993). Obviously, the functioning of LVA channels here bears no relation to transmitter release. It has been shown directly in experiments on cultured Helisoma neurones that they are able to release transmitter only at the stage when solely HVA Ca^{2+} channels are left in the membrane (Haydon and Man-Son-Hing, 1989). Activity of LVA channels might be crucial for the initiation of the outgrowth of neurites and the development of growth cones; early expression of HVA channels (Gottmann, et al., 1991) as well as continuous increase in $[Ca^{2+}]_i$ (Garyantes and Regehr, 1992) are not necessary for these processes. LVA channels may be also involved in the induction of long-term potentiation, as in kitten visual cortex the latter occurs only at developmental stages when these channels are present in neuronal membranes (Komatsu and Iwakiri, 1992).

Finally, a specific role of LVA Ca^{2+} channels in secretion has recently been suggested in a definite substrate: adrenal cortex. It has been shown that T-type channels are required for adrenocorticotrophin-stimulated cortisol production in adrenal zona fasciculata cells; other types of Ca^{2+} channels are absent here (Enyeart et al., 1993). Steroidogenesis in zona glomerulosa cells also demanded the activity of T-type channels and could be blocked with a specific T-type blocker—tetrandrine (Rossier et al., 1993a)—and also by thapsigargin, an inhibitor of endoplasmic Ca pumps, in micromolar concentrations (Rossier et al., 1993b).

HIGH-VOLTAGE-ACTIVATED Ca^{2+} CHANNELS AND TRANSMITTER RELEASE

It is obvious now that the crucial role of Ca^{2+} signals in transmitter release, detected in the classic experiments of Katz and Miledi (1967a, 1967b), is connected predominantly to the functioning of HVA Ca^{2+} channels. A general view about this role of HVA channels considers the inactivating (N- or P-type) channels as directly involved in transmitter release and the non-inactivating (L-type) ones as responsible for the triggering of more general cellular functions. ω-Aga-toxin sensitive P-type channels are shown to trigger transmitter release in crayfish excitatory and inhibitory (Araque et al., 1994) and mammalian excitatory neuromuscular terminals (Uchitel et al., 1992), glutamate release in rat brain synaptosomes (Turner, et al., 1992) and in transmitter release in rat cerebellar synapses (Momiyama and Takahashi, 1994), although in the latter case transmission is supported in part (about 29%) also by N-type channels (Regehr and Mintz, 1994). In mammalian sympathetic ganglia too the large initial transmitter release has been shown to be triggered by ω-Aga-IVA and sFTX-sensitive (P-type) channels, while other (N-type) channels participate during prolonged depolarization (Burgos et al., 1995). ω-Conotoxin-sensitive N-type channels are dominant in secretion in frog pituitary gland (Obaid et al., 1989), in mammalian autonomic neurotransmission (Altiere et al., 1992), synaptic transmission in the spinal cord of *Xenopus* (Wall and Dale, 1994), synaptic transmission between thalamic neurones in culture (Pfrieger et al., 1992a, b) and synaptic transmission between hippocampal neurones, although in the latter case a substantial component could be blocked only by the ω-conotoxin MVIIC, implying the participation of not well-identified Q-type Ca^{2+} channels (Wheeler et al., 1994). In identified *Aplysia* synapses ω-conotoxin-sensitive Ca^{2+} channels control only 50–60% of synaptic transmission, the rest being blocked by synthetic ω-Aga toxin (sFTX); however, only the N-type channels are a target for the neuromodulatory effect of endogenous peptides on synaptic transmission here (Trudeau et al., 1993; Fossier et al., 1994). In developing mammalian neuromuscular synapses L-type channels may be responsible for regulation of spontaneous transmitter release (Fu and Huang, 1994); experiments on large neurohypophyseal presynaptic terminals indicate that both N and L types of channel contribute to release, N-type channels being responsible for a large initial influx of Ca^{2+} and L-type channels for their steady influx (Nowycky, 1991; Wang et al., 1993b). Probably, the N-type channels here have specific properties: they open throughout long depolarizing pulses; some authors have designated them as N_t channels (Wang et al., 1993a). In adrenal chromaffin cells all three types of HVA channel can participate in triggering secretion (Pun et al., 1988; Artalejo et al., 1994), although here localized L-type channels may be of main importance for controlling exocytosis (Lopez et al., 1994). In human neuroblastoma and rat phaeochromocytoma cells ω-conotoxin-sensitive channels are responsible for the peak in intracellular Ca^{2+} transients whereas DHP-sensitive ones are responsible for their plateau (Sher et al., 1988). In goldfish retina transmitter release from bipolar cells is only DHP-sensitive (Tachibana et al., 1993). The relative importance of the channels may vary in different species: according to Lundy et al. (1991), in chick brain ACh release is triggered only by N-type channels, whereas in rat it is triggered by both types. In rat nodosum neurones transmitter release could be inhibited by neuropeptide Y; both N- and L-type channels were depressed during such inhibition (Wiley et al., 1990). Baclofen (a GABA receptor antagonist) suppressed both the ω-conotoxin- and DHP-sensitive components of HVA I_{Ca} in rat hippocampal pyramidal neurones and interneurones; after application of both Ca^{2+} channel blockers almost no effect of baclofen was observed. Thus, modulation of both N- and L-type channels may be responsible for presynaptic inhibition in these neurones (Scholz and Miller, 1991b).

Alterations in the functioning of Ca^{2+} channels involved in synaptic transmission definitely form an important component of the action of many substances, inducing deep changes in the functioning of the nervous system. Thus, it has been shown that ethanol directly modulates the gating of HVA (L-type) Ca^{2+} channels in neurohypophyseal terminals, reducing their open probability (Wang et al., 1994).

Cannabinoids inhibit N-type channels in neuroblastoma cells via a PTX-sensitive pathway (Mackie and Hille, 1992). Tricyclic antidepressants (amitriptyline) inhibited Ca^{2+} channels in rat brain cortex synaptosomes (Lavoie *et al.*, 1990); chlorpromazine and other psychotrophic drugs inhibited them in neuroblastoma cells (Ogata *et al.*, 1989), and carbamazepine in spinal ganglion neurones (Schirrmacher *et al.*, 1993); μ- and δ- opioid receptor agonists reversibly decreased HVA Ca^{2+} currents in human neuroblastoma cells (Reuveny and Narahashi, 1991), neostriatal neurones (Stefani *et al.*, 1994b) and in DRG neurones via a G_o-type GTP-binding protein (Moises *et al.*, 1994). On the other hand, nootrophic agents (nefiracetam) enhanced them in human neuroblastoma cells (Yoshii and Watanabe, 1994).

As Ca^{2+} ions entering the secretory site via different Ca^{2+} channels obviously have the same properties, all the above-mentioned peculiarities of the connections between channel activity and synaptic transmission depend on the differences in the spectrum of Ca^{2+} channels in different neuronal structures and their density and strategic location. The initiation of transmitter release is an extremely fast process (latency between Ca^{2+} entry and its beginning is in the range of 0.2 ms), and Ca^{2+} ions have time to diffuse only over a fraction of micrometres; thus there must be a close opposition of channels and release sites. Simon and Llinas (1985) proposed that several calcium domains must open simultaneously directly under the synaptic vesicle in order to trigger its exocytosis, with Ca^{2+} binding at each of several sites on the vesicle. However, if one assumes that Ca^{2+} acts linearly at each binding site, it is difficult to account for the facilitation of release during repetitive stimulation and for the highly non-linear dependence of release upon external Ca^{2+}. This difficulty can be overcome by the suggestion that the vesicular binding site is activated only if n Ca^{2+} ions are bound, and the vesicle is released only if it is activated by n ions at each of N binding sites. A corresponding model was developed independently by Fogelson and Zucker (1985); in this case Ca^{2+} ions were assumed to act cooperatively at a locus on a vesicle rather than at several independent sites, and the release was assumed to occur about 50 nm away from the calcium channel, consistent with experimental observations at neuromuscular junctions. In this model Ca^{2+}-binding sites are never exposed to intense Ca^{2+} concentration peaks immediately under the channel mouth, Ca^{2+} ions act cooperatively, and a non-linear dependence of release on macroscopic Ca^{2+} current can be explained (see Zucker, 1993 for review).

A particular question is whether Ca^{2+} released from intracellular stores can also participate in this process. Obviously, in synaptic terminals the amount of such stores is negligible; this has been directly shown on isolated neurohypophyseal nerve endings, in which no substantial ATP-dependent intracellular Ca^{2+} sequestration could be detected (Stuenkel, 1994). The situation can be different in neurosecretory cells like the chromaffin cell; however, even here the contribution of released Ca^{2+} might be not very large, taking into account that the release sites are located inside the cell and lack the spatial advantages of membrane Ca^{2+} channels. Substantial release of intracellular Ca^{2+} may occur here with intense long-term stimulation, such as with K^+ depolarization, but it is probably not associated with single action potentials (Neher and Augustine, 1992b).

The intrinsic mechanism of triggering the release of transmitter-containing vesicles by Ca^{2+} ions entering the release sites is still not wholly understood; definitely it

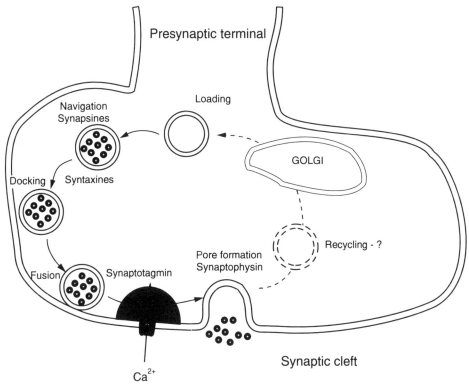

Figure 5.1. The general scheme of neurotransmitter release mechanisms in the nerve terminal (see text for explanation)

includes several successive steps represented by specific proteins connected to the vesicles (see reviews by Sudhof and Jahn, 1991; Bennett and Scheller, 1993; Sihra and Nichols, 1993). They include: a set of *synapsins* engaged in the navigation of synaptic vesicles along the cytoskeleton; *syntaxins* involved in the docking process of vesicles near the voltage-gated Ca^{2+} channels; and *synaptophysins* as candidates for the formation of the exocytotic pore complex. The most crucial of these is obviously the binding of entering Ca^{2+} ions to a specific Ca-binding protein, helping the synaptic vesicles to fuse with the cell membrane (*synaptotagmin*). This is a highly conserved protein (molecular weight 65 kDa) located at the vesicle surface, which binds Ca^{2+} at physiological concentrations and forms ternary complexes with negatively charged phospholipids. The binding causes rearrangement of membrane phospholipids into a perfusion state (Matthew *et al.*, 1981; Perin *et al.*, 1991). It should be especially noted that direct measurements of the relations between elevation of $[Ca^{2+}]_i$ and secretion in chromaffin cells (Augustine and Neher, 1992a) have shown no saturation of this process below concentrations of 10 μM, indicating that Ca^{2+} binding here is a low-affinity event; this explains why close spatial relations between the sources of Ca^{2+} ions and release sites are so important. A schematic presentation of different steps in the Ca^{2+}-induced exocytosis is given in Fig. 5.1.

It is not yet clear if the above-mentioned scheme can be applied to all types of synaptic vesicles, especially to the large dense-core ones (LDCV) secreting neuropeptides. LDCV exocytosis has been demonstrated at sites ectopic to the active zones, and the properties of Ca^{2+} binding here may be quite different, demanding higher affinity of the corresponding receptor sites (Zhu et al., 1986; Verhage et al., 1991).

Presynaptic repetitive stimulation induces an immediate short-term (decay time constant up to a few minutes) enhancement of synaptic transmission known as post-tetanic potentiation (PTP). An increase in resting $[Ca^{2+}]_i$ in the synaptic terminal as a residual process after tetanic stimulation has been suggested to account either wholly or partially for PTP. This suggestion has been tested on several synapses; in crayfish neuromuscular junction it has been shown that presynaptic Ca^{2+} levels in terminal boutons in fact rose to about 2 μM during tetanus and decayed first rapidly and then slowly back to initial levels; a 13-fold potentiation corresponded to a 500 nM elevation of Ca^{2+}. Probably, the submembrane Ca^{2+} elevation was even higher but could not be detected (Delaney, et al., 1989). The mechanism of such persistent elevation may be quite complex; for instance, accumulation of Na^+ in the terminal may play a role by slowing down the Na^+/Ca^{2+} exchange and thus keeping $[Ca^{2+}]_i$ and correspondingly PTP prolonged (Mulkey and Zucker, 1992).

CONTROL OF SYNAPTIC PLASTICITY

In parallel with short-term potentiation, much more prolonged changes (decay time constants of tens of minutes) in the effectiveness of synaptic transmission occur in some synaptic junctions, and they are of special interest because of possible connections with such long-lasting plastic changes in neuronal functions as learning and memory. The question to what extent modulation of Ca^{2+} signalling is connected with long-lasting changes in synaptic transmission is not yet clear.

In neonatal rat hippocampus low-frequency stimulation of presynaptic Schaffer collaterals induced long-term depression (LTD) in CA1 neurones which occurred specifically in the stimulated pathway and was thus homosynaptic; induction of LTD depended on postsynaptic Ca^{2+} entry through L-type channels paired with activation of metabotropic glutamate receptors. However, the immediate reason for the depression was a decrease in transmitter release from *presynaptic* terminals; obviously the events in the postsynaptic cell in some way stimulated the production of a diffusible retrograde messenger which diffused into the presynaptic terminals and altered here the mechanisms of transmitter release (Bolshakov and Siegelbaum, 1994). Probably, the depolarization of the postsynaptic neurone itself is not important for the effect. In the cerebellar network paired stimulation of parallel fibres and climbing fibres induces LTD of the responsiveness of the Purkinje neurone to stimulation of parallel fibres. According to Kasono and Hirano (1994), LTD could be induced here by direct elevation of $[Ca^{2+}]_i$ in the postsynaptic cell (using the photolabile Ca^{2+} chelator nitr-5) plus application of glutamate to it, but neither photolysis alone nor glutamate application induced LTD. The results indicate that activation of glutamate receptors, together with intracellular Ca^{2+} increase *without membrane depolarization*, is necessary and sufficient for this process.

Long-term potentiation (LTP) of synaptic transmission is also connected with changes in intracellular Ca^{2+} as one of the components of a complicated mechanism. The immediate reason for increased synaptic transmission is an increase in the release probability of the presynaptic terminals, as shown by quantal analysis (cf. Voronin, 1993). However, injection of Ca^{2+} ions into the postsynaptic element is an obligatory step in this process, as intracellular injection of Ca^{2+} chelators blocks LTP. Because NMDA receptors are predominantly located on dendritic spines, it is believed that spines may act to localize the Ca^{2+} signal by restricting the diffusion of Ca^{2+}. At the same time, they may be the site of liberation of some retrograde messenger which induces changes in the presynaptic release mechanism. Nitric oxide (NO) is a possible candidate for this role, although evidence collected so far seems to be far from conclusive (see Bekkers and Stevens, 1990; Bliss and Collingridge, 1993). It is important that potentiation of release is expressed even in the absence of Ca^{2+} entry into the presynaptic terminals due to application of Ca^{2+} -free external solution (Malgaroli and Tsien, 1992) or blocking of both P- and N-type Ca^{2+} channels mainly responsible for transmitter release (Castillo et al., 1994).

There is a question why the initiation of two opposing types of plasticity of excitatory synapses in hippocampus (LTD and LTP) should require the same receptor-operated Ca^{2+} triggering event. Probably, the direction of the change in synaptic strength is determined by a balance between phosphorylation and dephosphorylation processes regulated by protein kinases and phosphatases, which in turn are selectively controlled by different levels of $[Ca^{2+}]_i$ (Debanne and Thompson, 1994).

MODULATION OF NEURONAL EXCITABILITY

Besides the action on the membrane of synaptic vesicles triggering their exocytosis and transmitter liberation, Ca^{2+} ions injected into the cell also exert another fast action on cellular membranes from the cytosolic side: they modulate in a feedback manner their ionic permeability. Fluctuations of $[Ca^{2+}]_i$ can effectively control membrane excitability via alteration of functional activity of voltage- and ligand-gated plasmalemmal channels as well as via modulation of a variety of Ca^{2+}-dependent conductances. One of the well-defined plasmalemmal targets for intracellular Ca^{2+} is the voltage-gated calcium channel. Cytoplasmic calcium either binds to the intracellular portion of the Ca^{2+} channel or dephosphorylates Ca^{2+} channels via Ca^{2+}-dependent enzymes (see chapter 1); both these interventions effectively inactivate Ca^{2+} channels, thus limiting transmembrane Ca^{2+} entry and preventing cell overload by Ca^{2+} ions. Similarly, increase of $[Ca^{2+}]_i$ inactivates NMDA-gated channels in hippocampal neurones (Legendre et al., 1993), presumably via direct binding to the receptor molecule.

Another set of plasmalemmal channels sensitive to $[Ca^{2+}]_i$ is presented by Ca^{2+}-dependent potassium, chloride and non-selective conductances. As was shown first by Meech (1974) and by Meech and Standen (1975), influx of Ca^{2+} ions stimulates the appearance in the plasmalemma of a special type of K^+ conductance, later designated as $G_{K(Ca)}$. It is mediated by specific channels that combine voltage dependence with sensitivity to internal Ca^{2+} ions which serve as a cofactor in channel activation (Kostyuk, et al., 1980; Lux and Hofmeier, 1982a; 1982b); the effect of Ca^{2+} is rather specific: Ba^{2+} ions, conversely, block these channels (Gorman and Hermann,

1979; Adams and Gage, 1980). Their function, like that of HVA Ca^{2+} channels, is dependent on cAMP-mediated protein phosphorylation (Peyer *et al.*, 1982; Ewald and Eckert, 1983).

The functional importance of this conductance is determined by the fact that it has no threshold and no inactivation; thus it can participate both in the determination of membrane conductance at rest and in its stimulus-evoked changes. Several models of oscillatory membrane phenomena based on activation of $G_{K(Ca)}$ have been elaborated (Gorman *et al.*, 1981; Mironov, 1983 and others). Concerning the intimate mechanism of the action of Ca^{2+} ions, the existence of at least two different subtypes of $G_{K(Ca)}$ and corresponding channels should be kept in mind (Koketsu *et al.*, 1982; Hermann and Hartung, 1983; Pennefather *et al.*, 1985; Martynyuk, 1987; Lang and Ritchie, 1987; Schwindt *et al.*, 1992). One component (representing the activity of large conductance channels) activates quite rapidly, so that it can take part in repolarization after a single spike. It is well developed in brain (hippocampal) neurones, and its activation needs substantial elevation of Ca^{2+} near the cytosolic channel mouth; so close proximity of these channels and voltage-operated Ca^{2+} channels has been suggested (Lancaster and Nicoll, 1987; Lancaster *et al.*, 1991). Such co-localization has been demonstrated directly in saccular hair cells, where Ca^{2+} and K^+ channels lie within a 300 nm diameter area (Roberts *et al.*, 1990). Another slowly developing component (produced by small conductance channels) rises to a peak amplitude in about 0.5 s and has obviously a different mechanism for Ca^{2+} activation; slow diffusion of Ca^{2+} ions, participation of an enzymatic cascade and Ca^{2+}-induced Ca^{2+} release have been suggested (Schwindt *et al.*, 1992; Lancaster and Zucker, 1994).

In parallel with modulation of K^+ permeability, intracellular Ca^{2+} ions also modulate Cl^- permeability of the neuronal membrane. This was first shown in embryonic and neonatal rat DRG neurones, in which a large persistent inward tail current could be recorded when the patch pipette was filled with KCl or CsCl (Mayer, 1985). The reversal potential of this current coincided with the chloride equilibrium potential. The Cl^- current could be activated by both Ca^{2+} and Ba^{2+} ions and increased by intracellular administration of GTPγS, indicating the participation of G proteins in this process (Dolphin *et al.*, 1987). Similar currents were recorded in other neuronal structures: rabbit pelvic parasympathetic neurones (Akasu *et al.*, 1990a); bovine chromaffin cells (Doroshenko, 1991; Doroshenko *et al.*, 1991); mouse pituitary cells (Korn *et al.*, 1991); and cone photoreceptors (Barnes and Bui, 1991). A potent $I_{Cl(Ca)}$ can be recorded in frog oocytes (Miledi *et al.*, 1989; Stuhmer, 1994), where it can be induced by InsP$_3$ injections in Ca^{2+}-free external solutions and abolished by injection of EGTA; this feature has to be kept in mind during oocyte channel expression experiments, as the appearance of such endogenous current might distort the induced currents. The functional meaning of $I_{Cl(Ca)}$ is still in question; it might help to maintain the membrane potential at a depolarized level, thus enhancing Ca^{2+} influx through Ca^{2+} channels

Fig. 5.2 summarizes the modulatory actions of $[Ca^{2+}]_i$ on membrane ionic channels.

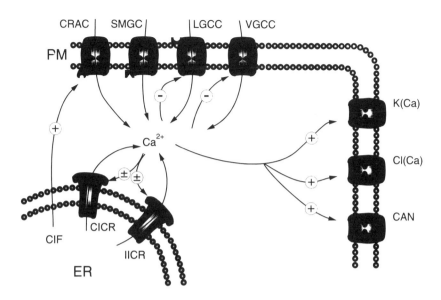

Figure 5.2. Interaction of $[Ca^{2+}]_i$ and ionic channels. The scheme shows the signalling pathways (+, positive; −, negative; ±, positive and negative feedback) involved in $[Ca^{2+}]_i$ regulation of ionic permeabilities. VGCC; LGCC; SMGC and CRAC; voltage-gated calcium channels, ligand-gated calcium channels, second-messenger-gated calcium channels; calcium-release activated calcium channels. K(Ca); Cl(Ca) and CAN: Ca^{2+}-dependent potassium, chloride and non-selective channels, respectively; CIF: 'calcium influx factor', generated upon depletion of ER calcium stores; it is believed to activate CRAC Ca^{2+} channels

NEURONAL–GLIAL INTERACTIONS

HOW CAN GLIA SENSE NEURONAL ACTIVITY?

As was discussed in chapter 4, glial cells are endowed with many types of neurotransmitter receptors, which underlie the generation of both membrane (ionic currents) and intracellular ($[Ca^{2+}]_i$ rises) signals. This leads to the obvious suggestion that glial cells may respond to the neuromediators, which are released from nerve cells. In a way, the acceptance of this assumption was not easy, due to the fact that for many years neurotransmission was believed to be exclusively restricted to the synaptic regions. However, this paradigm changed considerably over recent years; and it seems that neurotransmitters can act through the whole brain, even in regions lacking morphologically distinct synapses.

The first observation of direct neuronal-to-glial interaction was made by Villegas at the beginning of the 1970s (Villegas, 1972, 1973, 1978). He found that stimulation of the squid axon induced a clear biphasic membrane response in neighbouring Schwann cells; this response comprised initial fast depolarization followed by a prolonged hyperpolarization. Originally, Villegas suggested the involvement of cholinergic receptors in this phenomenon; later, however, the key role of glutamate-triggered Ca^{2+} release from InsP$_3$-releasable stores was found (Lieberman and Sanzenbacher

1992). Subsequently, the $[Ca^{2+}]_i$ increase following electrical stimulation of motor nerve was directly observed in perisynaptic Schwann cells in frog neuromuscular junction (Reist and Smith, 1992; Jahromi *et al.*, 1992). This $[Ca^{2+}]_i$ elevation was mimicked by muscarine and was presumably a result of IICR generation. The functional meaning of calcium signal in perisynaptic Schwann cells is as yet unclear; in squid axon it was proposed to affect membrane K^+ permeability, thus increasing the ability of Schwann cells to control extracellular potassium; in vertebrates, $[Ca^{2+}]_i$ elevation may trigger release of neuroactive substances which may modulate synaptic efficacy.

Later, similar examples of direct axonal-to-glial interactions were found in video-imaging experiments on rat optic nerve (Kriegler and Chiu, 1993; Chiu and Kriegler, 1994). In these experiments calcium green-based confocal microscopy revealed a prominent $[Ca^{2+}]_i$ rise in glial cells in response to electrical stimulation of the nerve. The mechanisms of glial $[Ca^{2+}]_i$ response in this case appeared to be quite complicated. By modifying transmembrane Na^+ and K^+ gradients, Kriegler and Chiu (1993) discovered that axonal electrical activity disturbs the ionic microenvironment with subsequent release of glutamate from axons and/or glial cells via Na^+-glutamate transporter. Released glutamate, in turn, acts on glial receptors, which initiate the generation of $[Ca^{2+}]_i$ response. Apart from glutamate, nerve axons may also release in a non-vesicular fashion other neuroactive ligands (e.g. purine nucleotides; Maire *et al.*, 1984) which can also trigger the calcium signal in periaxonal glial cells.

In the grey matter the preferential pathway for neuronal-to-glial communications is presumably via synaptically released neurotransmitters and changes in the ionic interstitial microenvironment following neuronal electrical activity, although the generation of glial $[Ca^{2+}]_i$ responses in brain tissue *in situ* has not yet been directly demonstrated.

Intracellular Ca^{2+} release may be involved in realization of contact-dependent signals originating from neurones. It is clear that growing oligodendrocytes migrate to nerve fibres in order to start myelinization; contact with neuronal membranes or with oligodendrocytes which have already started myelinization may induce intracellular Ca^{2+} transients serving as a trigger for myelinization. Indeed, it was shown recently that myelin extracts trigger $[Ca^{2+}]_i$ elevation in oligodendrocytes as a result of Ca^{2+} release from internal stores (Moorman and Hume, 1994).

HOW MAY GLIA INFLUENCE NEURONES?

Neuronal function is strongly influenced by changes in the interstitial microenvironment. Glial cells are heavily involved in maintaining chemical homeostasis in the interstitium and glial cytoplasmic calcium is probably one of the key factors in this glial function. One of the most important roles of glial cells is control of the ionic composition of the interstitial space. As has already been mentioned, neuronal electrical activity is associated with massive potassium efflux. Even under normal conditions nerve activity may increase interstitial K^+ concentration substantially, which obviously will affect neuronal electrogenesis. The excessive potassium is taken up by glial cells, and this uptake is crucially dependent on glial $[Ca^{2+}]_i$. Glial Ca^{2+}-activated K^+ channels obviously underlie the control of interstitial K^+. These channels have been found in several glial subtypes, including astrocytes and Schwann cells (cf. Sontheimer, 1994). The open probability of glial $K_{(Ca)}$ channels increases substantially (Tas et al., 1988; Barres et al., 1990a) while increasing $[Ca^{2+}]_i$, with half-activation at 0.4–1 μM Ca^{2+}. The causal relationship between $[Ca^{2+}]_i$ and activation of $K_{(Ca)}$ channels has been demonstrated in perineural crayfish glial cells, where KCl depolarization induces a large increase in K^+ permeability blocked either by removal of extracellular Ca^{2+} or treatment with Ca^{2+} channel antagonists (Butt et al., 1990).

The second important glial-dependent step in regulation of the interstitial microenvironment is associated with Ca^{2+}-dependent volume regulation of glial cells. It was confirmed by several groups that brain astrocytes undergo swelling, thereby changing the interstitium volume, and $[Ca^{2+}]_i$ plays an important role in this process (cf. O'Connor and Kimelberg, 1993).

Third, an important determinant of the brain microenvironment which has not been experimentally confirmed yet is associated with the control of extracellular Ca^{2+} concentration. It is known that electrical stimulation of the brain structures may induce a substantial drop in extracellular Ca^{2+} concentration: in hippocampus, for example, electrical stimulation decreased $[Ca^{2+}]_o$ from 2 mM to 1.4 mM (Benninger et al., 1980); spreading depression caused an even more pronounced fall in $[Ca^{2+}]_o$, bringing it from 2.2 mM to 0.8 mM (Kraig and Nicholson, 1987). Certainly, the drop in interstitial Ca^{2+} concentration will affect neuronal function dramatically. One speculation is that glial $[Ca^{2+}]_i$ may be used for replenishment of the interstitial calcium content.

Finally, glial cells were reported to accumulate and release a number of neuroligands, and once more $[Ca^{2+}]_i$ is probably involved in the regulation of these processes. The crucial role of $[Ca^{2+}]_i$ was suggested for glia-derived release of taurine (Philibert et al., 1988), purine nucleotides (Ballerini et al., 1992) and nerve growth factor (NGF) (Carman-Krzan et al., 1991). Glial cells also express an elaborate system for transmembrane glutamate transport, thereby regulating interstitial glutamate concentration and synaptic efficacy. Glutamate uptake/release is mediated by an $Na^+/K^+/$glutamate electrogenic transporter which translocates three Na^+ ions in and one K^+ ion out for each molecule of glutamate transported into the cell. This type of glutamate transporter was demonstrated in cultured oligodendrocytes (Oka et al., 1993) and astrocytes (Wyllie et al., 1991). The activity of glutamate uptake by cultured astrocytes is enhanced by Ca^{2+} ions, due to both Na^+/K^+ and Ca^{2+}-dependent glutamate uptake systems (Flott and Seifert, 1991). The direct activation of glutamate transporter (as measured by appearance of transporter current in astrocytes) was demonstrated in neuronal–glial 'micro-island' co-cultures following autaptic excitation of adjacent neurones (Mennerick and Zorzumski, 1994). These experiments suggest that glial glutamate uptake is indeed involved in removal of glutamate from synaptic clefts, thus contributing to the regulation of synaptic transmission in hippocampus.

The activity of glutamate transporter in glial cells may be dually controlled by $[Ca^{2+}]_i$: the latter exerts not only positive but also negative feedback on glutamate transport. Increase in $[Ca^{2+}]_i$ could activate phospholipase A_2, with subsequent formation of arachidonic acid. The latter is reported to inhibit glial glutamate transport, thus increasing the amount of glutamate in the synapse and the efficacy of neurotransmission (Glowinski et al., 1994).

In addition to neurotransmitter glial–neuronal communications, there is evidence favouring the existence of direct neuronal–astrocytic connections through octanol-sensitive junction-like structures; astrocytic $[Ca^{2+}]_i$ waves could thus propagate to neurones (Nedergaard, 1994).

Glial calcium signalling may be involved not only in the physiological behaviour of brain structures but also in pathological reactions in the nervous system. Experiments on cultured glial cells demonstrated that after periods of ischaemia they lose the ability to maintain $[Ca^{2+}]_i$ homeostasis and become Ca^{2+} overloaded (Kim-Lee et al., 1992). Similarly to nerve cells, glia may respond by irreversible $[Ca^{2+}]_i$ elevation following massive exposure to excitatory amino acids, which accompanies ischaemic or epileptic brain damage. This kind of excitotoxicity was demonstrated for cultured astrocytes, which responded to prolonged glutamate administration with Ca^{2+}-dependent swelling and cytoskeletal damage (Koyama et al., 1991). The sensitivity of astroglia to excitotoxic influences is, however, considerably less as compared to neurones: glutamate or aspartate exposure sufficient to kill neurones did not affect astrocytes (Regan and Choi, 1991), although this was not the case for oligodendrocytes (Oka et al. 1993). This led to speculation that astrocytes act as a save system against excitotoxicity in the brain, eliminating, to some extent, excessive glutamate released during brain failure.

It is now becoming more and more obvious that glia represents a meaningful and important signalling system which not only feeds neurones but may also be involved in brain information flow. Several mechanisms (see Fig. 5.3) have been proposed in order to explain how glial cells may communicate with neurones. However, the current state of our knowledge is only at the beginning of understanding glial–neuronal cross-talk. Although we imagine how neurones may influence glia, we still lack experimental data concerning mechanisms of glial-to-neuronal communication. The forthcoming years will bring new excitement in the understanding of the role of glial cells in brain functioning.

MODULATION OF GENE EXPRESSION, CELL DIFFERENTIATION AND PROGRAMMED DEATH

Besides the above-described rapid effects of intracellular Ca^{2+} signals, they exert extensive long-lasting effects, determining in fact the whole live cycle of the cell. The elucidation of the intimate mechanisms of this role of Ca^{2+} ions is just at the beginning, and the available data are often controversial. Obviously, the main pathway to induce such long-lasting changes would be the modulation of the expression of the corresponding genes. One of the important determinants of gene expression is the transcription of the immediate early genes (e.g. c-fos and c-jun), which are also called primary response genes. The proteins encoded by these genes are, in fact, transcription activators, which transduce intracellular signals into later long-term gene expression changes (cf. Kerr et al., 1992). The induction of immediate early gene transcription is extremely rapid and, as was shown by a number of investigators, it may be controlled by cytoplasmic Ca^{2+} perturbations. Among primary response genes members of fos and jun families were found to be $[Ca^{2+}]_i$-inducible (see Roche and Prentki, 1994 for review). The $[Ca^{2+}]_i$ dose dependence of c-fos genes was clearly bell-shaped, with

151

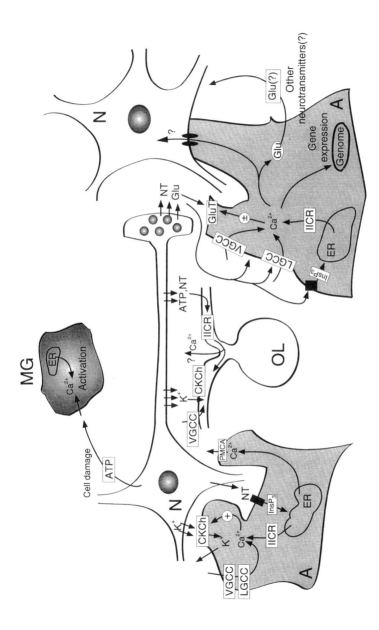

Figure 5.3. Mechanisms of neuronal–glial interactions. N, neurones; A, astrocytes; OL, oligodendrocyte, MG, microglial cell. Glial $[Ca^{2+}]_i$ is disturbed by Ca^{2+} entry via voltage- and ligand-operated Ca^{2+} channels (VGCC and LGCC) and by neurotransmitter (NT)-induced $InsP_3$-mediated Ca^{2+} release (IICR). Both astro- and oligodendrocytes are involved in regulation of interstitial K^+ concentration via Ca^{2+}-activated K^+ channels (CKCh); they may also supply the interstitial space by Ca^{2+} ions released from the stores by a still unknown mechanism (involving for example plasmalemmal Ca^{2+} pumps—PMCA). Glial cell can also participate in uptake and release of neurotransmitters, (e.g. via glutamate-transporter-GLuT) thus modulating synaptic efficacy. Astrocytic $[Ca^{2+}]_i$ waves may possibly penetrate into neighbouring neurones via gap junction-like pathways

maximal transcription activation at about 250 nM (as revealed by ionophore-clamp technique applied to HL-60 leukaemia cells—Werlen et al., 1993). Interestingly that even a very short (~1 min) $[Ca^{2+}]_i$ elevation was sufficient to exert the maximal effect on c-fos transcription. Similarly, in the glial cell line 1321N1 carbachol-induced $[Ca^{2+}]_i$ rise was reported to stimulate expression of c-fos and c-jun (Trejo and Brown, 1991). In cultured hypothalamic neurones stimulation of c-fos is increased within 1.5–2 h after cell depolarization with 50 mM KCl. The effect is obviously due to Ca^{2+} signalling and is combined with cAMP-dependent activation of PK-A, as it could be inhibited by Ca channel blockers and increased by forskolin (Sim et al., 1994). Calmodulin and Ca^{2+}/calmodulin-dependent protein kinases also presumably serve as an intermediate step in coupling $[Ca^{2+}]_i$ rise and gene transcription. The most striking observation, made by Greenberg and his colleagues (Banding et al., 1993) stressed the point that the way Ca^{2+} enters the cell may be critically important for inducing primary response gene expression. Working with hippocampal neurones they found that KCl depolarization, but not NMDA-evoked $[Ca^{2+}]_i$ elevation, is responsible for c-fos transcription stimulation. This may mean that both the level of $[Ca^{2+}]_i$ and mode of Ca^{2+} entry (e.g. spatial differences) may activate distinct Ca^{2+}-dependent signalling pathways. It would be of great importance to follow the functioning of these pathways during cell development and differentiation. Certainly new experimental approaches, combining $[Ca^{2+}]_i$ recordings and molecular biological techniques (e.g. single-cell PCR), may highlight unknown events in $[Ca^{2+}]_i$–gene expression coupling mechanisms.

It has been shown that inhibition of Ca^{2+} influx, as well as depletion of Ca^{2+} stores, affect neuronal differentiation during a particular period of development (Bixby and Spitzer, 1994; Holliday and Spitzer, 1990). The period of sensitivity to depletion corresponds to the period of sensitivity to removal of extracellular Ca^{2+} and to the period of most frequent spontaneous $[Ca^{2+}]_i$ elevations. These elevations diminish with neuronal maturation, and depletion of Ca^{2+} stores at early times affects neuronal differentiation in a manner similar to the prevention of influx (Holliday et al., 1991). Different Ca^{2+} channels may have a specific role in this process because of their strategic location. Thus, L-type channels in the somatic membrane are often concentrated at the base of major dendrites (Westenbroek et al., 1990; Sher et al., 1991) which may be a strategically important site for influencing such functions.

The importance of Ca^{2+} signalling at the early stages of ontogenetic development of brain functions has also been demonstrated in our recent experiments, showing the possibility of their grave disturbances related to a long-lasting depression of HVA Ca^{2+} channels in the somatic membrane. It has been demonstrated on phaeoch-romocytoma cells that intracellular administration of L-tyrosine stabilizes the functioning of HVA channels; α-methyl-D,L-tyrosine (a tyrosine hydroxylase blocker) exerted a similar effect. Conversely, L phenylalanine (a precursor of L-tyrosine) accelerated the 'washout' of the corresponding currents. As tyrosination of α-tubulin is an important step in its metabolism, these effects may indicate that some interaction of tubulin with HVA Ca^{2+} channels may be important for normal functioning of these channels (Kostyuk et al., 1991).

In view of these data, model experiments were made on newborn rats in which chronic elevation of the plasma level of L-phenylalanine had been induced by its intraperitoneal injection; the situation was similar to that observed in phenylketonuria,

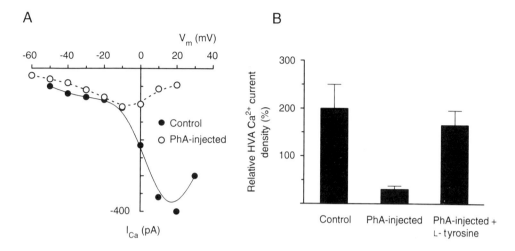

Figure 5.4. Changes in HVA Ca^{2+} current densities in experimentally modelled phenylketonuria in hippocampal neurones (own observations). (A) I–V curves of I_{Ca} measured from control neurones and neurones obtained from phenylalanine-injected (PhA) animals. (B) Relative densities of HVA I_{Ca} in controls, after phenylalanine injection and in neurones obtained from PhA-injected animals which were kept in L-tyrosine-enriched media

a congenital disease characterized by severe impairment of brain function. It has been found that in the soma of hippocampal neurones isolated from such rats the amplitude of HVA $I_C{}^a$ was largely depressed; no changes in LVA currents were observed (Fig. 5.4). The decrease remained during several days of culturing of the neurones; however, addition of L-tyrosine to the culture medium could partly restore the HVA current (Martynyuk *et al.*, 1991). Thus it seems that further investigations of the relations between Ca^{2+} signalling and development of the cytoskeleton in the early period of ontogenesis might be quite important.

An obligatory stage in the development of the nervous system is the elimination of excessive neuronal elements (their programmed death). A special point here is the possible involvement of Ca^{2+} channels in the process of cellular death. In mouse motoneurones during the period of cell death and elimination of supernumbering synapses the density of HVA Ca^{2+} channels increased significantly (Mynlieff and Beam, 1992). Conversely, data are available indicating that developmental neuronal death depends on NGF, which promotes survival by suppressing programmed death; elevation of [Ca^{2+}]$_i$ by membrane depolarization and Ca^{2+} influx through DHP-sensitive Ca^{2+} channels in this case promoted survival, probably by diminishing this NGF dependence (Franklin and Johnson, 1992; Johnson and Deckwerth, 1993). Pharmacological reduction of [Ca^{2+}]$_i$ or depletion of ER stores kills early NGF-independent neurones, but has a negligible effect on older neurones growing in the presence of brain-derived neurotrophic factors. Shortly before they become dependent on NGF, neurones express L-type calcium channels and their survival can be enhanced by depolarization-induced Ca^{2+} influx (Larmet *et al.*, 1992). Developmentally associated increase in [Ca^{2+}]$_i$ may also underline the decrease in trophic factor dependence of nerve cells with maturation.

[Ca^{2+}]$_i$ HOMEOSTASIS AND AGEING

Disturbances in [Ca^{2+}]$_i$ homeostasis seem to be deeply involved in neuronal dysfunction associated with ageing. The age-dependent changes in [Ca^{2+}]$_i$ handling comprise (1) alteration of the resting [Ca^{2+}]$_i$ level, (2) changes in stimulus-evoked [Ca^{2+}]$_i$ transients and (3) disturbances in Ca^{2+} extrusion from the cytoplasm (see Khachaturian, 1994; Verkhratsky et al., 1994 for review). The first clues pointing out the disturbances in [Ca^{2+}]$_i$ homeostasis in ageing came from experiments on brain synaptosomes, which demonstrated the elevation of resting [Ca^{2+}]$_i$ in aged neurones (Gibson and Petersen, 1987; Martinez-Serrano et al., 1988, 1992). Subsequently, the constant elevation of resting [Ca^{2+}]$_i$ in neurones was directly confirmed in microfluorimetric experiments. Initially, an age-associated rise in resting [Ca^{2+}]$_i$ was found in cultured DRG neurones: in cells isolated from aged (30 months) rats the cytoplasmic free calcium was significantly higher as compared with adult values (207 ± 37 nM versus 96 ± 23 nM; Kirischuk et al., 1992). Similarly, resting [Ca^{2+}]$_i$ was significantly higher in granule neurones studied in acutely isolated cerebellar slices of old mice as compared with young and adult mice (Kirischuk et al., 1995f). Apart from the increase in resting [Ca^{2+}]$_i$, indo-1 and fura-2 experiments performed on both cultured DRG neurones and neurones in cerebellar slices revealed a strong reduction in the amplitudes of depolarization-triggered [Ca^{2+}]$_i$ transients in cells from old rats and mice. At least in the case of DRG neurones, the age-dependent attenuation of depolarization-triggered [Ca^{2+}]$_i$ elevation reflected the remarkable decrease in the number of voltage-gated plasmalemmal Ca^{2+} channels (Kostyuk et al., 1993; Verkhratsky et al., 1994). In central neurones the age-dependent changes in plasmalemmal Ca^{2+} currents are less clear. Radioisotope experiments revealed a decrease in K$^+$-stimulated ^{45}Ca^{2+} influx in brain synaptosomes isolated from old animals (Martinez-Serrano et al., 1989). In line with these data, decrease in HVA Ca^{2+} currents was observed in hippocampal granular neurones (Reynolds and Carlen, 1989). In contrast, Landfield and his colleagues (Landfield, 1994; Landfield et al., 1989; Pitler and Landfield, 1990) found prolongation of the calcium spike in hippocampal slice neurones from aged rats and increase in Ca^{2+} currents in aged hippocampal CA1 neurones; moreover, they described the appearance of unusually long Ca^{2+} tail currents in aged neurones, which would further increase voltage-activated Ca^{2+} influx. The reason for such controversial data remains unclear, and certainly more precise experiments are still necessary.

Surprisingly, our experiments on [Ca^{2+}]$_i$ homeostasis in aged neurones (cf. Verkhratsky et al., 1994) revealed that reduction of the amplitude of [Ca^{2+}]$_i$ rise in old neurones is associated with prominent deceleration of the recovery of [Ca^{2+}]$_i$ transients. The slowing down of [Ca^{2+}]$_i$ clearance following depolarization was also consistently observed in experiments on synaptosomes from old brain (cf. Michaelis, 1994). These disturbances in calcium signal recovery presumably reflect the alteration of Ca^{2+} extrusion systems within ageing. Indeed, marked reduction of Ca^{2+} extrusion through Na$^+$/Ca^{2+} exchange and plasmalemmal calcium pumps was observed in synaptosomes obtained from old brain (Martinez-Serrano et al., 1992). Other systems involved in calcium signal termination, including mitochondrial Ca^{2+} uptake (Vitorica and Satrustegui, 1986), cytoplasmic Ca^{2+} buffering (Villa et al., 1994) and ER calcium accumulation (Verkhratsky *et al.*, 1994) are also reported to undergo age-associated changes.

In our opinion, changes in Ca^{2+} homeostasis with ageing may have a complex mechanism which is initiated by decrease in the effectiveness of cytoplasmic Ca^{2+} buffering and clearing, subsequent elevation of resting $[Ca^{2+}]_i$ and recurrent downregulation of HVA Ca^{2+} channels. The functional meaning of the age-dependent elevation of $[Ca^{2+}]_i$ is not obvious. It may be one of the causes of cellular death; however, moderate elevation may be considered also as a kind of compensatory mechanism preventing disaster, as it happens during neuronal elimination in early ontogenesis. In any case, our data together with studies performed in other laboratories certainly suggest that the system of $[Ca^{2+}]_i$ homeostasis is altered in ageing neurones. Presumably these alterations underlie increased vulnerability of the old brain to various types of brain failures, first of all ischaemic, which are associated with excessive Ca^{2+} entry into neuronal cells.

CALCIUM SIGNALLING AND BRAIN PATHOLOGY

Because of its participation in triggering or modulation of all aspects of nerve cell functioning, changes in Ca^{2+} signalling are always involved in grave pathological states of the brain. In this respect they often resemble changes already described during ageing, being more severe and generalized (cf. Disterhoft *et al.*, 1994). A detailed description of the cellular mechanisms of brain pathology is beyond the scope of this book, and only the main findings concerning such widely occurring pathology as Alzheimer's disease, AIDS-related dementia, amyotrophic lateral sclerosis and diabetic neuropathy will be discussed.

ALZHEIMER'S DISEASE

The changes in calcium homeostasis during Alzheimer's disease are probably the most obvious because of profound changes in neuronal membrane conductance induced by β-amyloid (Aβ), a small peptide (about 42 amino acids) accumulating in the brain during its course. The molecules of this peptide aggregate in solution and become neurotoxic. They insert themselves into the lipid bilayer and form ionic channels selective for Ca^{2+} but permeable also for other monovalent cations; thus an additional pathway for injection of Ca^{2+} into nerve cells is created (cf. Arispe *et al.*, 1994). In fact, neurones exposed to Aβ show a rapid rise in $[Ca^{2+}]_i$ level (over a period of several hours) and signs of neuronal degeneration ending with apoptosis; this rise may be a direct reason for such pathological changes or a signal that Aβ makes neurones more sensitive to deleterious changes in the extracellular environment. Interestingly, the presence of DHP Ca^{2+} channel blockers (nimodipine) substantially attenuated the injury, indicating that Ca^{2+} influx through L-type Ca^{2+} channels may also be an important component in cell injury (Cotman *et al.*, 1994). A special feature of this pathology is its expression predominantly in neurones with a high density of glutamate receptors (hippocampus, entorhinal cortex). It has been demonstrated in cultured hippocampal and cortical neurones that a close parallelism exists between loss of neurones and sustained elevation of $[Ca^{2+}]_i$ after exposure to glutamate (excitotoxicity; see Ogura et al., 1988; Choi, 1994 and others). Notably, influx of Ca^{2+} through NMDA receptor-gated channels was potentially more detrimental than influx through other channels. When both glutamate and K^+-induced depolarization were used to increase the $[Ca^{2+}]_i$ level, only the former was toxic (Tymianski et al. 1993). Thus the site of Ca^{2+} entry also has to be taken into account in explaining the damage; neurones vulnerable towards the disease may also be selectively vulnerable under conditions of metabolic compromise (cf. Mattson, 1994; Siesjo, 1994).

AIDS-RELATED DEMENTIA

A substantial number of adults and children with AIDS develop neurological manifestations of the disease connected with substantial injury to brain neurones. The latter is related to the action of the virus envelope protein gp120 which in picomolar concentrations induces neuronal loss in hippocampal cultures (cf. Lipton, 1994). An excessive rise in neuronal Ca^{2+} triggered by gp120 is thought to contribute to a final common pathway of neurotoxic events leading to free radical formation, cellular necrosis and possibly apoptosis; these events may include overactivation of neuronal Ca^{2+}-dependent enzymes. Concurrent activation of NMDA receptors is also needed for neuronal injury by gp120, as in Alzheimer's disease.

AMYOTROPHIC LATERAL SCLEROSIS

Early studies of amyotrophic lateral sclerosis (ALS) focused on glutamate excitotoxicity and ligand-gated Ca^{2+} channels as the main course of neuronal damage. Later it was shown that ALS IgG inhibits skeletal L-type Ca^{2+} channels, being one of the reasons for changes in muscle functioning. Conversely, the same immunoglobulins increased Ca^{2+} entry in motoneurones, probably inducing their vulnerability and finally leading to cell death (Appel et al., 1994). The question why in the case of this illness spinal motoneurones are selectively damaged is still unclear.

DIABETIC NEUROPATHY

Another illness with more localized damage of neuronal functioning related to alterations in Ca^{2+} homeostasis is insulin-dependent diabetes mellitus (IDDM), which is often followed by severe alterations in sensory function in the form of hyperalgesia (increased pain sensitivity). As has been mentioned in chapter 3, there are substantial differences in the mechanisms of Ca^{2+} homeostasis in different sensory neurones: in neurones of small size, responsible mainly for nociception, no functional intracellular stores were detected, and the termination of Ca^{2+} signals is therefore dependent mostly on Ca^{2+} extrusion by the plasmalemmal Ca^{2+} pump (Shmigol et al., 1994b). If experimental IDDM was induced in rats by injection of streptozotocin, no definite changes in the amplitude and time course of Ca^{2+} transients were observed in large DRG sensory neurones transmitting exteroceptive signals; however, in small ones the decay of Ca^{2+} transients became substantially prolonged. This prolongation was probably induced by the action of chronic hyperglycaemia depressing the activity of the plasmalemmal Ca pump by excessive glycosylation (Vlassara *et al.*, 1994). As such activity in small neurones is absolutely necessary for the termination of calcium signals, the latter are obviously especially vulnerable during IDDM, and the prolongation of residual $[Ca^{2+}]_i$ transients in them may be the reason for potentiation of the transmission of nociceptive signals (Kostyuk *et al.*, 1995).

CONCLUSIONS

Calcium signals generated in neuronal and glial cells by the complex system analysed in the preceding chapters exert a powerful triggering and modulatory action on all aspects of cellular functioning, the detailed mechanisms of which are far from being understood yet. Definitely, this action can be separated into immediate and sustained components. The *immediate* effects are exerted by Ca^{2+} binding to specific intracellular proteins which trigger the corresponding function (release of synaptic vesicles, opening of ionic channels, etc.). As the amount of Ca^{2+} ions injected into the cytosol during calcium signal generation is quite small and the affinity of the binding not very high, special prerequisites are necessary for reliable initiation of these effects (close opposition of Ca^{2+} channels and Ca^{2+} binding sites, clustering of Ca^{2+}-injecting channels, etc.). The *sustained* effects involve a complex chain of intracellular intermediate processes as well as neuronal–glial interactions, differently affected by Ca^{2+} ions; they might include modulation of gene expression and processing of the synthesized protein molecules. These effects determine all stages of the nerve cell life cycle, including its ageing and death; correspondingly they are subjected to profound alterations during severe pathological states of the brain like Alzheimer's disease, AIDS-induced dementia, amyotrophic lateral sclerosis and others.

References

Abe, Y., Sorimachi, M., Itoyama, Y., Furukawa, K., Akaike, N. (1995) ATP responses in the embryo chick ciliary ganglion cells. *Neuroscience* **64**, 547–551.

Adams, B.A, Beam, K.G. (1989) A novel calcium current in dysgenic skeletal muscle. *J. Gen. Physiol.* **94**, 429–444.

Adams, D.J., Gage, P.W. (1980) Divalent ion currents and the delayed potassium conductance in an *Aplysia* neurone. *J. Physiol. (Lond.)* **304**, 297–313.

Ahmed, Z., Lewis, C.A., Faber, D.S. (1990) Glutamate stimulates release of Ca^{2+} from internal stores in astroglia. *Brain Res.* **516**, 165–169.

Akaike, N., Tsuda, Y., Oyama, Y. (1988) Separation of current- and voltage-dependent inactivation of calcium current in frog sensory neuron. *Neurosci. Lett.* **84**, 46–50.

Akaike, N., Kostyuk, P.G., Osipchuk, Y.V. (1989) Dihydropyridine-sensitive low-threshold calcium channels in isolated rat hypothalamic neurones. *J. Physiol. (Lond.)* **412**, 181–195.

Akaike, N., Krishtal, O.A., Maruyama, T. (1990) Proton-induced sodium current in frog isolated dorsal root ganglia cells. *J. Neurophysiol.* **63**, 805–813.

Akasu, T., Nisimura, T., Tokimasa, T. (1990a) Calcium-dependent chloride current in neurones of the rabbit pelvic parasympathetic ganglia. *J. Physiol. (Lond.)* **422**, 303–320.

Akasu, T., Tsurusaki, M., Tokimasa, T. (1990b) Reduction of the N-type calcium current by noradrenaline in neurones of rabbit vesical parasympathetic ganglia. *J. Physiol. (Lond.)* **426**, 439–452.

Alford, S., Fenguelli, B.G., Collingridge, G.L. (1993) Characterization of Ca^{2+} signals induced in hippocampal CA1 neurones by the synaptic activation of NMDA receptors. *J. Physiol. (Lond.)* **469**, 693–716.

Allen, C.N., Brady, R., Swan, J., Hori, N., Carpenter, D.O. (1988) N-methyl-d-aspartate (NMDA) receptors are inactivated by trypsin. *Brain Res.* **458**, 147–150.

Allsup, D.J., Boarder, M.R. (1990) Comparison of P_2-purinergic receptors of aortic endothelial cells with those of the adrenal medulla: Evidence for heterogeneity of receptor subtype and inositol phosphate response. *Mol. Pharmacol.* **38**, 84–91.

Altiere, R.J., Diamond, L., Thompson, D.C. (1992) Omega-conotoxin-sensitive calcium channels modulate autonomic neurotransmission in guinea pig airways. *J. Pharmacol. Exp. Ther.* **260**, 98–103.

Amedee, T., Ellie, E., Dupouy, B., Vincent, J.D. (1991) Voltage-dependent calcium and potassium channels in Schwann cells cultured from dorsal root ganglia of the mouse. *J. Physiol. (Lond.)* **441**, 35–56.

Amundsen, J., Clapham, D. (1993) Calcium waves. *Curr. Opinion Neurobiol.* **3**, 375–382.

Anderson, K., Lai, F.A., Liu, Q.Y., Rousseau, E., Erickson, H.P., Meissner, G. (1989) Structural and functional characterization of the purified cardiac ryanodine receptor–Ca^{2+} release channel complex. *J. Biol. Chem.* **264**, 1329–1335.

Andreeva, N., Khodorov, B., Stelmashook, E., Cragoe, E., Victorov, I. (1991) Inhibition of Na^+/Ca^{2+} exchange enhances delayed neuronal death elicited by glutamate in cerebellar granule cell cultures. *Brain Res.* **548**, 322–325.

Andressen, C., Blumcke, I., Celio, M.R. (1993) Calcium-binding proteins: selective markers of nerve cells. *Cell Tissue Res.* **271**, 181–208.

Appel, S.H., Smith, R.G., Alexianu, M. *et al.* (1994) Neurodegenerative disease: autoimmunity involving calcium channels. *Ann. NY Acad. Sci.* **747**, 183–194.

Aramori, I., Nakanishi, S. (1992) Signal transduction and pharmacological characteristics of a metabotropic glutamate receptor, mGluR1, in transfected CHO cells. *Neuron* **8**, 757–765.

Araque, A., Clarac, F., Buno, W. (1994) P-type Ca^{2+} channels mediate excitatory and inhibitory synaptic transmitter release in crayfish muscle. *Proc. Natl Acad. Sci. USA* **91**, 4224–4228.

Arbones, L., Picatoste, F., Garsia, A. (1988) Histamine H_1 receptors mediate phosphoinositide hydrolysis in astrocyte-enriched primary cultures. *Brain Res.* **450**, 144–152.

Arispe, N., Pollard, H.B. Rojas, E. (1994) The ability of amyloid β-protein /AβP(1–40)/ to form Ca^{++} channels provides a mechanism for neuronal death in Alzheimer's disease. *Ann. NY Acad. Sci.* **747**, 256–266.

Armstrong, C.M, Neyton, J. (1991) Two-site' behavior from a one site model of the calcium channel. *Biophys. J.* **59**, 275a.

Artalejo, C.R, Mogul, D.J, Perlman, R.L, Fox, A.P. (1991a) Three types of bovine cell Ca channels: facilitation increases the opening probability of a 27 pS channel. *J. Physiol. (Lond.)* **444**, 213–240.

Artalejo, C.R, Perlman, R.L, Fox, A.P. (1991b) ω-Conotoxin inhibits a Ca current in bovine chromaffin cells that does not seem to be N-type. *Biophys. J.* **59**, 369a.

Artalejo, C.R., Adams, M.E., Fox, A.P. (1994) Three types of Ca^{2+} channels trigger secretion with different efficacies in chromaffin cells. *Nature* **367**, 72–76.

Asher, P., Nowak, L. (1988) The role of divalent cations in the N-methyl-d-aspartate response of mouse central neurones in culture. *J. Physiol. (Lond.)* **399**, 247–266.

Ashley, R.H. (1989) Activation and conductance properties of ryanodine-sensitive calcium channels from brain microsomal membranes incorporated into planar lipid bilayers. *J. Membrane Biol.* **111**, 179–189.

Astrup, J., Norberg, K. (1976) Potassium activity in cerebral cortex in rats during progressive severe hypoglycemia. *Brain Res.* **103**, 418–423.

Augustine, G.J., Neher, E. (1992a) Calcium requirements for secretion in bovine chromaffin cells. *J. Physiol. (Lond.)* **450**, 247–271.

Augustine, G.J., Neher, E. (1992b) Neuronal Ca^{2+} signalling takes the local route. *Curr. Opinion Neurobiol.* **2**, 302–307.

Baimbridge, K.G., Celio, M.R., Rogers, J.H. (1992) Calcium-binding proteins in the nervous system. *Trends Neurosci.* **15**,303–308.

Ballerini,P., Cicarelli, R., DiNapoli, M. *et al.* (1992) Cytosolic calcium influence on purine release from cultured rat astrocytes. *Pharmacol. Res.* **2**, 323–324.

Banding, H., Ginty, D.D., Greenberg, M.E. (1993) Regulation of gene expression in hippocampal neurones by distinct calcium signaling pathways. *Science* **260**, 181–186.

Bargas, J., Surmeier, D.J., Kitai, S.T. (1991) High-and low-voltage activated calcium currents are expressed by neurons cultured from embryonic rat neostriatum. *Brain Res.* **541**, 70–74.

Bargas, J., Howe, A., Eberwine, J., Cao Y., Surmeier, D.J. (1994) Cellular and molecular characterization of Ca^{++} currents in acutely isolated adult rat neostriatal neurons. *J. Neurosci.* **14**, 6667–6686.

Barger, S.W., Van Eldick, L.J. (1992) S100β stimulates calcium fluxes in glial and neuronal cells. *J. Biol. Chem.* **267**, 9689–9694.

Barish, M.E. (1991) Increases in intracellular calcium ion concentration during depolarization of cultured embryonic *Xenopus* spinal neurones. *J. Physiol. (Lond.)* **444**, 545–565.

Barnes, S., Bui, Q. (1991) Modulation of calcium-activated chloride current via pH-induced changes of calcium channel properties in cone photoreceptors. *J. Neurosci.* **11**, 4015–4023.

Barnes, S., Haynes, L.W. (1992) Low-voltage-activated calcium channels in human retinoblastoma cells. *Brain Res.* **598**, 19–22.

Barres, B.A., Chun, L.L.Y., Corey, D.P. (1988) Ion channel expression by white matter glia. *Glia* **1**, 10–30.

Barres, B.A., Chun, L.L.Y., Corey, D.P. (1989) Calcium current in cortical astrocytes: Induction by cAMP and neurotransmitters and permissive effect of serum factors. *J. Neurosci.* **9**,3169–3175.

Barres, B.A., Chun, L.L.Y., Corey, D.P. (1990a) Ion channels in vertebrate glia. *Annu. Rev. Neurosci.* **13**, 441–474.

Barres, B.A., Koroshetz, W.J., Chun, L.L.Y., Corey, D.P. (1990b) Ion channel expression by white mater glia: the type-1 astrocyte. *Neuron* **5**, 527–544.

Bean, B.P. (1991) Pharmacology of calcium channels in cardiac muscle, vascular muscle, and neurons. *Am. J. Hypertens.* **4**, 406S–411S.

Bean, B.P. (1992) Pharmacology and electrophysiology of ATP-activated ion channels. *Trends Pharmacol. Sci.* **13**, 87–91.

Bean, B.P., Rios, E. (1989) Nonlinear charge movement in mammalian cardiac ventricular cells: components from Na and Ca channel gating. *J. Gen. Physiol.* **94**, 65–93.

Bean, B.P., Williams, C.A., Ceelen, P.W. (1990) ATP-activated channels in rat and bull-frog sensory neurones: current–voltage relation and single-channel behaviour. *J. Neurosci.* **10**, 11–19.

Bekkers, J.M., Stevens, C.F. (1990) Presynaptic mechanism for long-term potentiation in the hippocampus. *Nature* **46**, 724–729.

Belan, P., Kostyuk, P.G., Snitsarev, V., Tepikin, A. (1993a) Calcium clamp in isolated neurones of the snail *Helix pomatia*. *J. Physiol. (Lond.)* **462**, 47–58.

Belan, P.V., Kostyuk, P.G., Snitsarev, V.A., Tepikin, A.V. (1993b) Calcium clamp in single nerve cells. *Cell Calcium* **14**, 419–425.

Benham, C.D., Evans, M.L., McBain, C.J. (1992) Ca^{2+} efflux mechanisms following depolarization evoked calcium transients in cultured rat sensory neurones. *J. Physiol. (Lond.)* **455**, 567–583.

Bennett, M.K., Scheller, R.H. (1993) The molecular machinery for secretion is conserved from yeast to neurons. *Proc. Natl Acad. Sci. USA* **90**, 1559–2563.

Benninger, C., Kadis, J., Prince, D.A. (1980) Extracellular calcium and potassium changes in hippocampal slices. *Brain Res.* **187**, 165–182.

Berger, A.J, Takahashi, T. (1990) Serotonin enhances a low-voltage activated calcium current in rat spinal motoneurones. *J. Neurosci.* **10**, 1922–1928.

Berger, T., Schnitzer, J., Orkand, P.M., Kettenmann, H. (1991) Sodium and calcium currents in glial cells of the mouse corpus callosum slices. *Eur. J. Neurosci.* **4**, 1277–1284.

Berger, T., Walz, W., Schnitzer, J., Kettenmann, H. (1992) GABA- and glutamate-activated currents in glial cells of the mouse corpus callosum slice. *J. Neurosci. Res.* **31**, 21–27.

Bernardi, P., Vassanelli, S., Veronese, P. et al. (1992) Modulation of the mitochondrial permeability transition pore: effect of protons and divalent cations. *J. Biol. Chem.* **267**, 2934–2939.

Berridge, M.J. (1993) Inositol trisphosphate and calcium signalling. *Nature* **361**, 315–325.

Bevan, S. (1990) Ion channels and neurotransmitter receptors in glia. *Semin. Neurosci.* **2**, 467–481.

Bezprozvannaya, S., Bezprozvanny, I., Ehrlich, B.E. (1994) Caffeine induced inhibition of inositol 1,4,5-trisphosphate-gated Ca channels. *Biophys. J.* **66**, A146.

Bezprozvanny, I., Ehrlich, B.E. (1993) ATP modulates the function of inositol 1,4,5-trisphosphate-gated channels at two sites. *Neuron* **10**, 1175–1184.

Bezprozvanny, I., Watras, J., Ehrlich, B.E. (1991) Bell-shaped calcium-response curves of Ins(1,4,5)P₃ and calcium-gated channels from endoplasmic reticulum of cerebellum. *Nature* **351**, 751–754.

Biagi, B.A, Enyeart, J.J. (1991) Multiple calcium currents in a thyroid C-cell line: biophysical properties and pharmacology. *Am. J. Physiol.* **260**, C1253–C1263.

Bindokas, V.P., Brorson, J.R., Miller, R.J. (1993) Characteristics of voltage sensitive calcium channels in dendrites of cultured rat cerebellar neurons. *Neuropharmacology* **32**, 1213–1220.

Birch, B.D., Eng, D.L., Kocsis, J.D. (1992) Intranuclear calcium transients during neurite regeneration of an adult mammalian neuron. *Proc. Natl Acad. Sci. USA* **89**, 7978–7982.

Bird, G.S.J., Burgess, G.M., Putney, J.W. (1993) Sulfhydril reagents and cAMP-dependent kinase increase the sensitivity of the inositol 1,4,5-trisphosphate receptor in hepatocytes. *J. Biol. Chem.* **268**, 17917–17923.

Birnbaumer, L., Campbell, K.P., Catterall, W.A. et al. (1994) The naming of voltage-gated calcium channels. *Neuron* **13**, 505–506.

Bito, H., Nakamura, M., Honda, Z. et al. (1992) Platelet-activating factor (PAF) receptor in rat brain: PAF mobilizes intracellular Ca^{2+} in hippocampal neurones. *Neuron* **9**, 285–294.

Bixby, J.L., Spitzer, N.C. (1994) Early differentiation of vertebrate spinal neurons in the absence of voltage-dependent Ca^{++} and Na^+ influx. *Dev. Biol.* **106**, 89–96.

Blackstone, C.D., Supattapone, S., Snyder, S.H. (1989) Inositol phospholipid-linked glutamate receptors mediate cerebellar parallel-fiber–Purkinje-cell synaptic transmission. *Proc. Natl*

Acad. Sci. USA **86**, 4316–4320.

Blank, W.F., Kirschner, H.S. (1977) The kinetics of extracellular potassium changes during hypoxia and anoxia in the rat cerebral cortex. *Brain Res.* **123**, 113–124.

Blankenfeld, G., Kettenmann, H. (1992) Glutamate and GABA receptors in vertebrate glial cells. *Mol. Neurobiol.* **5**, 31–43.

Blankenfeld, G., Trotter, J., Kettenmann, H. (1991) Expression and developmental regulation of a GABA$_A$ receptor in cultured murine cells of the oligodendrocyte lineage. *Eur. J. Neurosci.* **3**, 310–316.

Blankenfeld, G., Verkhratsky, A., Kettenmann, H. (1992) Ca^{2+} channel expression in the oligodendrocyte lineage. *Eur. J. Neurosci.* **4**, 1035–1048.

Blaustein, M.P., Goldman, W.F., Fontana, G. *et al.* (1991) Physiological role of the sodium–calcium exchanger in nerve and muscle. *Ann. NY Acad. Sci.* **639**, 254–274.

Blaxter, T.J, Carlen, P.L, Nielsen, C. (1989) Pharmacological and anatomical separation of calcium currents in rat dentate granule neurones in vitro. *J. Physiol. (Lond).* **412**, 93–112.

Bleakman, D., Roback, J.D., Wainer, B.H., Miller, R.J., Harrison, N.L. (1993) Calcium homeostasis in rat septal neurones in tissue culture. *Brain Res.* **600**, 257–267.

Blinks, J.R., Olson, C.B., Jewell, B.R., Bravery, P. (1972) Influence of caffeine and other methylxanthines on mechanical properties of isolated mammalian heart muscle. *Circ. Res.* **30**, 367–392.

Bliss, T.V.P., Collingridge, G.L. (1993) A synaptic model of memory: long-term potentiation in the hippocampus. *Nature* **361**, 31–39.

Blondel, O., Takeda, J., Janssen, H., Seino, S., Bell, G.I. (1993) Sequence and functional characterization of a third inositol trisphosphate receptor subtype, IP$_3$R-3 expressed in pancreatic islets, kidney, gastrointestinal tract and other tissues. *J. Biol. Chem.* **268**, 11356–11363.

Boitano, S., Dirksen, E.R., Sanderson, M.J. (1992) Intercellular propagation of calcium waves mediated by inositol trisphosphate. *Science* **258**, 292–295.

Boland, L.M., Bean, B.P. (1993) Modulation of N-type calcium channels in bullfrog sympathetic neurons by luteinizing hormone-releasing hormone: kinetics and voltage dependence. *J. Neurosci.* **13**, 516–533.

Boland, L.M., Motrill, J.A., Bean, B.P. (1994) ω-Conotoxin block of N-type calcium channels in frog and rat sympathetic neurons. *J. Neurosci.* **14**, 5011–5027.

Bolshakov, V.Y., Siegelbaum, S.A. (1994) Postsynaptic induction and presynaptic expression of hippocampal long-term depression. *Science* **264**, 1148–1152.

Bookman, R.J, Liu, Y. (1990) Analysis of calcium channel properties in cultured leech Retzius cells by internal perfusion, voltage-clamp and single-channel recording. *J. Exp. Biol.* **149**, 223–237.

Bootman, M.D. (1994) Quantal Ca^{2+} release from InsP$_3$-sensitive intracellular Ca^{2+} stores. *Mol. Cell. Endocrinol.* **98**, 157–166.

Borges, K., Ohlemeyer, C., Trotter, J., Kettenmann, H. (1994) AMPA/kainate receptor activation in murine oligodendrocyte precursor cells leads to activation of a cation conductance: calcium influx and blockade of delayed rectifying K$^+$ channels. *Neuroscience* **63**, 135–149.

Bormann, J. (1988) Electrophysiology of GABA$_A$ and GABA$_B$ receptor subtypes. *Trends Neurosci.* **11**, 112–116.

Bossu, J.-L., DeWaard, M., Feltz, A. (1991a) Inactivation characteristics reveal two calcium currents in adult bovine chromaffin cells. *J. Physiol. (Lond.)* **437**, 603–620.

Bossu, J.-L., DeWaard, M., Feltz, A. (1991b) Two types of calcium channels are expressed in adult bovine chromaffin cells. *J. Physiol. (Lond.)* **437**, 621–634.

Bouron, A., Reber, B.F.X. (1994) Differential modulation of pharmacologically distinct components of Ca^{2+} currents by protein kinase C activators and phosphatase inhibitors in nerve growth-factor-differentiated rat pheochromocytoma (PC12) cells. *Pflugers Arch.* **427**, 510–516.

Bovolin, P., Santi, M.R., Puia, G., Costa, E., Grayson, D. (1992) Expression patterns of γ-aminobutyric acid type A receptor subunit mRNAs in primary cultures of granule neurones and astrocytes from neonatal rat cerebella. *Proc. Natl Acad. Sci. USA* **89**, 9344–9348.

Bragadin, M., Pozzan, T., Azzone, G.F. (1979) Kinetics of Ca^{2+} carrier in rat liver mitochondria. *Biochemistry* **18**, 5972–5978.

Brake, A.J., Wagenbach, M.J., Julius, D. (1994) New structural motif for ligand-gated ion channels determined by an ionotropic ATP receptor. *Nature* **371**, 519–523.

Brandl, C.J., Green, N.M., Korczak, B., MacLennan, D.H. (1986) Two Ca^{2+} ATPase genes: homologies and mechanistic implications of deducted amino acid sequences. *Cell* **44**, 597–607.

Broadwell, R.D., Cataldo, A.M. (1983) The neuronal endoplasmic reticulum: its cytochemistry and contribution to the endomembrane system. I. Cell bodies and dendrites. *J. Histochem. Cytochem.* **31**, 1077–1088.

Broadwell, R.D., Cataldo, A.M. (1984) The neuronal endoplasmic reticulum: its cytochemistry and contribution to the endomembrane system. II. Axons and terminals. *J. Comp. Neurol.* **230**, 231–248.

Brorson, J.R., Bleakman, D., Gibbons, S.J., Miller, R.J. (1991) The properties of intracellular calcium stores in cultured rat cerebellar neurons. *J. Neurosci.* **11**, 4024–4043.

Brorson, J.R., Manzolillo, P.A., Miller, R.J. (1994) Ca^{2+} entry via AMPA/KA receptors and endotoxicity in cultured cerebellar Purkinje cells. *J. Neurosci.* **14**, 187–197.

Brown, A.M., Sayer, R.J., Schwindt, P.C., Crill, W.E. (1994) P-type calcium channels in rat neocortical neurones. *J. Physiol. (Lond.)* **475**, 197–205.

Bruner, G., Murphy, S. (1993) UTP activates multiple second messenger systems in cultured rat astrocytes. *Neurosci. Lett.* **162**, 105–108.

Brust, P.T., Simerson, S., McCue, A.F. *et al.* (1993) Human neuronal voltage-dependent calcium channels: studies on subunit structure and role in channel assembly. *Neuropharmacology* **32**, 1089–1102.

Burgos, G.R.G., Biali, F.I., Cherskey, B.D. *et al.* (1995) Different calcium channels mediate transmitter release evoked by transient or sustained depolarization at mammalian sympathetic ganglia. *Neuroscience* **64**, 117–123.

Burk, S.E., Lytton, J., MacLennan, D.H., Shull, G.E. (1989) cDNA cloning, functional expressing, and mRNA tissue distribution of a third organellar Ca^{2+} pump. *J. Biol. Chem.* **164**, 18561–18568.

Burnashev, N. (1993a) Recombinant ionotropic glutamate receptors: functional distinctions impaired by different subunits. *Cell Physiol. Biochem.* **3**, 318–331.

Burnashev, N.A. (1993b) Structure and function of ionotropic glutamate receptors. Dr Sci. thesis, Kiev, pp. 1–48.

Burnashev, N., Khodorova, A., Jonas, P. *et al.* (1992) Calcium-permeable AMPA-kainate receptors in fusiform cerebellar glial cells. *Science* **256**, 1566–1570.

Burnashev, N., Zhou, Z., Neher, E., Sakmann, B. (1995) Fractional calcium currents through recombinant GluR channels of the NMDA, AMPA and kainate receptor subtypes. *J. Physiol. (Lond.)* **485**, 403–418.

Burnstock, G. (1972) Purinergic nerves. *Pharmacol. Rev.* **24**, 509–581.

Butt, A.M., Hargittai, P.T., Lieberman, E.M. (1990) Calcium-dependent regulation of potassium permeability in the glial perineurium (blood–brain barrier) of the crayfish. *Neuroscience* **38**, 175–185.

Byerly, L, Hagiwara, S. (1982) Calcium currents in internally perfused nerve cell bodies of *Limnea stagnalis*. *J. Physiol. (Lond).* **322**, 503–528.

Carafoli, E. (1992) Calcium pump of the plasma membrane. *Physiol. Rev.* **71**, 129–153.

Carafoli, E., Crompton, M. (1976) Calcium ion and mitochondria. *Symp. Soc. Exp. Biol.* **30**, 89–115.

Carbone, E., Lux, H.D. (1984) A low voltage-activated, fully inactivating Ca channel in vertebrate sensory neurones. *Nature* **310**, 501–503.

Carbone, E., Lux, H.D. (1987) Single low-voltage-activated calcium channels in chick and rat sensory neurones. *J. Physiol. (Lond.)* **386**, 571–601.

Carbone, E., Lux, H.D. (1988) ω-Conotoxin blockade distinguishes Ca from Na permeable states in neuronal calcium channels. *Pflugers Arch.* **413**, 14–22.

Carman-Krzan, M., Vige, X., Wise, B.C. (1991) Regulation by interleukin-1 of nerve growth factor secretion and nerve growth factor mRNA expression in rat primary astroglial cultures. *J. Neurochem.* **56**, 636–643.

Castellano, A., Wei, X., Birnbaumer, L., Perez-Reyes, E. (1993) Cloning and expression of a neuronal calcium channel β subunit. *J. Biol. Chem.* **268**, 12359–12366.

Castillo, P.E., Weisskopf, M.G., Nicoll, R.A. (1994) The role of Ca^{2+} channels in hippocampal mossy fiber synaptic transmission and long-term potentiation. *Neuron* **12**, 261–169.

Catterall, W.A., Seagar, M.J, Takahashi, M. (1988) Molecular properties of dihydropyridine-sensitive calcium channels in skeletal muscle. *J. Biol. Chem.* **263**, 3533–3538.

Cavalie, A., Ochi, R., Pelzer, D., Trautwein, W. (1983) Elementary currents through Ca channels in guinea-pig myocytes. *Pflugers Arch.* **398**, 284–297.

Cena, V., Brocklehurst, K.W., Pollard, H.B., Rojas, E. (1991) Pertussis toxin stimulation of catecholamine release from adrenal medullary chromaffin cells: mechanism may be by direct activation of L-type and G-type calcium channels. *J. Membrane Biol.* **122**, 23–31.

Chard, P.S., Bleakman, D., Christakos, S., Fullmer, C.S., Miller, R.J. (1993) Calcium buffering properties of calbindin D_{28k} and parvalbumin in rat sensory neurones. *J. Physiol. (Lond.)* **472**, 341–357.

Charles, A.C., Merril, J.E., Dirksen, E.R., Sanderson, M.J. (1991) Intercellular signalling in glial cells: calcium waves and oscillations in response to mechanical stimulation and glutamate. *Neuron* **6**, 983–992.

Charles, A.C., Dirksen, E.R., Merrill, J.E., Sanderson, M.J. (1993) Mechanisms of intercellular calcium signaling in glial cells studied with dantrolene and thapsigargin. *Glia* **7**, 134–145.

Charlton, M.P., Augustine, G.J. (1990) Classification of presynaptic calcium channels at the squid giant synapse: neither T-, L- nor N-type. *Brain Res.* **525**, 133–139.

Cheeck, T.R., Moreton, R.B., Berridge, M.J. *et al.* (1993) Quantal Ca^{2+} release from caffeine-sensitive stores in adrenal chromaffin cells. *J. Biol. Chem.* **268**, 27076–27083.

Chen, C., Hess, P. (1990) Mechanism of gating of T-type calcium channels. *J. Gen. Physiol.* **96**, 603–630.

Chen, C., Schofield, G.G. (1993) Nitric oxide modulates Ca^{2+} channel current in rat sympathetic neurons. *Eur. J. Pharmacol.* **243**, 83–86.

Chen, C., Zhang, J., Vincent, J.-D., Israel, J.-M. (1990) Two types of voltage-dependent calcium currents in rat somatotrophs are reduced by somatostatin. *J. Physiol. (Lond.)* **425**, 29–42.

Chen, S.R.W., Vaughan, D.M., Airey, J.A., Coronado, R., MacLennan, D.H. (1993) Functional expression of cDNA encoding the Ca^{2+} release channel (ryanodine receptor) of rabbit skeletal muscle sarcoplasmic reticulum in COS-1 cells. *Biochemistry* **32**, 3743–3753.

Chen, Z.P., Levy, A., Lightman, S.L. (1994) Activation of specific ATP receptors induces a rapid increase in intracellular calcium ions in rat hypothalamic neurones. *Brain Res.* **641**, 249–256.

Chernevskaya, N.I., Obukhov, A.G., Krishtal, O.A. (1991) NMDA receptor agonists selectively block N-type Ca channels in rat hippocampal neurons. *Biophys. J.* **59**, 83a.

Cherubini, E., Gaiarsa, J.L., Ben-Ari, Y. (1991) GABA: an excitatory transmitter in early postnatal life. *Trends Neurosci.* **14**, 515–519.

Chiu, S.Y., Kriegler, S. (1994) Neurotransmitter-mediated signaling between axons and glial cells. *Glia* **11**, 191–200.

Choi, D.W. (1994).Calcium and excitotoxic neuronal injury. *Ann. NY Acad. Sci.* **747**, 162–171.

Clapper, D.L., Walseth, T.F., Dargie, P.J., Lee, H.C. (1987) Pyridine nucleotide metabolites stimulate calcium release from sea urchin egg microsomes desensitized to inositoltrisphosphate. *J. Biol. Chem.* **262**, 9561–9568.

Clarke, D.M., Loo, T.W., Inesi, G., MacLennan, D.H. (1989a) Location of high affinity Ca^{2+} binding sites within the predicted transmembrane domain of the sarcoplasmic reticulum Ca^{2+}-ATPase. *Nature* **339**, 476–478.

Clarke, D.M., Maruyama, K., Loo, T.W., Leberer, E., Inesi, G., MacLennan, D.H. (1989b) Functional consequences of glutamate, aspartate, glutamine, and asparagine mutations in the stalk sector of the Ca^{2+}-ATPase of sarcoplasmic reticulum. *J. Biol. Chem.* **264**, 11246–11251.

Collingridge, G.L., Lester, R.A.J. (1989) Excitatory amino acid receptors in the vertebrate central nervous system. *Pharmacol. Rev.* **40**, 143–210.

Connor, J.A., Tseng, H.Y., Hockberger, P.E. (1987) Depolarization- and transmitter-induced changes in intracellular Ca^{2+} of rat cerebellar granule cells in explant culture. *J. Neurosci.* **7**, 1384–1400.

Connor, J.A., Pozzo Miller, L.D., Petrozzino, J., Muller, W. (1994) Calcium signaling in dendritic spines of hippocampal neurones. *J. Neurobiol.* **25**, 234–242.

Coppola, T., Waldmann, R., Borsollo, M. *et al.* (1994) Molecular cloning of a murine N-type calcium channel α_1 subunit: evidence for isoforms, brain distribution and chromosomal localization. *FEBS Lett.* **338**, 1–5.

Coraboeuf, E., Otsuka, M. (1956) L'action des solutions hyposodiques sur les potentiels cellulaires de tissu cardiaque de mammiferes. *CR Acad. Sci.* **243**, 441–444.

Cornell-Bell, A.H., Finkbeiner, S.M. (1991) Ca^{2+} waves in astrocytes. *Cell Calcium* **12**, 185–204.

Cornell-Bell, A.H., Finkbeiner, S., Cooper, M.S., Smith, S.J. (1990) Glutamate induces calcium waves in cultured astrocytes: long-range glial signalling. *Science* **247**, 470–473.

Corriveau, R.A., Berg, D.K. (1993) Coexpression of multiple acetylcholine receptor genes in neurons: quantification of transcripts during development. *J. Neurosci.* **13**, 2662–2671.

Corvalan, V., Cole, R., DeVillis, J., Hagiwara, S. (1990) Neuronal modulation of calcium channel activity in cultured rat astrocytes. *Proc. Natl Acad. Sci. USA* **87**, 4345–4348.

Cotman, C.W., Whittemore, E.R., Watt, J.A., Anderson, A.J., Loo, D.T. (1994). Possible role of apoptosis in Alzheimer's disease. *Ann. NY Acad. Sci.* **747**, 36–49.

Coulter, D.A., Huguenard, J.R., Prince, D.A. (1989) Calcium currents in rat thalamocortical relay neurones: kinetic properties of the transient, low-threshold current. *J. Physiol. (Lond.)* **414**, 587–604.

Coulter, D.A., Huguenard, J.R., Prince, D.A. (1990) Differential effects of petit mal anticonvulsants and convulsants on thalamic neurones: calcium current reduction. *Br. J. Pharmacol.* **100**, 800–806.

Currie, K.P.M., Swann, K., Galione, A., Scott, R.H. (1993) Activation of Ca^{2+}-dependent currents in cultured rat dorsal root ganglion neurones by a sperm factor and cyclic ADP-ribose. *Mol. Biol. Cell.* **3**, 1415–1425.

Daly, J.W. (1993) Mechanisms of action of caffeine. In: *Caffeine, Coffee, and Health*, ed. by Garattini, S. Raven Press, New York, pp. 97–150.

Dani, J.W., Chernjavsky, A., Smith, S.J. (1992) Neuronal activity triggers calcium waves in hippocampal astrocyte networks. *Neuron* **8**, 429–440.

Danko, S., Kim, D.H., Sreter, F.A., Ikemoto, N. (1985) Inhibitors of Ca^{2+} release from the isolated sarcoplasmic reticulum. II. The effects of dantrolene on Ca^{2+} release induced by caffeine, Ca^{2+} and depolarization. *Biochem. Biophys. Acta* **816**, 18–24.

Danoff, S.K., Supattapone, S., Snyder, S.H. (1988) Characterization of a membrane protein from brain mediating the inhibition of inositol 1,4,5-trisphosphate receptor binding by calcium. *Biochem. J.* **254**, 701–705.

Dave, V., Gordin, G.W., McCarthy, K.D. (1991) Cerebral type-2 astroglia are heterogeneous with respect to their ability to respond to neuroligands linked to calcium mobilization. *Glia* **4**, 440–447.

Davies, N.W., Lux, H.D. (1989) The effect of noradrenaline on Ca channels of cultured chick dorsal root ganglion neurones requires external divalent cations. *J. Physiol. (Lond.)* **410**, 87P.

Davies, N.W., Lux, H.D., Morad, M. (1988) Site and mechanism of inactivation of proton-induced sodium current in chick dorsal root ganglion neurones. *J. Physiol. (Lond.)* **400**, 159–187.

De Jongh, K.S., Colvin, A.A., Wang, K.K., Catterall, W.A. (1994) Differential proteolysis of the full-length form of the L-type calcium channel alpha 1 subunit by calpain. *J. Neurochem.* **63**, 1558–1564

De Waard, M., Pragnell, M., Campbell, K.P. (1994a) Ca^{2+} channel regulation by a conserved β-subunit domain. *Neuron* **13**, 495–503.

De Waard, M., Witcher, D.R., Campbell, K.P. (1994b) Functional properties of the purified N-type Ca++ channel form rabbit brain. *J. Biol. Chem.* **269**, 6716–6724.

De Weille, J.R., Scweeitz, H., Maes, P., Tartar, A., Lazdunski, M. (1991) Calciseptine, a peptide isolated from black mamba venom, is a specific blocker of the L-type calcium channel. *Proc. Natl Acad. Sci. USA* **88**, 2437–2440.

Debanne, D., Thompson, S.M. (1994) Calcium: a trigger for long-term depression and potentiation in the hippocampus. *News Physiol. Sci.* **9**, 256–260.

Decker, E.R., Dani, J.A. (1990) Calcium permeability of the nicotinic receptor: the single-channel calcium influx is significant. *J. Neurosci.* **10**, 3413–3420.

Delaney, K.R., Zucker, R.S., Tank, D.W. (1989) Calcium in motor nerve terminals associated with posttetanic potentiation. *J. Neurosci.* **9**, 2558–3567.

Delumeau, J.C., Petitet, F., Cordier, J., Glowinski, J., Premont, J. (1991a) Synergistic regulation of cytosolic Ca^{2+} concentration in mouse astrocytes by NK1 tachykinin and adenosine agonists.

J. Neurochem. **57**, 2026–2035.

Delumeau, J.C., Tence, M., Marin, P., Cordier, J., Glowinski, J., Premont, J. (1991b) Synergistic regulation of cytosolic Ca^{2+} concentration by adenosine and α1-adrenergic agonists in mouse striatum astrocytes. *Eur. J. Neurosci.* **3**, 539–550.

Desole, M.S., Kim, W.-K., Rabin, R.A., Laychock, S.G. (1994) Nitric oxide reduces depolarization-induced calcium influx in PC12 cells by a cyclic GMP-mediated mechanism. *Neuropharmacology* **33**, 193–198.

Disterhoft, J.F., Moyer, J.R. Jr, Thompson, L.T. (1994) The calcium rationale in aging and Alzheimer's disease: evidence from an animal model of normal aging. *Ann. NY Acad. Sci.* **747**, 382–406.

Dolphin, A.C. (1990) Ca channel currents in rat sensory neurones: interaction between guanine nucleotides, cyclic AMP and Ca channel ligands. *J Physiol. (Lond.)* **432**, 23–43.

Dolphin, A.C., McGuirk, S., Scott, R.H. (1987) Barium-activated tail currents in cultured rat dorsal root ganglion neurones are modified by GTP-γ-S and BAY K 8644. *J. Physiol. (Lond.)* **390**, 87P.

Doroshenko, P. (1991) Second messengers mediating activation of chloride current by intracellular GTP-γ-S in bovine chromaffin cells. *J. Physiol. (Lond.)* **436**, 725–738.

Doroshenko, P., Penner, R., Neher, E. (1991) Novel chloride conductance in the membrane of bovine chromaffin cells activated by intracellular GTP-γ-S. *J. Physiol. (Lond.)* **436**, 711–724.

Dossi, R.C, Nunez, A., Steriade, M. (1992) Electrophysiology of a slow (0.5–4 Hz) intrinsic oscillation of cat thalamocortical neurones in vitro. *J. Physiol. (Lond.)* **447**, 215–234.

Droogmans, G, Nilius, B. (1989) Kinetic properties of the cardiac T-type calcium channel in the guinea-pig. *J. Physiol. (Lond).* **419**, 627–650.

Dryer, S.E., Dourado, M.M., Wisgirda, M. (1991) Properties of Ca currents in acutely dissociated neurons of the chick ciliary ganglion: inhibition by somatostatin-14 and somatostatin-28. *Neuroscience* **44**, 663–672.

Dubel, S.J., Starr, T.V.B., Hell, J. *et al.* (1992) Molecular cloning of the α 1 subunit of an ω-conotoxin-sensitive calcium channel. *Proc. Natl Acad. Sci. USA* **89**, 5058–5062.

Dubyak, G.R., El-Moatassim, C. (1993) Signal transduction via P_2-purinergic receptors for extracellular ATP and other nucleotides. *Am. J Physiol.* **265**, C577–C606.

Duchen, M.R., Valdeomillos, M., O'Neill, S.C., Eisner, D.A. (1990) Effect of metabolic blockade on the regulation of intracellular calcium in dissociated mouse primary sensory neurones. *J. Physiol. (Lond.)* **424**, 411–426.

Duffy, S., MacVicar, B.A. (1994) Potassium-dependent calcium influx in acutely isolated hippocampal astrocytes. *Neuroscience* **61**, 51–61.

Durroux, T., Gallo-Payet, N., Payet, M.D. (1991) Effects of adrenocorticotropin action potential and calcium currents in cultured rat and bovine glomerulosa cells. *Endocrinology* **129**, 2139–2147.

Dyer, C.A., Benjamins, J.A. (1990) Glycolipids and transmembrane signaling: antibodies to galactocerebroside cause an influx of calcium in oligodendrocytes. *J. Cell Biol.* **111**, 625–633.

Dzhura, I.A., Kostyuk, P.G., Lyubanova, O., Naidyonov, V., Shuba, Ya. (1994) Expression of low-voltage activated Ca^{2+} channels from rat brain neurones in *Xenopus* oocytes. *NeuroReport* **5**, 283–286.

Edwards, F.A. (1994) ATP receptors. *Curr. Opinion Neurobiol.* **4**, 347–352.

Edwards, F.A., Gibb, A.J. (1993) ATP – A fast neurotransmitter. *FEBS Lett.* **325**, 86–89.

Ehrlich, B.E., Watras, J. (1988) Inositol 1,4,5-trisphosphate activates a channel from smooth muscle sarcoplasmic reticulum. *Nature* **336**, 583–586.

Ehrlich, B.E., Kaftan, E., Bezprozvannaya, S., Bezprozvanny, I. (1994) The pharmacology of intracellular Ca^{2+}-release channels. *Trends Pharmacol. Sci.* **15**, 145–149.

El-Hayek, R., Valdivia, C., Valdivia, H.H., Coronado, R. (1993) Activation of the Ca^{2+} release channel of skeletal muscle sarcoplasmic reticulum by palmitoyl carnitine. *Biophys. J.* **65**, 779–789.

Elmslie, K.S., Kammermeier, P.J., Jones, S.W. (1994) Reevaluation of Ca^{2+} channel types and their modulation in bullfrog sympathetic neurons. *Neuron* **13**, 217–228.

Engel, J., Althaus, H.H., Kristjansson, G.I. (1994) NGF increases $[Ca^{2+}]_i$ in regenerating mature oligodendroglial cells. *NeuroReport* **5**, 397–400.

Enkvist, M.O.K., Holopainen, I., Akerman, K.E. (1989a) α-Receptor and cholinergic receptor-linked changes in cytosolic Ca^{2+} and membrane potential in primary rat astrocytes. *Brain Res.* **500**, 46–54.

Enkvist, M.O.K., Holopainen, I., Akerman, K.E.O. (1989b) Glutamate-receptor-linked changes in membrane potential and intracellular Ca^{2+} in primary rat astrocytes. *Glia* **2**, 397–402.

Enkvist, M.O.K., McCarthy, K.D. (1992) Activation of protein kinase C blocks astroglial gap junction communication and inhibits the spread of calcium waves. *J. Neurochem.* **59**, 519–526.

Enyeart, J.J., Mlinar, B., Enyeart, J.A. (1993) T-type Ca^{2+} channels are required for adrenocorticotropin-stimulated cortisol production by bovine adrenal zona fasciculata cells. *Mol. Endocrinol.* **7**, 1031–1040.

Ewald, D., Eckert, R. (1983) Cyclic AMP enhances calcium-dependent potassium current in *Aplysia* neurons. *Cell. Mol. Neurobiol.* **3**, 345–354.

Ewald, D.A., Walker, M.W., Perney, T.M., Matthies, H.J.G., Miller, R.J. (1988) Neurotransmitter modulation of calcium currents in rat sensory neurons. In: *Calcium and Ion Channel Modulation*, ed. by Grinell, A.D., Armstrong, D., Jackson, M.B. Plenum Press, New York, pp. 263–273.

Fasolato C., Innocenti B., Pozzan T. (1994) Receptor-activated Ca^{2+} influx: how many mechanisms for how many channels? *Trends Neurosci.* **15**, 77–83.

Fatatis, A., Russel, J.T. (1992) Spontaneous changes in intracellular calcium concentration in type I astrocytes from rat cerebral cortex in primary cultures. *Glia* **5**, 95–104.

Fatt, P., Katz, B. (1953) The electrical properties of crustacean muscle fibres. *J. Physiol. (Lond.)* **120**, 431–446.

Fedulova, S.A., Kostyuk, P.G., Veselovsky, N.S. (1985) Two types of calcium channels in the somatic membrane of newborn rat dorsal root ganglion neurones. *J. Physiol. (Lond.)* **359**, 431–446.

Fedulova, S.A, Kostyuk, P.G., Veselovsky, N.S. (1986) Changes in ionic mechanisms of electrical excitability of the somatic membrane of rat dorsal root ganglion neurons during ontogenesis. Correlation between inward current densities. *Neurophysiology (Kiev)* **18**, 820–827.

Fedulova, S.A., Kostyuk, P.G., Veselovsky, N.S. (1994) Comparative analysis of ionic currents in the somatic membrane of sensory neurons from embryonic and newborn rats. *Neuroscience* **58**, 341–346.

Feiber, L.A., Adams, D.J. (1991) Acetylcholine-evoked currents in cultured neurones dissociated from the rat parasympathetic cardiac ganglia. *J. Physiol. (Lond.)* **434**, 215–238.

Ferris, C.D., Snyder, S.H. (1992) Inositol phosphate receptors and calcium disposition in the brain. *J. Neurosci.* **12**, 1567–1574.

Fesenko, E.E., Kolesnikov, S.S., Lyubarsky, A.L. (1985) Induction by cyclic GMP of cationic conductance in plasma membrane of retinal rod outer segment. *Nature* **313**, 310–313.

Fill, M., Coronado, R. (1988) Ryanodine receptor channel of sarcoplasmic reticulum. *Trends Neurosci.* **11**, 453–457.

Filloux, F., Karras, J. Impericl, J.S., Gray, W.R., Olivera, B.M. (1994) The distribution of omega-conotoxin MVIICnle-binding sites in rat brain measured by autoradiography. *Neurosci. Lett.* **178**, 263–266.

Finkbeiner, S.M. (1992) Calcium waves in astrocytes: filling in the gaps. *Neuron* **8**, 1101–1108.

Finkbeiner, S.M. (1993) Glial calcium. *Glia* **9**, 83–104.

Fisher, R., Johnson, D. (1990) Differential modulation of single voltage-gated calcium channels by cholinergic and adrenergic agonists in adult hippocampal neurons. *J. Neurophysiol.* **64**, 1291–1302.

Fisher, R.E., Gray, R., Johnston, D. (1990) Properties and distribution of single voltage-gated calcium channels in adult hippocampal neurons. *J. Neurophysiol.* **64**, 91–104.

Flott, B., Seifert, W. (1991) Characterization of glutamate uptake systems in astrocyte primary cultures from rat brain. *Glia* **4**, 293–304.

Fogelson, A.L., Zucker, R.S. (1985) Presynaptic calcium diffusion from various arrays of single channels: implications for transmitter release and synaptic facilitation. *Biophys. J.* **48**, 1003–1017.

Fomina, A.F., Kostyuk, P.G., Sedova, M.B. (1993) Glucocorticoids modulation of calcium currents in growth hormone 3 cells. *Neuroscience*, **55**, 721–725.

Formenti, A., Arrigoni, E., Mancia, M. (1992) Effects of nimodipine on LVA calcium channels in adult rat sensory neurons. In: *Abstracts of the 15th Annual Meeting of the European Neuroscience Association (Munich 1992)* Oxford University Press, Oxford, p. 60.

Formenti, A., Arrigoni, E., Mancia, M. (1993) Low-voltage activated calcium channels are differently affected by nimodipine. *NeuroReport* **5**, 145–147.

Forti, L., Tottene, A., Moretti, A., Pietrobon, D. (1994) Three novel types of voltage-dependent calcium channels in rat cerebellar neurons. *J. Neurosci.* **14**, 5243–5256.

Fossier, P., Baux, G., Tauc, L. (1994) N- and P-type Ca^{2+} channels are involved in acetylcholine release at a neuroneuronal synapse: only the N-type channel is the target of neuromodulators. *Proc. Natl Acad. Sci. USA* **91**, 4771–4775.

Fournier, F., Bourinet, E., Nargeot, J., Charnet, P. (1993) Cyclic AMP-dependent regulation of P-type calcium channels expressed in *Xenopus* oocytes. *Pflugers Arch.* **423**, 173–180.

Fox, A.P., Nowycky, M.C., Tsien, R.W. (1987) Kinetic and pharmacological properties distinguishing three types of calcium currents in chick sensory neurones. *J. Physiol. (Lond.)* **394**, 149–172.

Franklin, J.L., Johnson, E.M. (1992) Suppression of programmed neuronal death by sustained elevation of cytosolic calcium. *Trends Neurosci.* **12**, 501–507.

Fraser, D.D., MacVicar, B.A. (1991) Low-threshold transient calcium current in rat hippocampal lacunosum-moleculare interneurons: kinetics and modulation by neurotrasmitters. *J. Neurosci.* **11**, 2812–2820.

Fraser, D.D., Mudrick-Donnon, L.A., MacVicar, B.A. (1994) Astrocytic GABA receptors. *Glia* **11**, 83–93.

Fredholm, B.B., Abbracchio, M.P., Burnstock, G. *et al.* (1994) Nomenclature and classification of purinoreceptors. *Pharmacol. Rev.* **46**, 143–156.

Frenguelli, B.G., Potier, B., Slater, N.T., Alford, S., Collingridge, G.L. (1993) Metabotropic glutamate receptors and calcium signalling in dendrites of hippocampal CA1 neurones. *Neuropharmacology* **32**, 1229–1237.

Friel, D.D., Tsien, R.W. (1992a) A caffeine- and ryanodine-sensitive Ca^{2+} store in bullfrog sympathetic neurones modulates effects of Ca^{2+} entry on $[Ca^{2+}]_{in}$. *J. Physiol. (Lond.)* **450**, 217–246.

Friel, D.D., Tsien, R.W. (1992b) Phase-dependent contributions from Ca^{2+} entry and Ca^{2+} release to caffeine-induced $[Ca^{2+}]_i$ oscillations in bullfrog neurons. *Neuron* **8**, 1109–1125.

Friel, D.D., Tsien, R.W. (1994) An FCCP-sensitive Ca^{2+} store in bullfrog sympathetic neurones and its participation in stimulus evoked changes in $[Ca^{2+}]_i$. *J. Neurosci.* **14**, 4007–4024.

Fryer, M.W., Zucker, R.S. (1993) Ca^{2+}-dependent inactivation of Ca^{2+} current in *Aplysia* neurons: kinetic studies using photolabile Ca^{2+} chelators. *J. Physiol. (Lond.)* **464**, 501–528.

Fu, W.-M., Huang, F.-L. (1994) L-type Ca^{2+} channel is involved in the regulation of spontaneous transmitter release at developing neuromuscular synapses. *Neuroscience,* **58**, 131–140.

Fujita, Y., Mynliff, M., Dirksen, R.T. *et al.* (1993) Primary structure and functional expression of the ω-conotoxin-sensitive N-type calcium channel from rabbit brain. *Neuron* **10**, 586–598.

Fukui, H., Inagaki, N., Ito, S. *et al.* (1991) Histamine H_1-receptors on astrocytes in primary cultures: a possible target for histaminergic neurones. *Agents Action Suppl.* **33**, 161–180.

Furuichi, T., Furutama, D., Hakamata, Y., Nakai, J., Takeshima, H., Mikoshiba, K. (1994a) Multiple types of ryanodine receptor/Ca^{2+} release channels are differentially expressed in rabbit brain. *J. Neurosci.* **14**, 4794–4805.

Furuichi, T., Kohda, K., Miyawaki, A., Mikoshiba, K. (1994b) Intracellular channels. *Curr. Opinion Neurobiol.* **4**, 294–303.

Furuya, S., Ohmori, H., Shigemoto, T., Sugiyama, H. (1989) Intracellular calcium mobilization triggered by a glutamate receptor in rat cultured hippocampal cells. *J. Physiol. (Lond.)* **414**, 539–548.

Gabellini, N., Facci, L., Milani, D. *et al.* (1991) Differences in induction of c-fos transcription by cholera toxin-derived cyclic AMP and Ca^{2+} signals in astrocytes and 3T3 fibroblasts. *Exp Cell Res.* **194**, 210–217.

Galione, A. (1993) Cyclic ADP-ribose: a new way to control calcium. *Science* **259**, 325–326.

Galione, A. (1994) Cyclic ADP-ribose, the ADP-ribosyl cyclase pathway and calcium signalling. *Mol. Cell. Endocrinol.* **98**, 125–131.

Galione, A., Lee, H.C., Busa, W.B. (1991) Ca^{2+}-induced Ca^{2+} release in sea urchin egg homogenates: modulation by cyclic ADP ribose. *Science* **253**, 1143–1146.

Galione, A., White, A., Willmott, N., Turner, M., Potter, B.V., Watson, S.P. (1993) cGMP mobilizes intracellular calcium in sea urchin eggs by stimulating cyclic ADP-ribose synthesis. *Nature* **365**, 456–459.

Galli, A., DeFelice, L.J. (1994) Inactivation of L-type Ca channels in embryonic chick ventricle cells: dependence on cytoskeletal agents colchicine and taxol. *Biophys. J.* **67**, 2296–2304.

Gallo, V., Patneau, D.K., Mayer, M.L., Vaccarino, F.M. (1994) Excitatory amino acid receptors in glial progenitor cells: molecular and functional properties. *Glia* **11**, 94–101.

Gandhi, C.R., Ross, D.H. (1987) Inositol 1,4,5-trisphosphate induced mobilization of Ca^{2+} from rat brain synaptosomes. *Neurochem. Res.* **12**, 67–72.

Ganitkevitch, V.Y., Isenberg, G. (1992) Caffeine-induced release and reuptake of Ca^{2+} by Ca^{2+} stores in myocytes from guinea-pig urinary bladder. *J. Physiol. (Lond.)* **458**, 99–117.

Garyantes, T.K, Regehr, W.G. (1992) Electrical activity increases growth cone calcium but fails to inhibit neurite outgrowth from rat sympathetic neurons. *J. Neurosci.* **12**, 96–103.

Gerasimenko, O.V., Kostyuk, P.G., Lyubanova, O.P., Dzhura, I.A. (1995) Differential expression of calcium channels from rat cerebellum and the forebrain mRNAs in *Xenopus* oocytes. *Neurophysiology (Kiev)* **27**, No. 1.

Gerschenfeld, H.M., Paupardin-Tritsch. D., Yakel, J.L. (1991) Muscarinic enhancement of the voltage-dependent calcium current in an identified snail neuron. *J. Physiol. (Lond.)* **434**, 85–105.

Gerzon, K., Humerickhouse, R.A., Besch, H.K. *et al.* (1993) Amino- and guanidinoacylryanodines: basic ryanodine esters with enhanced affinity for the sarcoplasmic reticulum Ca^{2+}-release channel. *J. Med. Chem.* **36**, 1319–1323.

Giannini, G., Clementi, E., Ceci, R., Marziali, G., Sorrentino, V. (1992) Expression of ryanodine receptor-Ca^{2+} channel that is regulated by TGF-β. *Science* **257**, 91–94.

Gibson, G.E., Peterson. C (1987) Calcium and the ageing nervous system. *Neurobiol. Ageing* **8**, 329–343.

Gimpl, G., Walz, W., Ohlemeyer, C., Kettenmann, H. (1992) Bradykinin receptors in cultured astrocytes from neonatal rat brain are linked to physiological responses. *Neurosci. Lett.* **144**, 139–142.

Gimpl, G., Kirchhoff, F., Lang, R.E., Kettenmann, H. (1993) Identification of neuropeptide Y receptors in cultured astrocytes from neonatal rat brain. *J. Neurosci. Res.* **34**, 198–205.

Glaum, S.R., Scholz, W.K., Miller, R.J. (1990) Acute- and long-term glutamate-mediated regulation of $[Ca^{++}]_i$ in rat hippocampal pyramidal neurones *in vitro*. *J. Pharmacol. Exp. Ther.* **253**, 1293–1302.

Glossmann, H., Striessnig, J. (1988) Calcium channels. *Vitam. Horm.* **44**, 155–328.

Glowinski, J., Marin, P., Tence, M. *et al.* (1994) Glial receptors and their intervention in astrocyto-astrocytic and astrocyto-neuronal interactions. *Glia* **11**, 201–208.

Goldman, R.S., Finkbeiner, S.M., Smith, S.J. (1991) Endothelin induces a sustained rise in intracellular calcium in hippocampal astrocytes. *Neurosci. Lett.* **123**:4–8.

Goldman, W.F., Yarowsky, P.J., Juhaszova, M., Krueger, B.K., Blaustein, M.P. (1994) Sodium/calcium exchange in rat cortical astrocytes. *J. Neurosci.* **14**, 5834–5843.

Gorman, A.L.F., Hermann, A. (1979) Internal effects of divalent cations on potassium permeability in molluscan neurones. *J. Physiol. (Lond.)* **296**, 393–410.

Gorman, A.L.F., Thomas, M.V. (1980) Intracellular calcium accumulation during depolarization in mollusc neurone. *J. Physiol. (Lond.)* **308**, 259–285.

Gorman, A.L.F., Hermann, A., Thomas, M.V. (1981) Intracellular calcium and the control of neuronal pacemaker activity. *Fed. Proc.* **40**, 2233–2239.

Gottmann, K., Rohrer, H., Lux, H.D. (1991) Distribution of Ca and Na conductance during neuronal differentiation of chick DRG precursor cells. *J. Neurosci.* **11**, 3371–3378.

Grantham, C.J., Bowman, D., Bath, C.P., Bell, D.C., Bleakman, D. (1994) ω-Conotoxin MVIIC reversibly inhibits a human N-type calcium channel and calcium influx into chick synaptosomes. *Neuropharmacology* **33**, 255–258.

Greengard, P. (1978) *Cyclic Nucleotides, Phosphorylated Proteins, and Neuronal Function*. Raven Press, New York.

Gross, R.A., Uhler, M.D., Macdonald, R.L. (1990a) The reduction of neuronal calcium currents by ATP-γ-S is mediated by a G protein and occurs independently of cyclic AMP-dependent protein kinase. *Brain Res.* **535**, 214–220.

Gross, R.A., Uhler, M.D., Macdonald, R.L. (1990b) The cyclic AMP-dependent protein kinase catalytic subunit selectively enhances calcium currents in rats nodose neurons. *J. Physiol. (Lond.)* **429**, 483–496.

Gruner, W., Silva, L.R. (1994) ω-Conotoxin sensitivity and presynaptic inhibition of glutamatergic sensory neurotransmission in vitro. *J. Neurosci.* **14**, 2800–2808.

Grynkiewicz, G., Poenie, M., Tsien, R.Y. (1985) A new generation of Ca^{2+} indicators with greatly improved fluorescent properties. *J. Biol. Chem.* **260**, 3440–3450.

Guthrie, P.B., Segal, M., Kater, S.B. (1991) Independent regulation of calcium revealed by imaging dendritic spines. *Nature* **354**, 76–80.

Hadley, R.W., Lederer, W.J. (1991) Ca and voltage inactivate Ca channels in guinea-pig ventricular myocytes through independent mechanisms. *J. Physiol. (Lond.)* **444**, 257–268.

Hagiwara, S., Naka, K.I. (1964) The initiation of spike potential in barnacle muscle fibres under low intracellular Ca^{++}. *J. Gen. Physiol.* **48**, 141–162.

Hagiwara, S., Nakajima, S. (1966) Effects of intracellular Ca ion concentration upon the excitability of the muscle fiber membrane of a barnacle. *J. Gen. Physiol.* **49**, 807–818.

Hakamata, Y., Nakai, J., Takeshima, H., Imoto, K. (1992) Primary structure and distribution of a novel ryanodine receptor/calcium release channel from rabbit brain. *FEBS Lett.* **312**, 229–235.

Hamill, O.P., Marty, A., Neher, E., Sakmann, B., Sigworth, F.J. (1981) Improved patch clamp techniques for high-resolution current recording from cell and cell-free membrane patches. *Pflugers Arch.*, **391**, 85–100.

Hamlyn, J.M., Blaistein, M.P., Bova, S. *et al.* (1991) Identification and characterization of a ouabain-like compound from human plasma. *Proc. Natl Acad. Sci. USA* **81**, 6259–6263.

Han, S., Schiefer, A., Isenberg, G. (1994) Ca^{2+} load of guinea-pig ventricular myocytes determines efficacy of brief Ca^{2+} currents as trigger for Ca^{2+} release. *J. Physiol. (Lond.)* **480**, 411–421.

Harper, A.A., Lawson, S.N. (1985) Conduction velocity is related to morphological cell type in rat dorsal root ganglion neurones. *J. Physiol (Lond.)* **359**, 31–46.

Hart, I.K., Ricgardson, W.D., Bolsover, S.R., Raff, M.C. (1989) PDGF and intracellular signalling in the timing of oligodendrocyte differentiation. *J. Cell Biol.* **109**, 3411–3417.

Hartzell, H.C., Fischmeister, R. (1992) Direct regulation of cardiac Ca^{2+} channels by G proteins: neither proven nor necessary? *Trends Pharmacol. Sci.* **13**, 380–385.

Hatton, G.I., Bicknell, R.J., Hoyland, J., Buntig, R., Mason, W.T. (1992) Arginine vasopressin mobilizes intracellular calcium via V_1-receptor activation in astrocytes (pituicytes) cultured from adult rat neural lobes. *Brain Res.* **588**, 367–370.

Hayakawa, N., Morita, T., Yamaguchi, T. *et al.* (1990) The high affinity receptor for ω-conotoxin represents calcium channels different from those sensitive to dihydropyridines in mammalian brain. *Biochem. Biophys. Res. Commun.* **173**, 483–490.

Haydon, P.G., Man-Son-Hing, H. (1989) Low- and high-voltage-activated calcium currents: their relationship to the site of neurotransmitter release in an identified neuron of *Helisoma*. *Neuron* **1**, 919–927.

Haymes A., Kwan Y.W., Arena J.P., Kass R.S., Hinkle P.M. (1992) Activation of protein kinase C reduces L-type calcium channel activity of GH_3 pituitary cells. *Am. J. Physiol.* **262**, C1211–C1219.

Haynes, L.W., Yau, K.-W., (1985) Cyclic GMP-sensitive conductance in outer segment membrane of catfish cones. *Nature* **317**, 61–64.

Heizmann, C.W., Hunziker, W. (1991) Intracellular calcium-binding proteins: more sights than insights. *Trends Biochem. Sci.* **16**, 98–103.

Hell, J.W., Westenbrock, R.E., Warner, C. *et al.* (1993) Identification and differential subcellular localization of the neuronal class C and class D L-type calcium channel alpha-1 subunit. *J. Cell Biol.* **123**, 949–962.

Henzi, V., MacDermott, A.B. (1992) Characteristics and function of Ca^{2+} and inositol 1,4,5-trisphosphate-releasable stores of Ca^{2+} in neurones. *Neuroscience* **46**, 251–274.

Hermann, A., Hartung, K. (1983) Ca^{2+}-activated K^+ conductance in molluscan neurones. *Cell Calcium* **4**, 387–405.

Hernandez-Cruz, A., Sala, F., Adams, P.R. (1990) Subcellular calcium transients visualized by confocal microscopy in a voltage-clamped vertebrate neuron. *Science* **247**, 858–862.

Hernandez-Cruz, A., Sala, F., Connor, J.A. (1991) Stimulus-induced nuclear calcium signals in fura-2 loaded amphibian neurones. *Ann. NY Acad. Sci.* **635**, 416–420.

Herrman-Frank, A., Darling, E., Meissner, G. (1991) Functional characterization of the Ca²⁺-gated Ca²⁺ release channel of vascular smooth muscle sarcoplasmic reticulum. *Pflugers Arch.* **418**, 353–359.

Hescheler, J., Miekes, G., Ruegg, J.C., Takai, A., Trautwein, W. (1988) Effects of a protein phosphatase inhibitor okadaic acid on membrane currents of isolated guinea-pig cardiac myocytes. *Pflugers Arch.* **412**, 248–252.

Hill, D.T., Berggren, P.O., Boynton, A.L. (1987) Heparin inhibits inositol trisphosphate induced calcium release in permeabilized rat liver cells. *Biochim. Biophys. Acta* **149**, 879–901.

Hillman, D., Chen, S., Aung, T.T. *et al.* (1991) Localization of P-type calcium channels in the central nervous system. *Proc. Natl Acad. Sci. USA* **88**, 7076–7080.

Hoehn, K., Watson, T.W.J., MacVicar, B.A. (1993) Multiple types of calcium channels in acutely isolated rat neostriatal neurons. *J. Neurosci.* **13**, 1244–1257.

Hofmann, F., Flockerzi, V., Nastainczyk, W. *et al.*, (1990) The molecular structure and regulation of muscular calcium channels. *Curr. Top. Cell. Regul.* **31**, 223–239.

Hofmann, F., Biel, M., Flockerzi, V. (1994a) Molecular basis for Ca²⁺ channel diversity in brain measured by autoradiography. *Neurosci. Lett.* **178**, 263–266.

Hofmann, F., Biel, M. Flockerzi, V. (1994b) Molecular basis for Ca²⁺ channel diversity. *Annu. Rev. Neurosci.* **17**, 399–418.

Holliday, J., Spitzer, N.C. (1990) Spontaneous calcium influx and its roles in differentiation of spinal neurons in culture. *Dev. Biol.* **141**, 13–23.

Holliday, J., Adams, R.J., Sejnowski, T.J., Spitzer, N.C. (1991) Calcium-induced release of calcium regulates differentiation of cultured spinal neurons. *Neuron* **7**, 787–796.

Hollman, M., Heinemann, S. (1994) Cloned glutamate receptors. *Annu. Rev. Neurosci.* **17**, 31–108.

Hollman, M.E. (1958) Membrane potentials recorded with high-resistance microelectrodes and the effects of changes in ionic environment on the electrical and mechanical activity of the smooth muscle of the taenia coli of the guinea-pig. *J. Physiol. (Lond.)* **141**, 464–488.

Holopainen, I., Enkvist, M.O.K., Akerman, K.E.O. (1989) Glutamate receptor agonists increase intracellular Ca²⁺ independently of voltage-gated Ca²⁺ channels in rat cerebellar granule cells. *Neurosci. Lett.* **98**, 57–62.

Holopainen, I., Enkvist, M.O.K., Akerman, K.E.O. (1990) Coupling of glutamatergic receptors to changes of intracellular Ca²⁺ in rat cerebellar granule cells in primary culture. *J. Neurosci. Res.* **25**, 187–193.

Holzwarth, J.A., Gibbons, S.J., Brorson, J.R., Philipson, L.H., Miller, R.J. (1994) Glutamate receptor agonists stimulate diverse calcium responses in different types of cultured rat cortical glial cells. *J. Neurosci.* **14**, 1879–1891.

Hosli, E., Hosli, L. (1993) Receptors for neurotransmitters on astrocytes in the mammalian central nervous system. *Prog. Neurobiol.* **40**, 477–506.

Hoth, M., Penner, R. (1992) Depletion of intracellular calcium stores activates a calcium current in mast cells. *Nature* **355**, 353–356.

Hoth, M., Penner, R. (1993) Calcium release-activated calcium current in rat mast cells. *J. Physiol. (Lond.)* **465**, 359–386.

Hua, S.Y., Nohmi, M., Kuba, K. (1993) Characteristics of Ca²⁺ release induced by Ca²⁺ influx in cultured bullfrog sympathetic neurones. *J. Physiol. (Lond.)* **464**, 245–272.

Hua, S.Y., Tokimas, T., Takasawa, S. *et al.* (1994) Cyclic ADP-ribose modulates Ca²⁺ release channels for activation by physiological Ca²⁺ entry in bullfrog sympathetic neurones. *Neuron* **12**, 1073–1079.

Huettner, J.E. (1991) Competitive antagonism of glycine at the N-methyl-d-aspartate (NMDA) receptor. *Biochem. Pharmacol.* **41**, 9–16.

Huguenard, J.R, Prince, D.A. (1992) A novel T-type current underlies prolonged Ca²⁺-dependent burst firing in GABAergic neurons of rat thalamic reticular nucleus. *J. Neurosci.* **12**, 3804–3817.

Hui, A., Ellinor, P.T., Krizanova, O. *et al.* (1991) Molecular cloning of multiple subtypes of a novel rat brain isoform of the α₁ subunit of the voltage-dependent calcium channel. *Neuron* **7**, 35–44.

Hullin, R., Singer-Lahat, D., Freichel, M. *et al.* (1992) Calcium channel beta subunit heterogeneity:

Functional expression of cloned cDNA from heart, aorta and brain. *EMBO J.* **11**, 885–890.

Hymel, L.J., Whitworth, A., Wang, S.N., Clarcson, C.W. (1994) Cardiac Ca^{2+} release channel is a high affinity receptor for cardiac glycosides. *Biophys. J.* **66**, A19.

Iino, M., Endo, M. (1992) Calcium-dependent immediate feedback control of inositol 1,4,5-trisphosphate-induced Ca^{2+} release. *Nature* **360**, 76–78.

Iino, M., Tsulioka, M. (1994) Feedback control of inositol trisphosphate signalling by calcium. *Mol. Cell. Endocrinol.* **98**, 141–146.

Iino, M., Ozawa, S., Tsuzuki, K. (1990) Permeation of calcium through excitatory amino acid receptor channels in cultured rat hippocampal neurones. *J. Physiol. (Lond.)* **424**, 151–165.

Ikemoto, N., Antoniu, B., Kang, J.-J., Meszaros, L.G., Ronjat, M. (1991) Intravesicular calcium transient during calcium release from sarcoplasmic reticulum. *Biochemistry* **30**, 5230–5237.

Imredy, J.P., Yue, D.T. (1994) Mechanism of Ca^{2+}-sensitive inactivation of L-type Ca++ channels. *Neuron* **12**, 1301–1318.

Inagaki, N., Wada, H. (1994) Histamine and prostanoid receptors on glial cells. *Glia* **11**, 102–109.

Inagaki, N., Fukui, H., Ito, S., Wada, H. (1991a) Type-2 astrocytes show intracellular Ca^{2+} elevation in response to various neuroactive substances. *Neurosci. Lett.* **128**, 257–260.

Inagaki, N., Fukui, H., Ito, S., Yamatodani, A., Wada, H. (1991b) Single type-2 astrocytes show multiple independent sites of Ca^{2+} signalling in response to histamine. *Proc. Natl Acad. Sci. USA* **88**, 4215–4219.

Irving, A.J., Collingridge, G.L., Schofield, J.G. (1992a) l-Glutamate and acetylcholine mobilise Ca^{2+} from the same intracellular pool in cerebellar granule cells using transduction mechanisms with different Ca^{2+} sensitivities. *Cell Calcium* **13**, 293–301.

Irving, A.J., Collingridge, G.L., Schofield, J.G. (1992b) Interaction between Ca^{2+} mobilizing mechanisms in cultured rat cerebellar granule cells. *J. Physiol. (Lond.)* **456**, 667–680.

Isenberg, G., Han, S. (1994) Gradation of Ca^{2+}-induced Ca^{2+} release by voltage-clamp pulse duration in potentiated guinea-pig ventricular myocytes. *J. Physiol. (Lond.)* **480**, 423–438.

Ishida, Y., Honda, H. (1993) Inhibitory action of 4-aminopyridine on Ca^{2+}-ATPase of the mammalian sarcoplasmic reticulum. *J. Biol. Chem.* **268**, 4021–4024.

Ito, S., Sugama, K., Inagaki, N. *et al.* (1992) Type-1 and type-2 astrocytes are distinct targets for prostaglandins D_2, E_2, and $F_{2\alpha}$. *Glia* **6**, 67–74.

Jaffe, D.B., Brown, T.H. (1994) Metabotropic glutamate receptors activation induces calcium waves within hippocampal dendrites. *J. Neurophysiol.* **72**, 471–474.

Jahromi, B.S., Robitaille, R., Charlton, M.P. (1992) Transmitter release increases intracellular calcium in perisynaptic Schwann cells in situ. *Neuron* **8**, 1069–1077.

Jenden, D.J., Fairhurst, A.S. (1969) The pharmacology of ryanodine. *Pharmacol. Rev.* **21**, 1–25.

Jensen, A.M., Chui, S.Y. (1990) Fluorescent measurement of changes in intracellular calcium induced by excitatory amino acids in cultured cortical astrocytes. *J. Neurosci.* **10**, 1165–1175.

Jensen, A.M., Chiu, S.Y. (1993) Expression of glutamate receptor genes in white matter: developing and adult rat optic nerve. *J. Neurosci.* **13**, 1664–1675.

Jensen, J.R., Rehder, V. (1991) FCCP releases Ca^{2+} from a nonmitochondrial store in an identified *Helisoma* neuron. *Brain Res.* **551**, 311–314.

Johnson, E.M., Deckwerth, T.L. (1993) Molecular mechanisms of developmental neuronal death. *Annu. Rev. Neurosci.* **16**, 31–46.

Johnson, J.W., Asher, P. (1987) Glycine potentiates the NMDA response in cultured mouse brain neurons. *Nature* **325**, 529–531.

Jonas, P., Racca, C., Sakmann, B., Seeburg, P.H., Monyer, H. (1994) Differences in Ca^{2+} permeability of AMPA-type glutamate receptor channels in neocortical neurones caused by differential GluR-B subunit expression. *Neuron* **12**, 1281–1289.

Jones, O.T, Kunze, D.L, Angelides, K.J. (1989) Localization and mobility of ω-conotoxin-sensitive Ca channels in hippocampal CA1 neurons. *Science* **244**, 1189–1193.

Jones, S.W., Jacobs, L.S. (1990) Dihydropyridine actions on calcium currents in frog sympathetic neurons. *J. Neurosci.* **10**, 2261–2267.

Jones, S.W., Marks, T.N. (1989) Calcium currents in bull frog sympathetic neurons. 1. Activation kinetics and pharmacology. *J. Gen. Physiol.* **94**, 151–167.

Kalman, D., O'Lague, P.H., Erxleben, C., Armstrong, D.L. (1988) Calcium-dependent inactivation of the dihydropyridine-sensitive calcium channels in GH cells. *J. Gen. Physiol.* **92**, 531–548.

Kaneda, M., Wakamori, M., Ito, C., Akaike, N. (1990) Low-threshold calcium current in isolated Purkinje cell bodies of rat cerebellum. *J. Neurophysiol.* **63**, 1046–1051.

Kang, Y., Kitai, S.T. (1993) A whole cell patch-clamp study on the pacemaker potential in dopaminergic neurons of rat substantia nigra compacta. *Neurosci. Res.* **18**, 209–221.

Kano, M., Satoh, R., Nakabayashi, Y. (1991) Developmental changes in voltage-dependent calcium and sodium channels during differentiation of embryonic chick skeletal muscle cells in culture. *Biomed. Res.* **12** (suppl.), 197–198.

Kano, M., Garaschuk, O., Verkhratsky, A., Konnerth, A. (1995) Ryanodine receptor-mediated intracellular calcium release in rat cerebellar Purkinje neurones. *J. Physiol. (Lond.)* **487**, 1.

Karlin, A. (1993) Structure of nicotinic acetylcholine receptors. *Curr. Opinion Neurobiol.* **3**, 299–309.

Karschin, A., Lipton, S.A. (1989) Calcium channels in solitary retinal ganglion cells from post-natal rat. *J. Physiol. (Lond.)* **418**, 379–396.

Karst, H., Joels, M., Wadman, W.J. (1993) Low threshold calcium current in dendrites of the adult rat hippocampus. *Neurosci. Lett.* **164**, 154–158.

Kasono, K., Hirano, T. (1994) Critical role of postsynaptic calcium in cerebellar long-term depression. *NeuroReport* **6**, 17–20.

Kass, R.S., Sanguinetti, M.C. (1984) Inactivation of calcium channel current in the calf cardiac Purkinje fiber: evidence for voltage-and calcium-mediated mechanisms. *J. Gen. Physiol.* **84**, 705–726.

Kass, R.S., Arena, J.P., Chin, S. (1991) Block of L-type calcium channels by charged dihydropyridines: sensitivity to side of application and calcium. *J. Gen. Physiol.* **98**, 63–75.

Kastritsis, C.H.C., McCarthy, K.D. (1993) Oligodendroglial lineage cells express neuroligand receptors. *Glia* **8**, 106–113.

Kastritsis, C.H.C., Salm, A.K., McCarthy, K. (1992) Stimulation of the P_{2y} purinergic receptor on type 1 astroglia results in inositol phosphate formation and calcium mobilization. *J. Neurochem.* **58**, 1277–1284.

Katz, B., Miledi, R. (1967a) The timing of calcium action during neuromuscular transmission. *J. Physiol. (Lond.)* **189**, 535–544.

Katz, B., Miledi, R. (1967b) A study of synaptic transmission in the absence of nerve impulses. *J. Physiol. (Lond.)* **192**, 407–436.

Kaupp, U.B. (1991) The cyclic nucleotide-gated channels of vertebrate photoreceptors and olfactory epithelium. *Trends Neurosci.* **14**, 150–157.

Kavalali, E.T., Plummer, M.R. (1994) Selective potentiation of a novel calcium channel in rat hippocampal neurones. *J. Physiol. (Lond.)* **480**, 475–484.

Kawano, S., DeHaan, R.L. (1990) Analysis of the T-type calcium channel in embryonic chick ventricular myocytes. *J. Membrane Biol.* **116**, 9–17.

Kawano. S., DeHaan, R.L. (1991) Developmental changes in the calcium currents in embryonic ventricular myocytes. *J. Membrane Biol.* **120**, 17–28.

Kawasaki, T., Kasai, M. (1994) Regulation of calcium channel in sarcoplasmic reticulum by calsequestrin. *Biochem. Biophys. Res. Commun.* **199**, 1120–1127.

Kay, A.R., Wong, R.K.S. (1987) Calcium current activation kinetics in isolated pyramidal neurones of the CA1 region of the mature guinea-pig hippocampus. *J. Physiol. (Lond.)* **392**, 603–616.

Keicher, E., Maggio, K., Hernandez-Nicaise, M.-L., Nicaise, G. (1991) The lacunar glial zone at the periphery of *Aplysia* giant neuron: volume of extracellular space and total calcium content of gliagrana. *Neuroscience* **42**, 593–601.

Keicher, E., Maggio, K., Hernandez-Nicaise, M.-L., Nicaise, G. (1992) The abundance of *Aplysia* gliagrana depends on Ca^{2+} and/or Na^+ concentrations in sea water. *Glia* **5**, 131–138.

Keinanen, K., Wisden, W., Sommer, B. *et al.* (1990) A family of AMPA-selective glutamate receptors. *Science* **249**, 556–560.

Keja, J.A., Kits, K.S. (1994) Single-channel properties of high- and low-voltage-activated calcium channels in rat pituitary melanotropic cells. *J. Neurophysiol.* **71**, 840–855.

Keja, J.A., Stoof, J.C., Kits, K.S. (1991) Voltage-activated currents through calcium channels in rat pituitary melanotropic cells. *Neuroendocrinology* **53**, 349–359.

Keja, J.A., Stoof, J.C., Kits, K.S. (1992) Dopamine D_2 receptor stimulation differentially affects voltage-activated calcium channels in rat pituitary melanotropic cells. *J. Physiol. (Lond.)* **450**, 409–435.

Kelly, J.S., Penington, N.J. (1989) 5-Hydroxytryptamine inhibits the voltage-dependent calcium current of acutely dissociated central neurones from the adult rat dorsal raphe nucleus. *J. Physiol. (Lond.)* **418**, 35P.

Kerr, L.D., Inoue, J., Verma, I.M. (1992) Signal transduction: the nuclear target. *Current Opin. Cell. Biol.* **4**, 496–501.

Kettenmann, H., Schachner, M. (1985) Pharmacological properties of GABA, glutamate and aspartate induced depolarization in cultured astrocytes. *J. Neurosci.* **5**, 3295–3301.

Kettenmann, H., Backus, K.H., Schachner, M. (1987) γ-Aminobutyric acid opens Cl⁻ channels in cultured astrocytes. *Brain Res.* **404**, 1–9.

Kettenmann, H., Banati, R., Walz, W. (1993) Electrophysiological behaviour of microglia. *Glia* **7**, 93–101.

Khachaturian, Z.S. (1994) Calcium hypothesis of Alzheimer's disease and brain ageing. *Ann. NY Acad. Sci.* **747**, 1–11.

Kiedrowski, L., Brooker, G., Costa, E., Wroblewski, J.T. (1994) Glutamate impairs neuronal calcium extrusion while reducing sodium gradient. *Neuron* **12**, 295–300.

Kim, W.T., Rioult, M.G., Cornell-Bell, A.H. (1994) Glutamate-induced calcium signalling in astrocytes. *Glia* **11**, 173–184.

Kim-Lee, M.H., Stokes, B.T., Yates, A.J. (1992) Reperfusion paradox: a novel mode of glial cell injury. *Glia* **5**, 56–64.

Kirchhoff, F., Kettenmann, H. (1992) GABA triggers a $[Ca^{2+}]_i$ increase in murine precursor cells of the oligodendrocyte lineage. *Eur. J. Neurosci.* **4**, 1049–1058.

Kirischuk, S., Verkhratsky, A. (1995) Mechanisms of calcium mobilization in cerebellar Bergmann glial cells. *J. Physiol. (Lond.)* **483P**, 62P.

Kirischuk, S.I., Pronchuk, N.F., Verkhratsky, A.N. (1992) Measurements of intracellular calcium in sensory neurones of adult and old rats. *Neuroscience* **90**, 947–951.

Kirischuk, S., Möller, T., Voileuko, N. Kettenmann, H., Verkhratsky, A. (1995a) ATP-induced cytoplasmic calcium mobilization in Bergmann glial cells. *J. Neurosci.* (in press).

Kirischuk, S., Neuhaus, J., Verkhratsky, A., Kettenmann, H. (1995b) Preferential localization of active mitochondria in process tips of immature retinal oligodendrocytes. *NeuroReport* **6** (in press).

Kirischuk, S., Sherer, J., Kettenmann, H., Verkhratsky, A. (1995c) Activation of P_2 purinoreceptors triggers Ca^{2+} release from InsP₃-sensitive internal stores in mammalian oligodendrocytes. *J. Physiol. (Lond.)* **483**, 41–57.

Kirischuk, S., Sherer, J., Müller, T., Kettenmann, H., Verkhratsky, A. (1995d) Subcellular heterogeneity of voltage-gated Ca^{2+} channels in cells of oligodendrocyte lineage. *Glia* **13**, 1–12.

Kirischuk, S., Voitenko, N., Kostyuk, P., Verkhratsky, A. (1995e) calcium signalling in granule neurones studied in cerebellar slice. *Cell Calcium* (in press).

Kirischuk, S., Voitenko, N., Kostyuk, P., Verkhratsky, A. (1995f) Age-associated changes of cytoplasmic calcium homeostasis in cerebellar granule neurones in situ: Investigation on thin cerebellar slices. *Exp. Gerontol.* (in press).

Klepper, M., Hans, M., Takeda, K. (1990) Nicotinic cholinergic modulation of voltage-dependent calcium current in bovine adrenal chromaffin cells. *J. Physiol. (Lond.)* **428**, 545–560.

Kobrinsky, E.M., Pearson, R.A., Dolphin, A.C. (1994) Low- and high-voltage-activated calcium channel currents and their modulation in the dorsal root ganglion cell line. *Neuroscience* **58**, 539–552.

Koch, R.A., Barish, M.E. (1994) Perturbation of intracellular calcium and hydrogen ion regulation in cultured mouse hippocampal neurones by reduction of the sodium ion concentration gradient. *J. Neurosci.* **14**, 2585–2593.

Koketsu, K., Akasu, T., Miyagawa, M. (1982) Identification of G_K systems activated by $[Ca^{2+}]_i$. *Brain Res.* **243**, 369–372.

Komatsu, Y., Iwakiri, M. (1992) Low-threshold Ca channels mediate induction of long-term potentiation in kitten visual cortex. *J. Neurophysiol.* **67**, 401–410.

Kondou, H., Inagaki, N., Fukui, H., Koyama, Y., Kanamura, A., Wada, H. (1991) Histamine-induced inositol phosphate accumulation in type-2 astrocytes. *Biochem. Biophys. Res. Commun.* **177**, 734–738.

Konishi, M., Kurihara, S. (1987) Effects of caffeine on intracellular calcium concentration in frog skeletal muscle fibers. *J. Physiol. (Lond.)* **383**, 269–283.

Konnerth, A., Lux, H.D., Morad, M. (1987) Proton-induced transformation of calcium channel in chick dorsal root ganglion cells. *J. Physiol. (Lond.)* **386**,603–633.

Kononenko, N.I., Kostyuk, P.G., Shcherbatko, A.D. (1983) The effect of intracellular cAMP injections on stationary membrane conductance and voltage- and time-dependent ionic currents in identified snail neurons. *Brain Res.* **268**, 321–328.

Kononenko, N.I., Kostyuk, P.G., Shcherbatko, A.D. (1986) Properties of cAMP-induced transmembrane current in mollusc neurons. *Brain Res.* **376**, 239–245.

Korczak, B., Zarain-Herzberg, A., Brandl, C.J., Ingles, C.J., Green, N.M., MacLennan, D.H. (1987) Structure of the rabbit fast-twitch skeletal muscle Ca^{2+}-ATPase. *Gene* **263**, 4813–4819.

Korn, S.J., Horn, R. (1991) Nordihydroguaiaretic acid inhibits voltage-activated Ca^{++} currents independently of lipoxygenase inhibition. *Mol. Pharmacol.* **38**, 524–530.

Korn, S.J., Bolden, A., Horn, R. (1991) Control of action potentials and Ca^{2+} influx by the Ca^{2+}-dependent chloride current in mouse pituitary cells. *J. Physiol. (Lond.)* **439**, 423–437.

Kostyuk, E.P., Pronchuk, N., Shmigol, A. (1995) Calcium signal prolongation in sensory neurons of mice with experimental diabetes. *NeuroReport* **6**, 1010–1012.

Kostyuk, P.G. (1992) *Calcium Ions in Nerve Cell Function.* Oxford University Press, Oxford.

Kostyuk, P.G., Kirischuk, S.I. (1993) Spatial heterogeneity of caffeine and inositol 1,4,5-trisphosphate-induced Ca^{2+} transients in isolated snail neurones. *Neuroscience* **53**, 943–947.

Kostyuk, P.G., Krishtal, O.A. (1977a) Separation of sodium and calcium currents in the somatic membrane of mollusc neurones. *J. Physiol. (Lond.)* **270**, 545–568.

Kostyuk, P.G., Krishtal, O.A. (1977b) Effects of calcium and calcium-chelating agents on the inward and outward currents in the membrane of mollusc neurones. *J. Physiol. (Lond.)* **270**, 569–580.

Kostyuk, P.G., Lukyanetz, E.A. (1993) Mechanisms of antagonistic action of internal Ca on serotonin-induced potentiation of calcium currents in *Helix* neurons. *Pflugers Arch.* **424**, 73–83.

Kostyuk, P.G., Mironov, S.L. (1986) Some predictions concerning the calcium channel model with different conformational states. *Gen. Physiol. Biophys.* **6**, 649–659.

Kostyuk, P., Verkhratsky, A. (1994) Calcium stores in neurones and glia. *Neuroscience* **63**, 381–404.

Kostyuk, P.G., Krishtal, O.A., Pidoplichko, V.I. (1975) Intracellular dialysis of nerve cells: effect of intracellular fluoride and phosphate on the inward current. *Nature* **257**, 691–693.

Kostyuk, P.G., Krishtal, O.A., Pidoplichko, V.I. (1977) Asymmetrical displacement currents in nerve cell membrane and effects of internal fluoride. *Nature* **267**, 70–72.

Kostyuk, P.G., Krishtal, O.A., Pidoplichko, V.I., Shakhovalov, Y.A. (1979) Kinetics of calcium inward current activation. *J. Gen. Physiol.* **73**, 675–677.

Kostyuk, P.G., Doroshenko, P.A., Tsyndrenko, A.Ya., (1980) Calcium-dependent potassium conductance studied on internally dialysed nerve cells. *Neuroscience* **5**, 2187–2192.

Kostyuk, P.G., Krishtal, O.A., Pidoplichko, V.I. (1981) Calcium inward current and related charge movements in the membrane of snail neurones. *J. Physiol. (Lond.)* **310**, 403–421.

Kostyuk, P.G., Mironov, S.L., Doroshenko, P.A. (1982) Energy profile of the calcium channel in the membrane of mollusc neurons. *J. Membrane Biol.* **70**, 181–189.

Kostyuk, P.G., Mironov, S.L., Shuba, Y.M. (1983) Two ion-selecting filters in the calcium channel of the somatic membrane of mollusc neurons. *J. Membrane Biol.* **76**, 83–93.

Kostyuk, P.G., Fedulova, S.A., Veselovsky, N.S. (1986) Changes in ionic mechanisms of electrical excitability of the somatic membrane of rat dorsal root ganglion neurons during ontogenesis: distribution of ionic channels of inward current. *Neurophysiology (Kiev)* **18**, 813–820.

Kostyuk, P.G., Shuba, Y.M., Savchenko, A.N. (1988a) Three types of calcium channels in the membrane of mouse sensory neurones. *Pflugers Arch.* **411**, 661–669.

Kostyuk, P.G., Shuba, Y.M., Savchenko, A.N., Teslenko, V.I. (1988b) Kinetic characteristics of different calcium channels in the neuronal membrane. In: *The Calcium Channel: Structure, Function and Implications,* ed. by Morad, M., Nayler, W., Kazda, S., Schramm, M. Springer-Verlag,

Berlin, pp. 442–464.

Kostyuk, P.G., Mironov, S.L., Tepikin, A.V., Belan, P.V. (1989) Cytoplasmic free calcium in isolated snail neurons as revealed by fluorescent probe fura-2: mechanisms of Ca recovery after Ca load and Ca release from intracellular stores. *J Membrane Biol.* **110**, 11–18.

Kostyuk, P.G., Lukyuanetz, E.A., Ter-Markosyan, A.S., Khudaverdyan, D.N. (1990) Stimulation of neuronal calcium conductance by parathyroid hormone. *Neurophysiology (Kiev)* **22**, 373–380.

Kostyuk, P.G., Martynyuk, A.E., Pogorelaya, N.Ch. (1991) Effects of intracellular administration of l-tyrosine and l-phenylalanine on voltage-operated calcium conductance in PC12 pheochromocytoma cells. *Brain Res.* **550**, 11–14.

Kostyuk, P.G., Molokanova, E.A., Pronchuk, N.F., Savchenko, A.N. Verkhratsky, A.N. (1992a) Different action of ethosuximide on low- and high-threshold calcium currents in rat sensory neurones. *Neuroscience* **91**, 755–758.

Kostyuk, P.G., Lukyanetz, E.A., Doroshenko, P.A. (1992b) Effects of serotonin and cAMP on calcium currents in different neurones of *Helix pomatia*. *Pflugers Arch.* **420**, 9–15.

Kostyuk, P.G., Lukyanetz, E.A., Ter-Markosyan, A.S. (1992c) Parathyroid hormone enhances calcium current in snail neurones: simulation of the effect by phorbol esters. *Pflugers Arch.* **420**, 146–152.

Kostyuk, P.G., Pronchuk, N.F., Savchenko, A.N., Verkhratsky, A.N. (1993) Calcium currents in aged dorsal root ganglion neurones. *J. Physiol. (Lond.)* **461**, 467–483.

Koyama, Y., Baba, A., Iwata, H. (1991) L-Glutamate-induced swelling of cultured astrocytes is dependent on extracellular Ca^{2+}. *Neurosci. Lett.* **122**, 210–212.

Kraig, R.T., Nicholson, C. (1987) Extracellular ionic variations during spreading depression. *Neuroscience* **3**, 1045–1059.

Kramer, R.H., Kaczmarek, L.K., Levitan, E.S. (1991) Neuropeptide inhibition of voltage-gated calcium channels mediated by mobilization of intracellular calcium. *Neuron* **6**, 557–563.

Kriegler, S., Chiu, S.Y. (1993) Calcium signaling of glial cells along mammalian axons. *J. Neurosci.* **13**, 4229–4245.

Krishtal, O.A., Pidoplichko, V.I. (1981) A receptor for protons in the membrane of sensory neurones may participate in nociception. *Neuroscience* **12**, 2599–2601.

Krishtal, O.A., Marchenko, S.M., Pidoplichko, V.I. (1983) Receptor for ATP in the membrane of mammalian sensory neurones. *Neurosci. Lett.* **35**, 41–45.

Kristipati, R., Nadasdi, L., Tarczy-Hornoch, K. *et al.* (1994) Characterization of the binding of omega-conopeptides to different classes of non-L-type neuronal calcium channels. *Mol. Cell. Neurosci.* **5**, 219–228.

Kuffler, S.W., Potter, D.D. (1964) Glia in the leech central nervous system: physiological properties and neuron–glia relationship. *J Neurophysiol.* **27**, 290–320.

Kuno, M., Maeda, N., Mikoshiba, K. (1994) IP3-activated calcium-permeable channels in the inside-out patches of cultured cerebellar Purkinje cells. *Biochem. Biophys. Res. Commun.* **199**, 1128–1135.

Kunze, D.L, Ritchie, A.K. (1990) Multiple conductance levels of the dihydropyridine-sensitive calcium channel in GH cells. *J. Membrane Biol.* **118**, 171–178.

Kuo, C.-C., Bean, B.P. (1993) G-protein modulation of ion permeation through N-type calcium channels. *Nature* **365**, 258–262.

Kuo, C.-C., Hess, P. (1992) A functional view of the entrances of L-type Ca^{2+} channels: estimates of the size and surface potential at the pore mouth. *Neuron* **9**, 515–526.

Kuo, C.-C., Hess, P. (1993a) Ion permeation through the L-type Ca^{2+} channel in rat pheochromocytoma cells: two sites of ion binding sites in the pore. *J. Physiol. (Lond.)* **466**, 629–655.

Kuo, C.-C., Hess P. (1993b) Characterization of the high-affinity Ca^{2+} binding sites in the L-type Ca^{2+} channel pore in rat phaeochromocytoma cells. *J. Physiol. (Lond.)* **466**, 657–682.

Kuo, C.-C., Hess, P. (1993c) Block of the L-type Ca^{2+} channel pore by external and internal Mg^{++} in rat phaeochromocytoma cells. *J. Physiol. (Lond.)* **466**, 683–706.

Kurahashi, T., Kaneko, A. (1993) Gating properties of the cAMP-gated channel in toad olfactory receptor cells. *J. Physiol. (Lond.)* **466**, 287–302.

Kuwajima, G., Futatsugi, A., Niinobe, M., Nakanishi, S., Mikoshiba, K. (1992) Two types of ryanodine receptors in mouse brain: skeletal muscle type exclusively in Purkinje cells and cardiac muscle type in various neurones. *Neuron* **9**, 1133–1142.

Lacerda, A.E., Kim, H.S., Ruth, P. *et al.* (1991) Normalization of current kinetics by interaction between the alpha-1 and beta subunits of the skeletal muscle dihydropyridine-sensitive Ca^{2+} channel. *Nature* **352**, 527–530.

Lacerda, A.E., Perez-Reyes, E., Wei, X., Castellano, A., Brown, A.M. (1994) T-type and N-type calcium channels of *Xenopus* oocytes: evidence for specific interactions with β subunits. *Biophys. J.* **66**, 1833–1843.

Lai, F.A., Dent, M., Wickenden, C. *et al.* (1992) Expression of a cardiac Ca^{2+}-release channel isoform in mammalian brain. *Biochem. J.* **288**, 553–564.

Lambert, N.A., Borroni, A.M., Grover, L.M., Teyler, T.J. (1991) Hyperpolarizing and depolarizing $GABA_A$ receptor-mediated dendritic inhibition in area CA1 of the rat hippocampus. *J. Neurophysiol.* **66**, 1538–1548.

Lampe, R.A., DeFeo, P.A., Davison, M.D. *et al.* (1993) Isolation and pharmacological characterization of ω-grammatoxin SIA, a novel peptide inhibitor of neuronal voltage-sensitive calcium channel responses. *Mol. Pharmacol.* **44**, 451–460.

Lancaster, B., Nicoll, R.A. (1987) Properties of two calcium-activated hyperpolarizations in rat hippocampal neurones. *J. Physiol. (Lond.)* **389**, 187–203.

Lancaster, B., Zucker, R.S. (1994) Photolytic manipulation of Ca^{2+} and the time course of slow, Ca^{2+}-activated K$^+$ current in rat hippocampal neurones. *J. Physiol. (Lond.)* **475**, 229–239.

Lancaster, B., Nicoll, R.A., Perkel, D.J. (1991) Calcium activates two types of potassium channels in rat hippocampal neurons in culture. *J. Neurosci.* **11**, 25–30.

Landfield, P.W. (1994) Increased hippocampal Ca^{2+} channel activity in brain ageing and dementia: hormonal and pharmacological modulation. *Ann. NY Acad. Sci.* **747**, 351–364.

Landfield, P.W., Campbell, L.W., Hao, S.-Y., Kerr, D.S.(1989) Aging-related increases in voltage-sensitive, inactivating calcium currents in rat hippocampus: implications for mechanisms of brain aging and Alzheimer's disease. *Ann. NY Acad. Sci.* **568**, 95–105.

Lang, D.G., Ritchie, A.K. (1987) Large and small conductance calcium-activated potassium channels in the GH$_3$ anterior pituitary cell line. *Pflugers Arch.* **410**, 614–622.

Lansman, J.B. (1990) Blockade of current through single calcium channels by trivalent lanthanide cations: effect of ionic radius on the rates of ion entry and exit. *J. Gen. Physiol.* **95**, 679–696.

Larmet, Y., Dolphin, A.C., Davies, A.M. (1992) Intracellular calcium regulates the survival of early sensory neurons before they become dependent on neurotrophic factors. *Neuron* **9**, 563–574.

Lavoie, P.-A., Beauchamp, G., Elie, R. (1990) Tricyclic antidepressants inhibit voltage-dependent calcium channels and Na^+–Ca^{2+} exchange in rat brain cortex synaptosomes. *Can. J. Physiol. Pharmacol.* **68**, 1414–1418.

Lazarewitch, J.W., Kanje, M., Sellstrom, A., Hamberger, A. (1977) Calcium fluxes in cultured and bulk isolated neuronal and glial cells. *J. Neurochem.* **29**, 495–502.

Lee, H.C., Walseth, T.F., Bratt, G.T., Hayes, R.N., Clapper, D.L. (1989) Structural determination of a cyclic metabolite of NAD$^+$ with intracellular Ca^{2+}-mobilizing activity. *J. Biol. Chem.* **264**, 1608–1615.

Lee, H.C., Zocchi, E., Guida, L., Franco, L., Benatti, U., de Flora, A. (1993) Production and hydrolysis of cyclic ADP-ribose at the outer surface of human erythrocytes. *Biochem. Biophys. Res. Commun.* **191**, 639–645.

Lee, H.C., Aarhus, R., Graeff, R., Gurnack, M.E., Walseth, T.F. (1994) Cyclic ADP ribose activation of the ryanodine receptor is mediated by calmodulin. *Nature* **370**, 307–309.

Lee, K.S., Marban, E., Tsien, R.W. (1985) Inactivation of calcium channels in mammalian heart cells: joint dependence on membrane potential and intracellular calcium. *J. Physiol. (Lond.)* **364**, 395–411.

Legendre, P., Rosemund, C., Westbrook, G.L. (1993) Inactivation of NMDA channels in cultured hippocampal neurones by intracellular calcium. *J. Neurosci.* **13**, 674–684.

Lemos, J.R., Nowycky, M.C. (1989) Two types of calcium channels coexist in peptide-releasing vertebrate nerve terminals. *Neuron* **2**, 1419–1426.

Levey, A.I., Kitt, C.A., Simonds, W.F., Price, C.L., Brann, M.R. (1991) Identification and localization of muscarinic acetylcholine receptor proteins in brain with subtype-specific antibodies. *J. Neurosci.* **11**, 3218–3226.

Lev-Ram, V., Ellisman, M.H. (1995) Axonal activation-induced calcium transients in myelinating Schwann cells, sources, and mechanisms. *J. Neurosci.* **15**, 2628–2637.

Levy, S. (1992) Effect of intracellular injection of inositol trisphosphate on cytosolic calcium and membrane currents in *Aplysia* neurones. *J. Neurosci.* **12**, 2120–2129.

Lieberman, E.M., Sanzenbacher, E. (1992) Mechanisms of glutamate-activation of axon-to-Schwann cell signaling in the squid. *Neuroscience* **47**, 931–939.

Lievano, A., Bolden, A. and Horn, R. (1994) Calcium channels in excitable cells: divergent genotypic and phenotypic expression of α_1-subunits. *Am. J. Physiol.* **267**, C411–C427.

Lin, W.-W., Kiang, J.G., Chuang, D.-M. (1992) Pharmacological characterization of endothelin-stimulated phosphoinositide breakdown and cytosolic free Ca^{2+} rise in rat C_6 glioma cells. *J. Neurosci.* **12**, 1077–1085.

Lipscombe, D., Madison, D.V., Poenie, M., Reuter, H., Tsien, R.W., Tsien, R.Y. (1988) Imaging of cytosolic Ca^{2+} transients arising from Ca^{2+} stores and Ca^{2+} channels in sympathetic neurons. *Neuron* **1**, 355–365.

Lipscombe, D., Kongsamut, S., Tsien, R.W. (1989) β-Adrenergic inhibition of sympathetic neurotransmitter release mediated by modulation of N-type calcium-channel gating. *Nature* **340**, 639–642.

Lipton, S.A. (1994) AIDS-related dementia and calcium homeostasis. *Ann. NY Acad. Sci.* **747**, 205–224.

Liu, P.S., Lin, Y.J., Kao, L.S. (1991) Caffeine-sensitive calcium stores in bovine adrenal chromaffin cells. *J. Neurochem.* **56**, 172–177.

Liu, Q.Y., Karpinski, E., Rao, M.R., Pang, P.K.T. (1991) Tetrandine: a novel anatagonist inhibits type I calcium channels in neuroblastoma cells. *Neuropharmacology* **30**, 1325–1331.

Llano, I., Dreessen, J., Kano, M., Konnerth, A. (1991) Intradendritic release of calcium induced by glutamate in cerebellar Purkinje cells. *Neuron* **7**, 577–583.

Llano, I., DiPolo, R., Marty, A. (1994) Calcium-induced calcium release in cerebellar Purkinje neurones. *Neuron* **12**, 663–673.

Llinas, R., Sugimori, M., Lin, J.-W, Cherksey, B. (1989) Blocking and isolation of a calcium channel from neurons in mammals and cephalopods utilizing a toxin fraction (FTX) from funnel-web spider poison. *Proc. Natl Acad. Sci. USA* **86**, 1689–1693.

Llinas, R., Sugimori, M., Silver, R.B. (1992) Microdomains of high calcium concentration in a presynaptic terminal. *Science* **256**, 674–679.

Loeb, J. (1906) *The Dynamics of Living Matter*. New York.

Lopez, M.G., Albillos, A., de la Fuente, M.T. *et al.* (1994) Localized L-type calcium channels control exocytosis in cat chromaffin cells. *Pflugers Arch.* **427**, 348–354.

Lovinger, D.M, White, G. (1989) Post-natal development of burst firing behavior and the low-threshold transient calcium current examined using freshly isolated neurons from rat dorsal root ganglia. *Neurosci. Lett.* **102**, 50–57.

Lucherini, M.J., Gruenstein, E. (1992) Histamine H_1 receptors in UC 11MG astrocytes and their regulation of cytoplasmic Ca^{2+}. *Brain Res.* **592**, 193–201.

Lückhoff, A., Clapham, D.E. (1994) Calcium channels activated by depletion of internal calcium stores in A431 cells. *Biophys. J.* **66**, A153.

Lundy, P.M., Frew, R., Fuller, T.W., Hamilton, M.G. (1991) Pharmacological evidence for an ω-conotoxin, dihydropyridine-insensitive neuronal Ca channel. *Eur. J. Pharmacol.* **206**, 61–68.

Lundy, P.M., Hamilton, M.G., Frew, R. (1994) Pharmacological identification of a novel Ca^{2+} channel in chicken brain synaptosomes. *Brain Res.* **643**, 204–210.

Lustig, K.D., Shiau, A.K., Brake, A.J., Julius, D. (1993) Expression cloning of an ATP receptor from mouse neuroblastoma cells. *Proc. Natl Acad. Sci. USA* **90**, 5113–5117.

Lux, H.D., Hofmeier, G. (1982a) Properties of a calcium- and voltage-activated potassium current in *Helix pomatia* neurons. *Pflugers Arch.* **394**, 61–69.

Lux, H.D., Hofmeier, G. (1982b) Activation characteristics of the calcium-dependent outward potassium current in *Helix*. *Pflugers Arch.* **394**, 70–77.

Lux, H.D., Carbone, E., Zucker, H. (1990) Na currents through low-voltage activated Ca channels of chick sensory neurones: block by external Ca and Mg. *J. Physiol. (Lond.)* **430**, 159–188.

Lyons, S.A., Morell, P., McCarthy, K.D. (1992) Subpopulations of Schwann cells respond to neuroligands with increases in intracellular calcium. *Soc. Neurosci. Abstr.* **18**, 626.2.

Lytton, J., Westlin, M., Hanley, M.R. (1991) Thapsigargin inhibits the sarcoplasmic or endoplasmic reticulum Ca-ATPase family of calcium pumps. *J. Biol. Chem.* **266**, 17067–17071.

MacDermott, A., Mayer, M.L., Westbrook, G.L., Smith, S.J., Barker, J.C. (1986) NMDA-receptor activation increases cytoplasmic calcium concentration in cultured spinal cord neurones. *Nature* **321**, 519–522.

Mackie, K., Hille, B. (1992) Cannabinoids inhibit N-type calcium channels in neuroblastoma-glioma cells. *Proc. Natl Acad. Sci. USA* **89**, 3825–3829.

MacLennan, D., Brandl, C.J., Korczak, B., Green, N.M. (1985) Amino-acid sequence of a Ca^{2+}–Mg^{2+}-dependent ATPase from rabbit muscle sarcoplasmic reticulum, deduced from its complementary DNA sequence. *Nature* **316**, 396–400.

MacVicar, B.A. (1984) Voltage-dependent calcium channels in glial cells. *Science* **226**, 1345–1347.

MacVicar, B.A., Tse, F.W.Y. (1988) Norepinephrine and cyclic adenosine-3-:5--cyclic mono-phosphate enhance a nifedipine-sensitive calcium current in cultured rat astrocytes. *Glia* **1**, 359–365.

MacVicar, B.A., Tse, F.W., Crichton, S.A., Kettenmann, H. (1989) GABA-activated Cl⁻ channels in astrocytes of hippocampal slices. *J. Neurosci.* **9**, 3677–3583.

MacVicar, B.A., Hochman, D., Delay, M.J., Weiss, S. (1991) Modulation of intracellular Ca^{++} in cultured astrocytes by influx through voltage-activated Ca^{++} channels. *Glia* **4**, 448–455.

Maeda, N., Niinobe, M., Inoue, Y., Mikoshiba, K. (1989) Developmental expression and intracellular location of P400 protein characteristic of Purkinje cells in the mouse cerebellum. *Dev. Biol.* **133**, 67–76.

Maeda, N., Niinobe, M., Mikoshiba, K. (1990) A cerebellar Purkinje cell marker P400 protein is an inositol 1,4,5-trisphosphate (InsP₃) receptor protein: purification and characterization of InsP₃ receptor complex. *Eur. Mol. Biol. Org.* **9**, 61–67.

Maeda, N., Kawasaki, T., Nakade, S. *et al.* (1991) Structural and functional characterization of inositol 1,4,5-trisphosphate receptor channel from mouse cerebellum. *J. Biol. Chem.* **266**, 1109–1116.

Magnusson, A., Haug, L.S., Walaas, S.I., Ostvold, A.C. (1993) Calcium-induced degradation of the inositol (1,4,5)-trisphosphate receptor/Ca^{2+} channel. *FEBS Lett.* **323**, 229–232.

Maire, J.C., Medilanski, J., Straub, R.W. (1984) Release of adenosine, inosine and hypoxanthine from rabbit non-myelinated nerve fibres at rest and during activity. *J. Physiol. (Lond.)* **357**, 67–77.

Malgaroli, A., Tsien, R.W. (1992) Glutamate-induced long-term potentiation of the frequency of miniature synaptic currents in cultured hippocampal neurones. *Nature* **357**, 134–139.

Marrion, N.V., Adams, P.R. (1992) Release of intracellular calcium and modulation of membrane currents by caffeine in bull-frog sympathetic neurones. *J. Physiol. (Lond.)* **445**, 515–535.

Marriot, D.R., Wilkin, S.P., Wood, J.N. (1991) Substance P-induced release of prostaglandins from astrocytes: regional specialization and correlation with phosphoinositol metabolism. *J. Neurochem.* **56**, 259–265.

Marshall, I.C., Taylor, C.W. (1993) Regulation of inositol 1,4,5 trisphosphate receptors. *J. Exp. Biol.* **184**, 161–182.

Martinez-Serrano, A. Satrustegui, J. (1989) Caffeine-sensitive calcium stores in presynaptic nerve endings: a physiological role? *Biochem. Biophys. Res. Commun.* **161**, 965–971.

Martinez-Serrano, A., Vitorica, E., Satrustegui, J. (1988) Cytosolic free calcium levels increase with age in rat brain synaptosomes. *Neurosci. Lett.* **88**, 336–342.

Martinez-Serrano, A., Bogonez, E., Vitorica, E., Satrustegui, J. (1989) Reduction of K⁺-stimulated ⁴⁵Ca^{2+} influx in synaptosomes with age involves inactivating and noninactivating calcium channels and is correlated with temporal modifications in protein dephosphorylation. *J. Neurochem.* **52**, 576–584.

Martinez-Serrano, A., Blanco, P., Satrustegui, J.(1992) Calcium binding to the cytosol and calcium extrusion mechanisms in intact synaptosomes and their alteration with ageing. *J. Biol. Chem.* **267**, 4672–4679.

Martynyuk, A.E. (1987) Two types of calcium-dependent channels of potassium outward current in the somatic membrane of *Helix pomatia* neurons. *Neurophysiology (Kiev)* **19**, 185–191.

Martynyuk, A.E., Savina, S., Skibo, G.G. (1991) Blocking effect of intraperitoneal injection of phenylalanine on high-threshold calcium currents in rat hippocampal neurons. *Brain Res.* **552**, 228–231.

Masters, S.B., Harden, T.K., Brown, J.H. (1984) Relationships between phosphoinositide and calcium responses to muscarinic agonists in astrocytoma cells. *Mol. Pharmacol.* **26**, 149–155.

Mathie, A., Bernheim, L., Hille, B. (1992) Inhibition of N- and L-type calcium channels by muscarinic receptor activation in rat sympathetic neurons. *Neuron* **8**, 907–914.

Matsushima, T., Tegner, J., Hill, R.H., Grillner, S. (1993) GABA$_B$ receptor activation causes a depression of low- and high-voltage-activated Ca^{2+} currents, postinhibitory rebound, and postspike afterhyperpolarization in lamprey neurons. *J. Neurophysiol.* **70**, 2606–2619.

Matteson, D.R., Armstrong, C.M. (1984) Evidence for two types of Ca channels in GH cells. *Biophys. J.* **45**, 36a.

Matthew, W.D., Tsavales, L., Reichardt, L.F. (1981) Identification of synaptic vesicle-specific membrane protein with a wide distribution in neuronal and neurosecretory tissue. *J. Cell Biol.* **91**, 257–269.

Mattson, M.P. (1994). Calcium and neuronal injury in Alzheimer's disease: contributions of β-amyloid precursor protein, mismetabolism, free radicals, and metabolic compromise. *Ann. NY Acad. Sci.* **747**, 50–76.

Mattson, M.P., Guthrie, P.B., Kater, S.B. (1989) A role for Na^+-dependent Ca^{2+} extrusion in protection against neuronal excitotoxicity. *FASEB J.* **3**, 2519–2526.

Matute, C., Miledi, R. (1993) Neurotransmitter receptors and voltage-dependent Ca^{2+} channels encoded by mRNA from the adult corpus callosum. *Proc. Natl Acad. Sci. USA* **90**, 3270–3274.

Mayer, M.L. (1985) Calcium-activated chloride current in rat dorsal root ganglion neurones. *J. Physiol. (Lond.)* **361**, 22P.

Mayer, M.L., Westbrook, G.L. (1987a) Permeation and block of N-methyl-d-aspartic acid receptor channel by divalent cations in mouse cultured central neurones. *J. Physiol. (Lond.)* **394**, 501–527.

Mayer, M.L., Westbrook, G.L. (1987b) The physiology of excitatory amino acids in the vertebrate central nervous system. *Prog. Neurobiol.* **28**, 197–276.

Mayer, M.L., Westbrook, G.L., Guthrie, P.B. (1984) Voltage-dependent block by Mg^{2+} of NMDA responses in spinal cord neurones. *Nature* **309**, 261–263.

McCarthy, K.D., Salm, A.K. (1991) Pharmacologically-distinct subsets of astroglia can be identified by their calcium response to neuroligands. *Neuroscience* **41**, 325–333.

McCobb, D.P., Beam, K.G. (1991) Action potential waveform voltage-clamp commands reveal striking differences in calcium entry via low and high-voltage-activated calcium channels. *Neuron* **7**, 119–127.

McDonough, P.M., Eubanks, J.H., Brown, J.H. (1988) Desensitization and recovery of muscarinic and histaminergic Ca^{2+} mobilization in 1321N1 astrocytoma cells. *Biochem. J.* **249**, 4672–4679.

McGrew, S.G., Wolleben, C., Siegl, P., Inui, M., Fleischer, S. (1989) Positive cooperativity of ryanodine binding to the calcium release channel of sarcoplasmic reticulum from heart and skeletal muscle. *Biochemistry* **28**, 1686–1691.

McMillan, M., Pritchard, G.A., Miller, L.G. (1990) Characterization of Ca^{2+}-mobilizing excitatory amino acid receptors in cultured chick cortical cells. *Eur. J. Pharmacol.* **189**, 253–266.

McPherson, P.S., Kim, Y.K., Valdivia, H. *et al.* (1991) The brain ryanodine receptor: a caffeine-sensitive calcium release channel. *Neuron* **7**, 17–25.

Meech, R.W. (1974) The sensitivity of *Helix aspersa* neurones to injected calcium ions. *J. Physiol. (Lond.)* **237**, 259–277.

Meech, R.W., Standen, N.B. (1975) Potassium activation in *Helix aspersa* neurones under voltage clamp: a component mediated by calcium influx. *J. Physiol. (Lond.)* **249**, 211–239.

Meissner, G. (1994) Ryanodine receptor/ Ca^{2+} release channels and their regulation by endogenous effectors. *Annu. Rev. Physiol.* **56**, 485–508.

Meldolesi, J., Madeddu, L., Pozzan, T. (1990) Intracellular Ca^{2+} storage organelles in non-muscle cells: heterogeneity and functional assignment. *Biochem. Biophys. Acta* **1055**, 130–140.

Mennerick, S., Zorzumski, C.F. (1994) Glial contributions to excitatory neurotransmission in cultured hippocampal cells. *Nature* **368**, 59–62.

Menon-Johansson, A.S., Berrow, N., Dolphin, A.C. (1993) G_o transduces $GABA_B$-receptor modulation of N-type calcium channels in cultured dorsal root ganglion neurons. *Pflugers Arch.* **425**, 335–343.

Meriney S.D., Gray D.B., Pillar G.R. (1994) Somatostatin-induced inhibition of neuronal Ca^{2+} current modulation by cGMP-dependent protein kinase. *Nature* **369**, 336–339.

Mery, P.-F., Lohmann, S.M., Walter, U., Fischmeister, R. (1991) Ca current is regulated by cyclic GMP-dependent protein kinase in mammalian cardiac myocytes. *Proc. Natl Acad. Sci. USA* **88**, 1197–1201.

Meszaros, L.G., Bak, J., Chui, A. (1993) Cyclic ADP-ribose as an endogenous regulator of the non-skeletal type ryanodine receptor Ca^{2+} channel. *Nature* **364**, 76–79.

Meves, H. (1994) Modulation of ion channels by arachidonic acid. *Prog. Neurobiol.* **43**, 175–186.

Michaelis, M.L. (1994) Ion transport systems and Ca^{2+} regulation in aging neurons. *Ann. NY Acad. Sci.* **747**, 407–418.

Michalak, M., Milner, R.E., Burns, K., Opas, M. (1992) Calreticulin. *Biochem. J.*, **285**, 681–692.

Mignery, G.A., Newton, C.L., Archer, B.T., Sudhof, T.C. (1990) Structure and expression of the rat inositol 1,4,5-trisphosphate receptor. *J. Biol. Chem.* **265**, 12679–12685.

Migneri, G.A., Johston, P.A., Sudhof, T.C. (1992) Mechanisms of Ca^{2+} inhibition of inositol 1,4,5-trisphosphate ($InsP_3$) binding to the cerebellar $InsP_3$ receptor. *J. Biol. Chem.* **267**, 7451–7455.

Mikami, A., Imoto, T., Tanabe, T. *et al.* (1989) Primary structure and functional expression of the cardiac dihydropyridine-sensitive calcium channel. *Nature* **340**, 230–233.

Mikoshiba, K., Okano, H., Tsukada, Y. (1985) P_{400} protein characteristic to Purkinje cells and related proteins in cerebella from neuropathological mutant mice: autoradiographic study by ^{14}C-leucine and phosphorylation. *Dev. Neurosci.* **7**, 179–187.

Milani, D., Facci, L., Guidolin, D., Leon, A., Skaper, S.D. (1989) Activation of polyphosphoinositide metabolism as a signal-transducing system coupled to excitatory amino acids receptors in astroglial cells. *Glia* **2**, 1246–1249.

Miledi, R., Parker, I., Woodward, R.M. (1989) Membrane currents elicited by divalent cations in *Xenopus* oocytes. *J. Physiol. (Lond.)* **417**, 173–195.

Mintz, I.M., Bean, B.P. (1993a) Block of calcium channels in rat neurons by synthetic ω-Aga-IVA. *Neuropharmacology* **32**, 1161–1169.

Mintz, I.M., Bean, B.P. (1993b) $GABA_B$ receptor inhibition of P-type Ca^{2+} channels in central neurons. *Neuron* **10**, 889–898.

Mintz, I.M., Venema, V.J., Adams, M.E., Bean, B.P. (1991) Inhibition of N- and L-type Ca^{2+} channels by the spider venom toxin ω-Aga-IIIA. *Proc. Natl Acad. Sci. USA* **88**, 6628–6631.

Mintz, I.M., Venema, V.J., Swiderek, K.M. *et al.* (1992) P-type calcium channels blocked by the spider toxin ω-Aga-IVA. *Nature* **355**, 827–829.

Mironov, S.L. (1983) Theoretical model of slow-wave membrane potential oscillations in molluscan neurons. *Neuroscience* **10**, 899–905.

Mironov, S.L. (1992) Conformational model for ion permeation in membrane channels: a comparison with multi-ion model and applications to calcium channel permeability. *Biophys. J.* **63**, 485–496.

Mironov, S.L. (1994a) Metabotropic ATP receptor in hippocampal and thalamic neurones: pharmacology and modulation of Ca^{2+} mobilizing mechanisms. *Neuropharmacology* **33**, 1–13.

Mironov, S.L. (1994b) Mechanisms of Ca^{2+} mobilization in chick sensory neurones. *NeuroReport* **5**, 445–448.

Mironov, S.L., Lux, H.D. (1991) Calmodulin antagonists and protein phosphatase inhibitor okadaic acid fasten the 'run-up' of high-voltage activated calcium current in rat hippocampal neurones. *Neurosci. Lett.* **133**, 175–178.

Mironov, S.L., Usachev, Y.M., Lux, H.D. (1993) Spatial and temporal control of intracellular free Ca^{2+} in chick sensory neurones. *Pflugers Arch.* **424**, 183–191.

Missiaen, L., Parys, J.B., De Smedt, H., Oike, M., Casteels, R. (1994) Partial calcium release in response to submaximal inositol 1,4,5-trisphosphate receptor activation. *Mol. Cell. Endocrinol.* **98**, 147–156.

Miyazaki, S. (1993) IP_3 receptor-mediated spatial and temporal Ca^{2+} signaling of the cell. *Jpn. J. Physiol.* **43**, 409–434.

Mlinar, B., Enyeart, J.J. (1993) Block of current through T-type calcium channels by trivalent metal cations and nickel in neural rat and human cells. *J. Physiol. (Lond.)* **469**, 639–652.

Mogul, D.J., Fox, A.P. (1991) Evidence for multiple types of Ca channels in acutely isolated hippocampal CA3 neurones of the guinea-pig. *J. Physiol. (Lond.)* **433**, 259–281.

Moises, H.C., Rusin, K.I., Macdonald, R.L. (1994) μ-Opioid receptor-mediated reduction of neuronal calcium current occurs via a G_o-type GTP-binding protein. *J. Neurosci.* **14**, 3842–3851.

Momiyama, A., Takahashi, T. (1994) Calcium channels responsible for potassium-induced transmitter release at rat cerebellar synapses. *J. Physiol. (Lond.)* **476**, 197–202.

Moorman, S.J., Hume, R.J. (1994) Contact with myelin evokes a release of calcium from internal stores in neonatal rat oligodendrocytes in vitro. *Glia* **10**, 202–210.

Mori, Y., Friedrich, T., Kim, M.-S. *et al.* (1991) Primary structure and functional expression from complementary DNA of a brain calcium channel. *Nature* **350**, 398–402.

Morrissette, J., Heisermann, G., Cleary, J., Ruoho, A., Coronado, R. (1993) Cyclic ADP-ribose induced Ca^{2+} release in rabbit skeletal muscle sarcoplasmic reticulum. *FEBS Lett.* **330**, 270–274.

Muallem, S., Pandol, S.J., Beeker, T.G. (1989) Hormone-evoked calcium release from intracellular stores is a quantal process. *J. Biol. Chem.* **264**, 205–212.

Mulkey, R.M., Zucker, R.S. (1992) Posttetanic potentiation at the crayfish neuromuscular junction is dependent on both intracellular calcium and sodium ion accumulation. *J. Neurosci.* **12**, 4327–4336.

Mulle, C., Choquet, D., Korn, H., Changeux, J.P. (1992) Calcium influx through nicotinic receptors in central neurones: its relevance to cellular regulation. *Neuron* **8**, 135–143.

Müller, T., Möller, T., Berger, T., Schnitzer, J., Kettenmann, H. (1992) Calcium entry through kainate receptors and resulting potassium-channel blockade in Bergmann glial cells. *Science* **256**, 1563–1566.

Müller, T., Grosche, J., Ohlemeyer, C., Kettenmann, H. (1993) NMDA-activated currents in Bergmann glial cells. *NeuroReport* **4**, 671–674.

Müller, T.H., Misgeld, U., Swandulla, D. (1992) Ionic currents in cultured rat hypothalamic neurones. *J. Physiol. (Lond.)* **450**, 341–362.

Müller, T.H., Partridge, L.D., Swandulla, D. (1993) Calcium buffering in bursting *Helix* pacemaker neurons. *Pflugers Arch.* **425**, 499–505.

Müller, W., Connor, J.A. (1991) Dendritic spines as individual neuronal compartments for synaptic Ca^{2+} responses. *Nature* **354**, 73–76.

Mundina-Weilenmann, C., Ma, J., Rios, E., Hosey, M.M. (1991) Dihydropyridine-sensitive skeletal muscle Ca channels in polarized planar bilayers. 2. Effects of phosphorylation by cAMP-dependent protein kinase. *Biophys. J.* **60**, 902–909.

Murphy, S.N., Miller, R.J. (1989a) Regulation of Ca^{2+} influx into striatal neurones by kainic acid. *J. Pharmacol. Exp. Ther.* **249**, 184–193.

Murphy, S.N., Miller, R.J. (1989b) Two distinct quisqualate receptors regulate Ca^{2+} homeostasis in hippocampal neurones *in vitro*. *Mol. Pharmacol.* **35**, 671–680.

Murphy, S.N., Thayer, S.A., Miller, R.J. (1987) The effects of excitatory amino acids on intracellular calcium in single mouse striatal neurons in vitro. *J. Neurosci.* **7**, 4145–4158.

Myazaki, S. (1994) IP_3 receptor-mediated spatial and temporal Ca^{2+} signalling of the cell. *Jpn. J. Physiol.* **43**, 409–434.

Mynlieff, M., Beam, K.G. (1992) Developmental expression of voltage-dependent calcium currents in identified mouse motoneurons. *Dev. Biol.* **152**, 407–410.

Mynlieff, M., Beam K.G. (1994) Adenosine acting at an A_1 receptor decreases N-type calcium current in mouse motoneurons. *J. Neurosci.* **14**, 3628–3634.

Nagasaki, K., Fleishner, S. (1988) Ryanodine sensitivity of the calcium release channel of sarcoplasmic reticulum. *Cell Calcium* **9**, 1–7.

Nakai, J., Imagawa, T., Hakamata, Y., Shigekawa, M., Takeshima, H., Numa, S. (1990) Primary structure and functional expression from cDNA of the cardiac ryanodine receptor/calcium release channel. *FEBS Lett.* **271**, 169–177.

Nakamura, T., Gold, G.H. (1987) A cyclic nucleotide-gated conductance in olfactory receptor cilia. *Nature* **325**, 442–444.

Nakanishi, N. (1992) Molecular diversity of glutamate receptors and implications for brain function. *Science* **258**, 597–603.

Nakatani, K., Yau, K.-W., (1988) Calcium and magnesium fluxes across the plasma membrane of the toad rod outer segments. *J. Physiol. (Lond.)* **395**, 695–729.

Nedergaard M. (1994) Direct signalling from astrocytes to neurones in cultures of mammalian brain cells. *Science* **263**, 1768–1771.

Neering, I.R., McBurney, R.N. (1984) Role for microsomal Ca storage in mammalian neurones? *Nature* **309**, 158–160.

Neher, E., Augustine, G.J. (1992) Calcium gradients and buffers in bovine chromaffin cells. *J. Physiol. (Lond.)* **450**, 273–301.

Nelson, E.J., Li, C.C.R., Bangalore, R. *et al.* (1994) Inhibition of L-type calcium channel activity by thapsigargin and 2,5-t-butylhydroquinone, but not by cyclopiasonic acid. *Biochem. J.* **302**, 147–154.

Netzer, R., Pflimlin, P., Trube, G. (1994) Tonic inhibition of neuronal calcium channels by G proteins removed during whole-cell patch-clamp experiments. *Pflugers Arch.* **426**, 206–213.

Newman, E.A. (1985) Voltage dependent calcium and potassium channels in retinal glial cells. *Nature* **317**, 809–811.

Nicholson, C., Bruggencate, G.T., Stockle, H., Steinberg, R. (1978) Calcium and potassium changes in extracellular microenvironment of cat cerebellar cortex. *J. Neurophysiol.* **41**, 1026–1039.

Nicoletti, F., Meek, J.L., Iadarola, M.J. *et al.* (1986a) Coupling of inositol phospholipid metabolism with excitatory amino acid recognition sites in rat hippocampus. *J. Neurochem.* **46**, 40–46.

Nicoletti, F., Wroblewski, J.T., Novelli, A. *et al.* (1986b) The activation of inositol phospholipid metabolism as a signal-transduction system for excitatory amino acids in primary cultures of cerebellar granule cells. *J. Neurosci.* **6**, 1905–1911.

Niidome, T., Mori, Y. (1993) Primary structure and tissue distribution of a novel calcium channel from rabbit brain. *Ann. NY Acad. Sci.* **707**, 368–372.

Niidome, T., Kim, M.S., Friedrich, T., Mori, Y. (1992) Molecular cloning and characterization of a novel calcium channel from rabbit brain. *FEBS Lett.* **308**, 7–13.

Nilsson, M., Eriksson, P.S., Ronnback, L., Hansson, E. (1993) GABA induces Ca^{2+} transients in astrocytes. *Neuroscience* **54**, 605–614.

Nishimura, S., Takeshima, H., Hofman, F. *et al.* (1993) Requirement of the calcium channels β subunit for functional conformation. *FEBS Lett.* **324**, 283–286.

Nohmi, M., Hua, S.Y., Kuba, K. (1992a) Basal Ca^{2+} and the oscillation of Ca^{2+} in caffeine-treated bullfrog sympathetic neurones. *J. Physiol. (Lond.)* **450**, 513–528.

Nohmi, M., Hua, S.Y., Kuba, K. (1992b) Intracellular calcium dynamics in response to action potentials in bullfrog sympathetic ganglion cells. *J. Physiol. (Lond.)* **458**, 171–190.

Nori, A., Villa, A., Podini, P., Witcher, D.R., Volpe, P. (1993) Intracellular Ca^{2+} stores of rat cerebellum: heterogeneity within and distinction from endoplasmic reticulum. *Biochem. J.* **291**, 199–204.

Noronha-Blob, L., Richard, C., U'Prichard, D.C. (1987) Calcium mobilization by muscarinic receptors in human astrocytoma cells: measurements with quin 2. *Biochem. Biophys. Res. Commun.* **147**, 182–188.

Nowycky, M.C. (1991) Kinetic properties of L and N-type Ca channels and their ability to promote exocytosis in neurohypophyseal terminals. *Biophys. J.* **59**, 276a.

Nowycky, M.C., Fox, A.P., Tsien, R.W. (1985) Three types of neuronal calcium channel with different calcium agonist sensitivity. *Nature* **316**, 440–443.

Nunn, D.L., Taylor, C.W. (1992) Luminal Ca^{2+} increases the sensitivity of Ca^{2+} stores to inositol 1,4,5-trisphosphate. *Mol. Pharmacol.* **41**, 115–119.

Obaid, A.L., Flores, R., Salzberg, B.M. (1989) Calcium channels that are required for secretion from intact nerve terminals of vertebrates are sensitive to ω-conotoxin and relatively insensitive to dihydropyridines: optical studies with and without voltage-sensitive dyes. *J. Gen. Physiol.* **93**, 715–729.

O'Connor, E.R., Kimelberg, H.K. (1993) Role of calcium in astrocyte volume regulation and in the release of ions and amino acids. *J. Neurosci.* **13**, 2638–2650.

O'Dell, T.J., Alger, B.E. (1991) Single calcium channels in rat and guinea-pig hippocampal neurones. *J. Physiol. (Lond.)* **436**, 739–767.

Ogata, N., Yoshii, M., Narahashi, T. (1989) Psychotropic drugs block voltage-gated ion channels in neuroblastoma cells. *Brain Res.* **476**, 140–144.

Ogata, T., Nakamura, Y., Tsuji, K. *et al.* (1994) Adenosine enhances intracellular Ca^{2+} mobilization in conjunction with metabotropic glutamate receptor activation by t-ACPD in cultured hippocampal astrocytes. *Neurosci. Lett.* **170**, 5–8.

Ogawa, Y. (1994) Role of ryanodine receptors. *Crit. Rev. Biochem. Mol. Biol.* **29**, 229–274.

Ogura, A., Ozaki, K., Kudo, Y., Amano, T. (1986) Cytosolic calcium elevation and cGMP production induced by serotonin in a clonal cell of glial origin. *J. Neurosci.* **6**, 2489–2494.

Ogura, A., Miyamoto, M., Kudo, Y. (1988) Neuronal death in vitro: parallelism between survivability of hippocampal neurones and sustained elevation of cytosolic Ca after exposure to glutamate receptor agonists. *Exp. Brain Res.* **73**, 447–459.

Ogura, A., Akita, K., Kudo, Y. (1990) Non-NMDA receptors mediate cytoplasmic Ca^{2+} elevation in cultured hippocampal neurones. *Neurosci. Res.* **9**, 103–113.

Ohta, T., Ohga, A. (1990) Inhibitory action of dantrolene on Ca^{2+}-induced Ca^{2+} release from sarcoplasmic reticulum in guinea pig skeletal muscle. *Eur. J. Pharmacol.* **178**, 11–19.

Oka, A., Belliveau, M.J., Rosenberg, P.A., Volpe, J.J. (1993) Vulnerability of oligodendroglia to glutamate: pharmacology, mechanisms and prevention. *J. Neurosci.* **13**, 1441–1453.

Oldershaw, K.A., Taylor, C.W. (1993) Luminal Ca^{2+} increases the affinity of inositol 1,4,5-trisphosphate for its receptor. *Biochem. J.* **292**, 631–633.

O'Malley, D.M. (1994) Calcium permeability of the neuronal nuclear envelope: evaluation using confocal volumes and intracellular perfusion. *J. Neurosci.* **14**, 5741–5758.

Ondrias, K., Borgatta, L., Kim, D.H., Ehrlich, B.E. (1990) Biphasic effects of doxorubicin on the calcium release channel from sarcoplasmic reticulum of cardiac muscle. *Circ. Res.* **67**, 1167–1174.

O'Neill, S.C., Donoso, P., Eisner, D.A. (1990) The role of $[Ca^{2+}]_i$ and $[Ca^{2+}]$ sensitization in the caffeine contracture of rat myocytes: measurement of $[Ca^{2+}]_i$ and $[caffeine]_i$. *J. Physiol. (Lond.)* **425**, 55–70.

Ono, K., Fozzard, H.A. (1992) Phosphorylation restores activity of L-type calcium channels after run-down in inside-out patches from rabbit cardiac cells. *J. Physiol. (Lond.)* **454**, 673–688.

Orkand, R.K., Nicholls, J.G., Kuffler, S.W. (1966) Effect of nerve impulses on the membrane potential of glial cells in the central nervous system of amphibia. *J. Neurophysiol.* **29**, 788–806.

Orrenius, S., McConkey, J., Bellomo, G., Nicotera, P. (1989) Role of Ca^{2+} in toxic cell killing. *Trends Pharmacol. Sci.* **10**, 281–285.

Otsu, K., Willard, H.F., Khanna, V.K., Zorzato, F., Green, N.M., MacLennan, D.H. (1990) Molecular cloning of cDNA encoding the Ca^{2+} release channel (ryanodine receptor) of rabbit cardiac muscle sarcoplasmic reticulum. *J. Biol. Chem.* **265**, 13472–13483.

Ouyang, Y., Deerinck, T.J., Walton, D.D., Airey, J.A., Sutko, J.L., Ellisman, M.H. (1993) Distribution of ryanodine receptors in the chicken central nervous system. *Brain Res.* **620**, 269–280.

Palade, P., Dettbarn, C., Alderson, B., Volpe, P. (1989) Pharmacological differentiation between inositol 1,4,5-trisphosphate-induced Ca^{2+} release and Ca^{2+}- or caffeine-induced Ca^{2+} release from intracellular membrane systems. *Mol. Pharmacol.* **36**, 673–680.

Pang, P.K.T., Wang, R., Shan, J., Karpinski, E., Benishin, C.G. (1990) Specific inhibition of long-lasting L-type calcium channels by synthetic parathyroid hormone. *Proc. Natl Acad. Sci. USA* **87**, 623–627.

Parekh, A.B., Terlau, H., Stühmer, W. (1993) Depletion of InsP₃ stores activates a Ca^{2+} and K^+ current by means of a phosphatase and a diffusible messenger. *Nature* **364**, 814–818.

Patneau, D.K., Wright, P.W., Winters, C., Mayers, M.L., Gallo, V. (1994) Glial cells of the oligodendrocyte lineage express both kainate- and AMPA-preferring subtypes of glutamate receptor. *Neuron* **12**, 357–371.

Paupardin-Tritsch, D., Hammond, C., Gerschenfeld, H.M. (1986) Serotonin and cyclic GMP both induce an increase of the calcium current in the same identified molluscan neurons. *J. Neurosci.* **6**, 2715–2723.

Pearce, B., Murphy, S. (1988) Neurotransmitter receptors coupled to inositol phospholipid turnover and Ca^{2+} flux: consequences for astrocyte function. In: *Glial Cell Receptors*, ed. by Kimelberg, H. Raven Press, New York, pp. 197–221.

Pearce, B.R., Cambray-Deakin, M.A., Morrow, C., Murphy, S. (1985) Activation of muscarinic and of α_1-adrenergic receptors on astrocytes results in the accumulation of inositol phosphates. *J. Neurochem.* **45**, 1534–1540.

Pearson, H.A., Dolphin, A.C. (1993) Inhibition of ω-conotoxin-sensitive Ca^{2+} channel currents by internal Mg^{2+} in cultured rat cerebellar granule neurones. *Pflugers Arch.* **425**, 518–527.

Pellegrini-Giampietro, D.E., Bennet, M.V.L., Zukin, R.S. (1992) Are Ca^{2+} permeable kainate/AMPA receptors more abundant in immature brain? *Neurosci. Lett.* **144**, 65–69.

Pelzer, S., Barhanin, J., Pauron, D. *et al.* (1989) Diversity and novel pharmacological properties of Ca channels in *Drosophila* brain membranes. *EMBO J.* **8**, 2365–2371.

Penington, N.J., Kelly, J.S., Fox, A.P. (1991) A study of the mechanism of Ca current inhibition produced by serotonin in rat dorsal raphe neurons. *J. Neurosci.* **11**, 3594–3609.

Pennefather, P., Lancaster, B., Adams, P.R., Nicoll, R.A. (1985) Two distinct Ca-dependent K currents in bullfrog sympathetic ganglion cells. *Proc. Natl Acad. Sci. USA* **82**, 3040–3044.

Penner, R., Fasolato, C., Hoth, M. (1993) Calcium influx and its control by calcium release. *Curr. Opinion Neurobiol.* **3**, 368–374.

Perez-Reyes, E., Kim, H.S., Lacerda, A.E. *et al.* (1989) Induction of calcium currents by the expression of the α_1-subunit of the dihydropyridine receptor from skeletal muscle. *Nature* **340**, 233–236.

Perin, M.S., Johnston, P.A., Ozcellik, T. (1991) Structural and functional conservation of synaptotagmin (p65) in *Drosophila* and humans. *J. Biol. Chem.* **266**, 615–622.

Peters, R. (1986) Fluorescence microphotolysis to measure nucleocytoplasmic transport and intracellular mobility. *Biochim. Biophys. Acta* **864**, 305–359.

Peters, S., Koh, J., Choi, D.W. (1987) Zinc selectively blocks the action of N-methyl-d- aspartate on cortical neurons. *Science* **236**, 589–593.

Petersen, O.H., Petersen, C.C.H., Kasai, H. (1994) Calcium and hormone action. *Annu. Rev. Physiol.* **56**, 297–319.

Peyer, J.E. de, Cachelin, A.B., Levitan, I.B., Reuter, H. (1982) Ca^{2+}-activated K^+ conductance in internally perfused snail neurons is enhanced by protein phosphorylation. *Proc. Natl Acad. Sci. USA* **79**, 4207–4211.

Pfeiffer-Linn, C., Lasater, E.M. (1993) Dopamine modulates in a differential fashion T- and L-type calcium currents in bass retinal horizontal cells. *J. Gen. Physiol.* **102**, 277–294.

Pfrieger, F.W., Veselovsky, N., Gottmann, K., Lux, H.D. (1992a) Presynaptic calcium channels mediating synaptic transmission between rat thalamic neurons *in vitro*. In: *Abstracts of the 15th Annual Meeting of the European Neuroscience Association (Munich 1992)*. Oxford University Press, Oxford, p 93.

Pfrieger, F.W., Veselovsky, N.S., Gottmann, K., Lux, H.D. (1992b) Pharmacological characterization of calcium currents and synaptic transmission between thalamic neurons in vitro. *J. Neuroscience* **12**, 4347–4357.

Pfrieger, F.W., Gottmann, K., Lux, H.D. (1994) Kinetics of $GABA_B$ receptor-mediated inhibition of calcium currents and excitatory synaptic transmission in hippocampal neurons in vitro. *Neuron* **12**, 97–107.

Philibert, R.A., Rogers, K.L., Allen, A.J., Dutton, G.R. (1988) Dose-dependent, K^+-stimulated efflux of endogenous taurine from primary astrocyte culture is Ca^{2+}-dependent. *J. Neurochem.* **51**, 122–126.

Pietrobon, D, Hess, P. (1990) Novel mechanism of voltage-dependent gating in L-type calcium channels. *Nature* **346**, 651–655.

Pietrobon, D., Di Virgilio, F., Pozzan, T. (1990) Structural and functional aspects of calcium homeostasis in eukaryotic cells. *Eur. J. Biochem.* **193**, 599–622.

Pintor J., Miras-Portugal, M.T. (1995) P_2 purinergic receptors for diadenosine polyphosphates in the nervous system. *Gen. Pharmacol.* **26**, 229–235.

Piser, T.M., Lampe, R.A., Keith, R.A., Thayer, S.A. (1994) ω-Grammotoxin blocks action-potential-induced Ca^{2+} influx and whole-cell Ca^{2+} current in rat dorsal-root ganglion neurons. *Pflugers Arch.* **426**, 214–220.

Pitler, T.A., Landfield, P.W. (1990) Aging-related prolongation of calcium spike duration in rat hippocampal neurons. *Brain Res.* **508**, 1–6.

Plessers, L., Eggermont, J.A., Wuytack, F., Casteels, R. (1991) A study of the organellar Ca^{2+} transport ATPase isozymes in pig cerebellar Purkinje neurones. *J. Neurosci.* **11**, 650–656.

Pochet, R., Lawson, D.E.M., Heizmann, C.W. (1990) Calcium-binding proteins in normal and transformed cells. *Adv. Exp. Med. Biol.* **269**, 1–223.

Pollack, H. (1928) Micrurgical studies in cell physiology. IV. Calcium ions in living cytoplasm. *J. Gen. Physiol.* **11**, 539–545.

Pollo, A., Taglialatela, M., Carbone, E. (1991) Voltage-dependent inhibition and facilitation of Ca channel activation by $GTP\gamma S$ and Ca-agonists in adult rat sensory neurons. *Neurosci. Lett.* **123**, 203–207.

Pollo, A., Lovallo, M., Sher, E., Carbone, E. (1992) Voltage-dependent noradrenergic modulation of ω-conotoxin-sensitive Ca^{2+} channels in human neuroblastoma IMR32 cells. *Pflugers Arch.* **422**, 75–83.

Pollo, A., Lovallo, M., Biancardi, E. *et al.* (1993) Sensitivity to dihydropyridines, ω-conotoxin and noradrenaline reveals multiple high-voltage-activated Ca^{++} channels in rat insulinoma and human pancreatic β-cells. *Pflugers Arch.* **423**, 462–471.

Post, G.R., Dawson, G. (1992) Regulation of carbachol- and histamine-induced inositol phospholipid hydrolysis in a human oligodendroglioma. *Glia* **5**, 122–130.

Pozzan, T., Rizzuto, R., Volpe, P., Meldolesi, J. (1994) Molecular and cellular physiology of intracellular calcium stores. *Physiol. Rev.* **74**, 595–636.

Przysienzniak, J., Spencer, A.N. (1992) Voltage-activated calcium currents in identified neurons from a hydrozoan jellyfish, *Polyorchis penicillatus. J. Neurosci.* **12**, 2065–2078.

Przywara, D.A., Bhave, S.V., Bhave, A., Wakade, T.D., Wakade, A.R. (1991) Stimulated rise in neuronal calcium is faster and greater in the nucleus than the cytosol. *FASEB J.* **5**, 217–222.

Publicover, N.G., Hammond, E.M., Sanders, K.M. (1993) Amplification of nitric oxide signalling by interstitial cells isolated from cat colon. *Proc. Natl Acad. Sci. USA* **90**, 2087–2091.

Pun, R.Y.K., Stauderman, K.A., Pruss, R.M. (1988) Characterization and regulation of multiple calcium channels mediating changes in calcium conductance, intracellular calcium, and neurotransmitter release in bovine adrenal medullary chromaffin cells. *J. Gen. Physiol.* **92**, 15a.

Puro, D.G. (1991a) Stretch-activated channels in human retinal Muller cells. *Glia* **4**, 456–460.

Puro, D.G. (1991b) A calcium-activated, calcium-permeable ion channel in human retinal glial cells: modulation by basic fibroblast growth factor. *Brain Res.* **548**, 329–333.

Puro, D.G., Mano, T. (1991) Modulation of calcium channels in human retinal glial cells by basic fibroblast growth factor: a possible role in retinal pathobiology. *J. Neurosci.* **11**, 1873–1880.

Putney, J.W. (1986) A model for receptor-regulated calcium entry. *Cell Calcium* **7**, 1–12.

Radermacher, M., Wagenknecht, T., Grassucci, R. *et al.* (1992) Cryo-EM of the native structure of the calcium release channel/ryanodine receptor from sarcoplasmic reticulum. *Biophys. J.* **61**, 936–940.

Rampe, D., Lacerda, A.E., Dage, R.C., Brown, A.M. (1991) Parathyroid hormone: an endogenous modulator of cardiac calcium channels. *Am. J. Physiol.* **261**, H1945–H1950.

Randriamampita, C. and Tsien, R.Y. (1993) Emptying of intracellular Ca^{2+} stores releases a novel small messenger that stimulates Ca^{2+} influx. *Nature* **364**, 809–814.

Ransom, B.R., Goldring, S. (1973) Ionic determinants of membrane potential of cells presumed to be glia in cerebral cortex of rat. *J Neurophysiol.* **36**, 855–868.

Reber, B.F.X., Stucki, J.W., Reuter, H. (1993) Unidirectional interaction between two intracellular calcium stores in rat phaeochromocytoma (PC12) cells. *J. Physiol. (Lond.)* **468**, 711–727.

Reed R.R. (1992) Signalling pathways in odorant detection. *Neuron* **8**, 205–209.

Regan, L.J., Sah, D.W.Y., Bean, B.P. (1991) Ca channels in rat central and peripheral neurons: high-threshold current resistant to dihydropyridine blockers and ω-conotoxin. *Neuron* **6**, 269–280.

Regan, R.F., Choi, D.W. (1991) Glutamate neurotoxicity in spinal cord cell culture. *Neuroscience* **43**, 585–591.

Regehr, W.G., Mintz, I.M. (1994) Participation of multiple calcium channel types in transmission at single climbing fiber to Purkinje cell synapses. *Neuron* **12**, 605–613.

Reichling, D.B., MacDermott, A.B. (1993) Brief calcium transients evoked by glutamate receptor agonists in rat dorsal horn neurones: fast kinetics and mechanisms. *J. Physiol. (Lond.)* **469**, 67–88.

Reichling, D.B., Kyrozis, A., Wang, J., MacDermott, A.B. (1994) Mechanisms of GABA and glycine depolarization-induced calcium transients in rat dorsal horn neurones. *J. Physiol. (Lond.)* **476**, 411–421.

Reist, N.E., Smith, S. J. (1992) Neurally evoked calcium transients in terminal Schwann cells at the neuromuscular junction. *Proc. Natl Acad. Sci. USA* **89**, 7625–7629.

Restrepo, D., Miyamoto, T., Bryant, B.P., Teeter, J.H. (1990) Odor stimuli trigger influx of calcium into olfactory neurons of the channel catfish. *Science* **249**, 1166–1168.

Reuter, H. (1974) Localization of beta adrenergic and cyclic nucleotides on action potentials, ionic currents and tension in mammalian cardiac muscle. *J. Physiol. (Lond.)* **242**, 429–451.

Reuveny, E., Narahashi, T. (1991) Specific inhibition of N-type calcium channels by μ-opioid receptor activation in human neuroblastoma cells. *Biophys. J.* **59**, 82a.

Reynolds, J.N., Carlen, P.L. (1989) Diminished calcium currents in aged hippocampal dentate gyrus granule neurones. *Brain Res.* **479**, 384–390.

Richard, S., Diochot, S., Nargeot, J., Baldy-Moulinier, M., Valmier, J. (1991) Inhibition of T-type calcium currents by dihidropyridines in mouse embryonic dorsal root ganglion neurons. *Neurosci. Lett.* **132**, 229–234.

Richardson, A., Taylor, C.W. (1993) Effects of Ca^{2+} chelators on purified inositol 1,4,5-trisphosphate (InsP$_3$) receptors and InsP$_3$-stimulated Ca^{2+} mobilization. *J. Biol. Chem.* **268**, 11528–11533.

Richter D.W., Champagnat J., Jacquin T., Benacka R. (1993) Calcium currents and calcium-dependent potassium currents in mammalian medullary respiratory neurones. *J. Physiol. (Lond.)* **470**, 23–33.

Ringer, S. (1883) A further contribution regarding the influence of the different constituents of the blood on the contraction of the heart. *J. Physiol. (Lond.)* **4**, 29–42.

Rios, E., Pizarro, C. (1991) Voltage-sensor of excitation-contraction coupling in skeletal muscle. *Physiol. Rev.* **76**, 849–908.

Ritchie, A.K. (1993) Estrogen increases low voltage-activated calcium current density in GH$_3$ anterior pituitary cells. *Endocrinology* **132**, 1621–1629.

Ritchie, J.M. (1992) Voltage-gated ion channels in Schwann cells and glia. *Trends Neurosci.* **15**, 345–351.

Rizzuto, R., Brini, M., Murgia, M., Pozzan, T. (1993) Microdomains with high Ca^{2+} close to IP$_3$-sensitive channels that are sensed by neighboring mitochondria. *Science* **262**, 744–747.

Robbins, J., Trouslard, J., Marsh, S.J., Brown, D.A. (1992) Kinetic and pharmacological properties of the M-current in rodent neuroblastoma glioma hybrid cells. *J. Physiol. (Lond.)* **451**, 159–185.

Roberts, W.M., Jacobs, R.A., Hudspeth, A.J. (1990) Colocalization of ion channels involved in frequency selectivity at synaptic active zones of hair cells. *J. Neurosci.* **10**, 3664–3684.

Robichaud, L.J., Wurster, S., Boxer, P.A. (1994) The voltage-sensitive Ca^{2+} channels (VSCC) antagonists ω-Aga-IVA and ω-CTX-MVIIC inhibit spontaneous epileptiform discharges in the rat cortical wedge. *Brain Res.* **643**, 352–256.

Robinson, I.M., Burgoyne, R.D. (1991) Characterization of distinct inositol 1,4,5-trisphosphate-sensitive and caffeine-sensitive calcium stores in digitonin-permeabilized adrenal chromaffin cells. *J. Neurochem.* **56**, 1587–1593.

Roche, E., Prentki, M. (1994) Calcium regulation of immediate-early response genes. *Cell Calcium* **16**, 331–338.

Rosenberg, R.L, Chen, X.-H. (1991) Characterization and localization of two ion-binding sites within the pore of cardiac L-type calcium channels. *J. Gen. Physiol.* **97**, 1207–1225.

Rossier, M.F., Putney, J.W. (1991) The identity of the calcium-storing, inositol 1,4,5-trisphosphate-sensitive organelle in non-muscle cells: calciosome, endoplasmic reticulum—or both? *Trends Neurosci.* **14**, 310–314.

Rossier, M.F., Python, C.P., Burnay, M.M. *et al.* (1993a) Thapsigargin inhibits voltage-activated calcium channels in adrenal glomerulosa cells *Biochem. J.* **296**, 309–312.

Rossier, M.F., Python, C.P., Capponi, A.M. *et al.* (1993b) Blocking T-type calcium channels with tetrandrine inhibits steroidogenesis in bovine adrenal glomerulosa cells. *Endocrinology* **132**, 1035–1043.

Rothe, T., Bigl, V., Grantyn, R. (1994) Potentiating and depressant effects of metabotropic glutamate receptor agonists on high-voltage-activated calcium currents in cultured retinal ganglion neurons from postnatal mice. *Pflugers Arch.* **426**, 161–170.

Rothman, S. (1984) Synaptic release of excitatory amino acids neurotransmitter mediated anoxic neuronal death. *J. Neurosci.* **4**, 1884–1891.

Rousseau, E., Smith, J.C., Henderson, J.S., Meissner, G. (1986) Single channel and $^{45}Ca^{2+}$ flux measurements of the cardiac sarcoplasmic reticulum calcium channel. *Biophys. J.* **50**, 1009–1014.

Rousseau, E., Smith, J.S., Meissner, G. (1987) Ryanodine modifies conductance and gating behavior of single Ca^{2+} release channel. Am. J. Physiol. **253**, C364–C368.

Roussier, M.F., Python, C.P., Burnay, M.M., Schlegel, W., Vallotton, M.B., Capponi, A.M. (1993) Thapsigargin inhibits voltage-activated calcium channels in adrenal glomerulosa cells. *Biochem J.* **296**, 309–312.

Ruth, P., Röhrkasten, A., Biel, M. *et al.* (1989) Primary structure of the β-subunit of the DHP-sensitive calcium channel from skeletal muscle. *Science* **245**, 1115–1118.

Ryu, P.D, Randic, M. (1990) Low- and high-voltage-activated calcium currents in rat spinal dorsal horn neurons. *J. Neurophysiol.* **73**, 273–285.

Sah, D.W. (1990) Neurotransmitter modulation of calcium current in rat spinal cord neurons. *J. Neurosci.* **10**, 136–141.

Sah, D.W., Bean, B.P. (1994) Inhibition of P-type and N-type calcium channels by dopamine receptor antagonists. *Mol. Pharmacol.* **45**, 84–92.

Sah, P., Fransis, K., McLachlan, E.M., Junankar, P. (1993) Distribution of ryanodine receptor-like immunoreactivity in mammalian central nervous system is consistent with its role in calcium-induced calcium release. *Neuroscience* **54**, 157–165.

Sahara, Y., Westbrook, G.L. (1993) Modulation of calcium currents by a metabotropic glutamate receptor involves fast and slow kinetic components in cultured hippocampal neurons. *J. Neurosci.* **13**, 3041–3050.

Sala, S., Matteson, D.R. (1990) Single-channel recordings of two types of calcium channels in rat pancreatic β-cells. *Biophys. J.* **58**, 567–571.

Saleh, M., Lang, R.J., Bartlett, P.F. (1988) Thy-I-mediated regulation of a low-threshold transient calcium current in cultured sensory neurons. *Proc. Natl Acad. Sci. USA* **85**, 4543–4547.

Salm, A.K., McCarthy, K.D. (1990) Norepinephrine-evoked calcium transients in cultured cerebral type 1 astroglia. *Glia* **3**, 529–538.

Salter, M.W., Hicks, J.L. (1994) ATP-evoked increases in intracellular calcium in neurones and glia from the dorsal spinal cord. *J. Neurosci.* **14**, 1563–1575.

Salter, M.W., Koninck, D.Y., Henry J.L. (1993) Physiological role for adenosine and ATP in synaptic transmission in the spinal dorsal horn. *Prog. Neurobiol.* **41**, 125–156.

Sanchez, J.A., Stefani, E. (1983) Kinetic properties of calcium channels of twitch muscle fibres of the frog. *J. Physiol. (Lond.)* **337**, 1–17.

Sather, W.A., Tanabe, T., Zhang, J.-F. *et al.* (1993) Distinctive biophysical and pharmacological properties of class A (BI) calcium channel α_1 subunits *Neuron* **11**, 291–303.

Sayer, R.J., Brown, A.M., Schwindt, P.C., Crill, W.E. (1993) Calcium currents in acutely isolated human neocortical neurons. *J. Neurophysiol.* **69**, 1596–1606.

Schatzmann, H.J. (1966) ATP-dependent Ca^{++} extrusion from human red cells. *Experientia* **22**, 364–368.

Schettini, G., Meucci, O., Grimaldi, M. *et al.* (1991) Dihydropyridine modulation of voltage-activated calcium channels in PC12 cells: effect of pertussis toxin pretreatment. *J. Neurochem.* **56**, 805–811.

Schirrmacher K., Mayer A., Walden J., Dusing R., Bingmann D. (1993) Effects of carbamazepine on action potentials and calcium currents in rat spinal ganglion cells in vitro. *Neuropsychobiology* **27**, 176–179.

Schmidt, A., Hescheler, J., Offermanns, S. *et al.* (1991) Involvement of pertussis toxin-sensitive G-proteins in the hormonal inhibition of dihydropyridine-sensitive Ca currents in an insulin-secreting cell line (RINm5F). *J. Biol. Chem.* **266**, 18025–18033.

Schmitt, H., Meves, H. (1994) Bovine serum albumin selectively increases the low-voltage-activated calcium current of HG108-15 neuroblastoma glioma cells. *Brain Res.* **656**, 375–380.

Schneggenburger, R., Zhou, Z., Konnerth, A., Neher, E. (1993) Fractional contribution of calcium to the cation current through glutamate receptor channels. *Neuron* **11**, 133–143.

Scholz, K.P., Miller, R.J. (1991a) Analysis of adenosine actions on Ca^{2+} currents and synaptic transmission in cultured rat hippocampal pyramidal neurones. *J. Physiol. (Lond.)* **435**, 373–393..

Scholz, K.P., Miller, R.J. (1991b) GABA receptor-mediated inhibition of Ca currents and synaptic transmission in cultured rat hippocampal neurones. *J. Physiol. (Lond.)* **444**, 669–686.

Schroeder, J.E., Fischbach, P.S., McCleskey, E.W. (1990) T-type calcium channels: heterogeneous expression in rat sensory neurons and selective modulation by phorbol esters. *J. Neurosci.* **10**, 947–951.

Schwindt, P.C., Spain, W.J., Crill, W.E. (1992) Calcium-dependent potassium currents in neurons from cat sensorimotor cortex. *J. Neurophysiol.* **67**, 216–226.

Scott, R.H., Dolphin, A.C. (1987) Activation of a G protein promotes agonist response to calcium channel ligands. *Nature* **330**, 760–762.

Scott, R.H., Dolphin, A.C., Bindokas, V.P., Adams, M.E. (1990a) Inhibition of neuronal Ca channel current by the funnel web spider toxin ω-Aga-IVA. *Mol. Pharmacol.* **38**, 711–718.

Scott, R.H., Wootton, J.F., Dolphin, A.C. (1990b) Modulation of neuronal T-type calcium channel currents by photoactivation of intracellular guanosine 5--O(3-thio)triphosphate. *Neuroscience* **38**, 285–294.

Scroggs, R.S., Fox, A.P. (1992a) Multiple Ca^{2+} currents elicited by action potential waveforms in acutely isolated adult rat dorsal root ganglion neurons. *J. Neurosci.* **12**, 1789–1801.

Scroggs, R.S., Fox, A.P. (1992b) Calcium current variation between acutely isolated adult rat dorsal root ganglion neurons of different size. *J. Physiol. (Lond.)* **445**, 639–658.

Seabrook, G.R., Knowles, M., Brown, N. (1994a) Pharmacology of high-threshold calcium currents in HGH_4C_1 pituitary cells and their regulation by activation of human D_2 and D_4 dopamine receptors. *Br. J. Pharmacol.* **112**, 728–734.

Seabrook, G.R., McAllister, G., Knowles, M.R. *et al.* (1994b) Depression of high-threshold calcium currents by activation of human D_2 (short) dopamine receptors expressed in differentiated HG108-15 cells. *Br. J. Pharmacol.* **111**, 1061–1066.

Segal, M. (1993) GABA induces a unique rise of $[Ca]_i$ in cultured rat hippocampal neurones. *Hippocampus* **3**, 229–238.

Segal, M., Manor, D. (1992) Confocal microscopic imaging of $[Ca^{2+}]_i$ in cultured rat hippocampal neurones following exposure to N-methyl-d-aspartate. *J. Physiol. (Lond.)* **448**, 655–676.

Seguela, P., Wadische, J., Dineley-Miller, K., Dani, J.A., Patrick, J.W. (1993) Molecular cloning, functional properties and distribution of rat brain α_7: a nicotinic cation channel highly permeable to calcium. *J. Neurosci.* **13**, 596–604.

Seidler, N.W., Jona, I., Vegh, M., Martonosi, A. (1989) Cyclopiazonic acid is a specific inhibitor of the Ca^{2+} ATPase of sarcoplasmic reticulum. *J. Biol. Chem.* **264**, 17816–17823.

Shao, Y., McCarthy, K.D. (1993) Regulation of astroglial responsiveness to neuroligands in primary culture. *Neuroscience* **55**, 991–1001.

Shao, Y., McCarthy, K.D. (1994) Plasticity of astrocytes. *Glia* **11**, 147–155.

Shao, Y., McCarthy, K.D. (1995) Receptor-mediated calcium signals in astroglia-multiple receptors, common stores and all-or-nothing responses. *Cell Calcium* **17**, 187–196.

Sharp, A.H., Dawson, T.M., Ross, C.A., Fotuhi, M., Mourey, R.J., Snyder, S.H. (1993a) Inositol 1,4,5-trisphosphate receptors: immunohistochemical localization to discrete areas of rat central nervous system. *Neuroscience* **53**, 927–942.

Sharp, A.H., McPherson, P.S., Dawson, T.M., Aoki, C., Campbell, K.P., Snyder, S.H. (1993b) Differential immunohistochemical localization of inositol 1,4,5-trisphosphate and ryanodine-sensitive Ca^{2+} release channels in rat brain. J. *Neuroscience* **13**, 3051–3063.

Sher, E., Pandiella, A., Clementi, F. (1988) ω-Conotoxin biding and effects on calcium channel function in human neuroblastoma and rat pheochromocytoma cell lines. *FEBS Lett.* **235**, 178–182.

Sher, E., Biancardi, E., Passafaro, M., Clementi, F. (1991) Physiopathology of neuronal voltage-operated calcium channels. *FASEB J.* **5**, 2677–2683.

Sherman, A., Keizer, J., Rinzel, J. (1990) Domain model for Ca^{2+}-inactivation of Ca^{2+} channels at low channel density. *Biophys. J.* **58**, 985–996.

Shimomura, O., Johnson, F.H., Saiga, Y. (1962) Extraction, purification and properties of aequiron, a bioluminescent protein from the luminous hydromedusan, *Aequorea*. *J. Cell. Comp. Physiol.* **59**, 233–239.

Shimomura, O., Misucki, B., Kishi, V. (1989) Semi-synthetic aequorines with improved sensitivity to Ca^{2+} ions. *Biochem. J.* **261**, 913–920.

Shirasaki, T., Harata, N., Akaike, N. (1994) Metabotropic glutamate response in acutely dissociated hippocampal CA1 pyramidal neurones of the rat. *J. Physiol. (Lond.)* **475**, 439–453.

Shmigol, A., Kirischuk, S., Kostyuk, P., Verkhratsky, A. (1994a) Different properties of caffeine-sensitive Ca^{2+} stores in peripheral and central mammalian neurones. *Pflugers Arch.* **426**, 174–176.

Shmigol, A., Kostyuk, P., Verkhratsky, A. (1994b) Role of caffeine–sensitive Ca^{2+} stores in Ca^{2+} signal termination in adult mouse DRG neurones. *NeuroReport* **5**, 2073–2076.

Shmigol, A., Kostyuk, P., Verkhratsky, A. (1995a) Dual action of thapsigargin on calcium mobilization in sensory neurones: inhibition of Ca^{2+} uptake by caffeine-sensitive pools and blockade of plasmalemmal Ca^{2+} channels. *Neuroscience* in press.

Shmigol, A., Verkhratsky, A., Isenberg, G. (1995b) Calcium induced calcium release in rat sensory neurones. *J. Physiol. (Lond.)* **65**, 1109–1118.

Shmigol, A., Eisber, D., Verkhratsky, A. (1995c) cyclic ADP-ribose enchances Ca^{2+}-induced Ca^{2+} release in isolated mouse sensory neurones. *J. Physiol. (Lond)* **483.P.** 63P–64P.

Shuba, Y.M., Savchenko, A.N. (1987) Two conductance states of single calcium channels in the membranes of dorsal root ganglion cells from mouse embryos. *Biol. Membrany (Moscow).* **4**, 374–378.

Shuba, Y.M., Teslenko, V.I. (1987) Kinetic model for activation of single calcium channels in mammalian sensory neurone membrane. *Biol. Membrany (Moscow).* **4**, 315–329.

Shuba, Y.M., Hesslinger, B., Trautwein, W., McDonald, T.F., Pelzer, D. (1990) Whole-cell calcium current in guinea-pig ventricular myocytes dialysed with guanine nucleotides. *J. Physiol. (Lond.)* **424**, 205–228.

Shuba, Y.M., McDonald, T.F., Trautwein, W., Pelzer, S., Pelzer, D. (1991a) Direct up-regulating effect of Gs on the whole-cell L-type Ca current in cardiac cells. *Gen. Physiol. Biophys.* **10**, 105–110.

Shuba, Y.M., Teslenko, V.I., Savchenko, A.N., Pogorelaya, N.H. (1991b) The effect of permeant ions on single calcium channel activation in mouse neuroblastoma cells: ion-channel interaction. *J. Physiol. (Lond.)* **443**, 25–44.

Siesjo, B.K. (1994) Calcium-mediated processes in neuronal degeneration. *Ann. NY Acad. Sci.* **747**, 140–161.

Sihra, T.S., Nichols, R.A. (1993) Mechanisms in the regulation of neurotransmitter release from brain nerve terminals: current hypotheses. *Neurochem. Res.* **18**, 47–58.

Sim, L.J., Selley, D.E., Tsai, K.P., Morris, M. (1994) Calcium and cAMP mediated stimulation of Fos in cultured hypothalamic tyrosine hydroxylase-immunoreactive neurons. *Brain Res.* **653**, 155–160.

Simon, S.M., Llinas, R.R. (1985) Compartmentalization of the submembrane calcium activity during calcium influx and its significance in transmitter release. *Biophys. J.* **48**, 485–498.

Simpson, P.B., Chaliss, R.A.J., Nahorski, S.R. (1993) Involvement of intracellular stores in the Ca^{2+} responses to N-methyl-d-aspartate and depolarization in cerebellar granule cells. *J. Neurochem.* **61**, 760–763.

Sitsapesan, R., Williams, A.J. (1990) Mechanisms of caffeine activation of single calcium-release channels of sheep cardiac sarcoplasmic reticulum. *J. Physiol. (Lond.)* **423**, 425–439.

Sitsapesan, R., McGarry, S.J., Williams, A.J. (1994) Cyclic ADP-ribose competes with ATP for the adenine nucleotide binding site on the cardiac ryanodine receptor Ca^{2+} release channel. *Circ. Res.* **75**, 596–600.

Sladeczek, F., Pin, J.-P., Recasens, M., Bockaert, J., Weiss, S. (1985) Glutamate stimulates inositol phosphate formation in striatal neurones. *Nature* **317**, 717–719.

Slesinger, P.A., Lansman, J.B. (1991) Inactivating and non-inactivating dihydropyridine-sensitive Ca channels in mouse cerebellar granule cells. *J. Physiol. (Lond.)* **439**, 301–323.

Smith, J.S., Coronado, R., Meissner, G. (1986) Single channel measurements of the calcium release channel from skeletal muscle sarcoplasmic reticulum: activation by Ca^{2+} and ATP and modulation by Mg^{2+}. *J. Gen. Physiol.* **88**, 573–588.

Smith, J.S., Imagawa, T., Ma, J., Fill, M., Campbell, K.P., Coronado, R. (1988) Purified ryanodine receptor from rabbit skeletal muscle is the calcium release channel of sarcoplasmic reticulum.

J. Gen. Physiol. **92**, 1–26.

Sommer, B., Köhler, M., Sprengel, R., Seeburg, P.H. (1991) RNA editing in brain controls a determinant of ion flow in glutamate-gated channels. *Cell* **67**, 11–19.

Sommer, I., Schachner, M. (1981) Monoclonal antibodies (O10 to O4) to oligodendrocyte surfaces: an immunocytological study in the central nervous system. *Dev. Biol.* **83**, 311–323.

Sommer, I., Schachner, M. (1982) Cells that are O4 antigen positive and O1-antigen negative differentiate into O1 antigen-positive oligodendrocytes. *Neurosci. Lett.* **29**, 183–188.

Sontheimer, H. (1994) Voltage-dependent ion channels in glial cells. *Glia* **11**, 156–172.

Sontheimer, H., Waxman, S.G. (1993) Expression of voltage-activated ion channels by astrocytes and oligodendrocytes in the hippocampal slice. *J. Neurophysiol.* **70**, 1863–1873.

Sontheimer, H., Trotter, J., Schachner, M., Kettenmann, H. (1989) Channel expression correlates with differentiation stage during the development of oligodendrocytes from their precursor cells in culture. *Neuron* **2**, 1135–1145.

Soong, T.W., Stea, A., Hodson, C.D. *et al.* (1993) Structure and functional expression of a new member of the low-voltage activated calcium channel family. *Science* **260**, 1133–1136.

Sorrentino, V., Volpe, P. (1993) Ryanodine receptors: how many, why and where? *Trends Pharmacol. Sci.* **14**, 98–103.

Spedding, M., Kenny, B. (1992) Voltage-dependent calcium channels: structure and drug-binding sites. *Biochem. Soc. Trans.* **20**, 147–153.

Spence, K.T., Plata-Salaman, C.R., ffrench-Mullen, J.M.H. (1991) The neurosteroids pregnenolone and pregnenolone-sulfate but not progesterone, block Ca^{++} currents in acutely isolated hippocampal CA1 neurons. *Life Sci.* **49**, PL-235–PL-239.

Stanley, E.F. (1991) Single calcium channels on a cholinergic presynaptic nerve terminal. *Neuron* **7**, 585–591.

Stanley, E.F., Atrakchi, A.H. (1990) Calcium currents recorded from a vertebrate presynaptic nerve terminal are resistant to the dihydropyridine nifedipine. *Proc. Natl Acad. Sci. USA* **87**, 9683–9687.

Stanley, E.F, Goping, G. (1991) Characterization of a calcium current in a vertebrate cholinergic presynaptic nerve terminal. *J. Neurosci.* **11**, 985–993.

Starr, T.V.B., Prystay, W., Snutch, T.P. (1991) Primary structure of a calcium channel that is highly expressed in the rat cerebellum. *Proc. Natl Acad. Sci. USA* **88**, 5621–5625.

Stauderman, K.A., Murawsky, M.M. (1991) The inositol 1,4,5-trisphosphate-binding agonist histamine activates a ryanodine-sensitive Ca^{++} release mechanism in bovine adrenal chromaffin cells. *J. Biol. Chem.* **266**, 19150–19153.

Stauderman, K.A., McKinney, A., Murawski, M.M. (1991) The role of caffeine-sensitive Ca^{2+} stores in agonist- and inositol 1,4,5-trisphosphate induced Ca^{2+} release from bovine adrenal chromaffin cells. *Biophys. J.* **278**, 643–650.

Stefani, A., Pisani, A., Mercuri, N.B., Bernardi, G., Calabresi, P. (1994a) Activation of metabotropic glutamate receptors inhibits calcium currents and GABA-mediated synaptic potentials in striatal neurons. *J. Neurosci.* **14**, 6734–6743.

Stefani, A., Surmeier, D.J., Bernardi, G. (1994b) Opioids decrease high-voltage activated calcium currents in acutely dissociated neostriatal neurons. *Brain Res.* **642**, 339–343.

Stein, P.G., Palade, P.T. (1988) Sarcoballs: direct access to sarcoplasmic reticulum Ca^{2+} channels in skinned frog skeletal muscle fibers. *Biophys. J.* **54**, 357–363.

Sternweis, P., Smrcka, A.V. (1992) G-protein regulation of phospholipase C. *Trends Biochem. Sci.* **17**, 502–506.

Storozhuk, M.V., Kostyuk, P.G., Kononenko, N.I. (1993) Patch-clamp recordings of cAMP-induced membrane current noise in *Helix pomatia* neurons. *Neurosci. Lett.* **154**, 203–205.

Strathmann, M., Simon, M.I. (1990) G-protein diversity: a distinct class of α subunits is present in vertebrates and invertebrates. *Proc. Natl Acad. Sci. USA* **87**, 9113–9117.

Strupish, J., Wojcikiewicz, R.J.H., Challis, R.A.J. *et al.* (1991) Is decavanadate a specific inositol 1,4,5-trisphosphate antagonist?. *Biochem. J.* **277**, 294.

Stuenkel, E.L. (1994) Regulation of intracellular calcium and calcium buffering properties of rat isolated neurohypophyseal nerve endings. *J. Physiol. (Lond.)* **481**, 251–271.

Stühmer, W. (1994) *Xenopus* oocytes as reporters for calcium influx. *J. Neurochem.* **63** (Suppl.1), S24.

Suarez-Isla, B.A., Alcayaga, C., Marengo, J.J., Bull, R. (1991) Activation of inositol trisphosphate-sensitive Ca^{++} channels of sarcoplasmic reticulum from frog skeletal muscle. *J. Physiol. (Lond.)* **441**, 575–591.

Sudhof, T.C., Jahn, R. (1991) Proteins of synaptic vesicles involved in exocytosis and membrane recycling. *Neuron* **7**, 665–677.

Sudhof, T.C., Newton, C.L., Archer, B.T., Ushkaryov, Y.A., Mignery, G.A. (1991) Structure of a novel InsP$_3$ receptor. *EMBO J.* **10**, 3199–3206.

Sudlow L.C., Huang. R.-C., Green, D.J., Gilette, R. (1993) cAMP-activated Na$^+$ current in molluscan neurones is resistant to kinase inhibitors and is gated by cAMP in the isolated patch. *J. Neurosci.* **13**, 5188–5193.

Supattapone, S., Worley, P.F., Baraban, J.M., Snyder, S.H. (1988) Solubilization, purification, and characterization of an inositol trisphosphate receptor. *J. Biol. Chem.* **263**, 1530–1534.

Supattapone, S., Simpson, A.W.M., Ashley, C.C. (1989) Free calcium rise and mitogenesis in glial cells caused by endothelin. *Biochem. Biophys. Res. Commun.* **165**, 1115–1122.

Surmeier, D.J., Seno, N., Kitai, S.T. (1994) Acutely isolated neurons of the rat globus pallidus exhibit four types of high-voltage-activated Ca^{2+} current. *J. Neurophysiol.* **71**, 1272–1280.

Swann, K. (1991) Thimerosal causes calcium oscillations and sensitizes calcium-induced calcium release in unfertilized hamster eggs. *FEBS Lett.* **278**, 175–178.

Swartz, K.J. (1993) Modulation of Ca^{2+} channels by protein kinase C in rat central and peripheral neurons: disruption of G protein-mediated inhibition. *Neuron* **11**, 305–320.

Swartz, K.J., Bean, B.P. (1992) Inhibition of calcium channels in rat CA3 pyramidal neurons by a metabotropic glutamate receptor. *J. Neurosci.* **12**, 4358–4371.

Swartz, K.J., Merritt, A., Bean, B.P., Lovinger, D.M. (1993) Protein kinase C modulates glutamate receptor inhibition of Ca^{++} channels and synaptic transmission. *Nature* **361**, 165–168.

Sykova, E. (1992) *Ionic and Volume Changes in the Microenvironment of Nerve and Receptor Cells.* Springer-Verlag, Berlin.

Tachibana, T., Okada, T., Arimura, T., Kobayashi, K., Piccolino, M. (1993) Dihydropyridine-sensitive calcium current mediates neurotransmitter release from bipolar cells of the goldfish retina. *J. Neurosci.* **13**, 2898–2909.

Taglialatela, M., Di Renzo, G., Annunziato, L. (1990) Na^{2+}–Ca^{2+} exchange activity in central nerve endings. I. Ionic conditions that discriminate ^{45}Ca^{2+} uptake through the exchanger from that occurring through voltage-operated Ca^{2+} channels. *Mol. Pharmacol.* **38**, 385–392.

Takahashi, K., Akaike, N. (1991) Calcium antagonist effects on low-threshold (T-type) calcium current in rat isolated hippocampal CA1 pyramidal neurons. *J. Pharmacol. Exp. Ther.* **256**, 169–175.

Takahashi, K, Ueno, S, Akaike, N. (1991) Kinetic properties of T-type Ca currents in isolated rat hippocampal CA1 pyramidal neurons. *J. Neurophysiol.* **65**, 148–155.

Takahashi, M., Tanzawa, K., Takahashi, S. (1993) Adenophostins, newly discovered metabolites of *Penicillium brevicompactum*, act as a potent agonists of the inositol 1,4,5-trisphosphate receptor. *J. Biol. Chem.* **269**, 369–372.

Takei, K., Stukenbrok, H., Metcalf, A. *et al.* (1992) Ca^{2+} stores in Purkinje neurons: endoplasmic reticulum subcompartments demonstrated by the heterogeneous distribution of the InsP$_3$ receptor, Ca$^{(2+)}$-ATPase, and calsequestrin. *J. Neurosci.* **12**, 489–505.

Takenoshita, M., Steinbach, J.H. (1991) Halothane blocks low-voltage-activated calcium currents in rat sensory neurons. *J. Neurosci.* **11**, 1404–1412.

Takesawa, S., Nata, K., Yonekura, H., Okamoto, H. (1993) Cyclic ADP-ribose in insulin secretion from pancreatic β cells. *Science* **259**, 370–373.

Takeshima, H., Nishimura, S., Matsumoto, T. *et al.* (1989) Primary structure and expression from complementary DNA of skeletal muscle ryanodine receptor. *Nature* **339**, 439–445.

Takeshima, H., Nishimura, S., Nishi, M., Ikeda, M., Sugimoto, T. (1993) A brain-specific transcript from the 3--terminal region of the skeletal muscle ryanodine receptor gene. *FEBS Lett.* **322**, 105–110.

Tallant, E.A., Jaiswal, N., Diz, D.I., Ferrario, C.M. (1991) Human astrocytes contain two distinct angiotensin receptor subtypes. *Hypertension* **18**, 32–39.

Tanabe, T., Takeshima, H., Mikami, A.(1987) Primary structure of the receptor for calcium channel blockers from skeletal muscle. *Nature* **328**, 313–318.

Tanabe, T., Mikami, A., Niidome, T., Numa S. (1993) Structure and function of voltage-dependent calcium channels from muscle. *Ann. NY Acad. Sci.* **707**, 81–86.

Tanabe, Y., Nomura, A., Masu, M., Shigemoto, R., Mizino, M., Nakanishi, S. (1993) Signal transduction, pharmacological properties, and expression patterns of two rat metabotropic glutamate receptors, mGluR3 and mGluR4. *J. Neurosci.* **13**, 1372–1378.

Tanaka, Y., Tashjian, H., Jr. (1994) Timerosal potentiates Ca^{2+} release mediated by both the inositol 1,4,5-trisphosphate and the ryanodine receptors in sea urchin eggs. *J. Biol. Chem.* **269**, 11247–11253.

Tarasenko, A.N., Loboda, A.P., Kostyuk, P.G. (1995) Developmental changes of voltage-operated Ca channels in rat visual cortical neurons. *Neurophysiology (Kiev)*, in press.

Tas, P.W.L., Koshel, K. (1990) Thrombin reverts the β-adrenergic agonist-induced morphological response in rat glioma C_6 cells. *Exp. Cell. Res.* **189**, 22–27.

Tas, P.W.L., Kress, H.G., Koschel, K. (1988) Presence of a charybdotoxin sensitive Ca^{2+}-activated K^+ channel in rat glioma C_6 cells. *Neurosci. Lett.* **94**, 279–284.

Tatebayashi, H., Ogata, N. (1992) Kinetic analysis of the $GABA_B$-mediated inhibition of the high-threshold Ca^{2+}-current in cultured rat sensory neurones. *J. Physiol. (Lond.)* **447**, 391–407.

Tatsumi, H., Katayama, Y. (1993) Regulation of the intracellular free calcium concentration in acutely dissociated neurones from rat nucleus basalis. *J. Physiol. (Lond.)* **464**, 165–181.

Taylor, C.W. (1992) Kinetics of inositol 1,4,5-trisphosphate stimulated Ca^{2+} mobilization. In: *Inositol Phosphates and Calcium Signalling*, ed. by Putney, J.W. Raven Press, New York, pp. 109–142.

Taylor, C.W., Potter, B.V.L. (1990) The size of inositol 1,4,5-trisphisphate-sensitive Ca^{2+} stores depends on inositol 1,4,5-trisphosphate concentration. *Biochem. J.* **266**, 189–194.

Tepikin, A.V., Kostyuk, P.G., Snitsarev, V.A., Belan, P.V. (1991) Extrusion of calcium from a single neuron of the snail *Helix pomatia*. *J. Membrane Biol.* **123**, 43–47.

Tepikin, A.V., Voronina, S.G., Gallacher, D.V., Petersen, O.H. (1992) Pulsatile Ca^{2+} extrusion from single pancreatic acinar cells during receptor-activated cytosolic Ca^{2+} spiking. *J. Biol. Chem.* **267**, 14073–14076.

Tepikin, A.V., Llopis, J., Snitsarev, V.A., Gallacher, D.V., Petersen, O.H. (1994) The droplet technique: measurement of calcium extrusion from single isolated mammalian cells. *Pflugers Arch.* **428**, 664–670.

Teramoto, T., Kuwada, M., Niidome, T. *et al.* (1993) A novel peptide from funnel web spider venom, ω-Aga-TK, selectively blocks P-type calcium channels. *Biochem. Biophys. Res. Commun.* **196**, 134–140.

Teraoka, H., Nakazato, Y., Ohga, A. (1991) Ryanodine inhibits caffeine-evoked Ca^{2+} mobilization and catecholamine secretion from cultured bovine adrenal chromaffin cells. *J. Neurochem.* **57**, 1884–1890.

Thastrup, O., Cullen, P.J., Drobak, B.K., Hanley, M.R., Dawson, A.P. (1990) Thapsigargin, a tumor promotor, discharges intracellular Ca^{2+} stores by specific inhibition of the endoplasmic reticulum Ca^{2+} ATPase. *Proc. Natl Acad. Sci. USA* **87**, 2466–2470.

Thayer, S.A., Miller, R.J. (1990) Regulation of the intracellular free calcium concentration in single rat dorsal root ganglion neurones in vitro. *J. Physiol. (Lond.)* **425**, 85–115.

Thayer, S.A., Perney, T.M., Miller, R.J. (1987) Regulation of calcium homeostasis in sensory neurones by bradykinin. *J. Neurosci.* **8**, 4089–4097.

Thayer, S.A., Hirning, L.D., Miller, R.J. (1988) The role of caffeine-sensitive calcium stores in the regulation of the intracellular free calcium concentration in rat sympathetic neurons in vitro. *Mol. Pharmacol.* **34**, 664–673.

Thompson, S.M., Wong, R.K.S. (1991) Development of calcium current subtypes in isolated rat hippocampal pyramidal cells. *J. Physiol. (Lond.)* **439**, 671–689.

Thorn, P., Petersen, O.H. (1991) Activation of voltage-sensitive Ca currents by vasopressin in an insulin-secreting cell line. *J. Membrane Biol.* **124**, 63–71.

Thorn, T., Gerasimenko, O., Petersen, O.H. (1994) Cyclic ADP-ribose regulation of adenosine receptors involved in agonist evoked cytosolic Ca^{2+} oscillations in pancreatic acinar cells. *EMBO J.* **13**, 2038–2043.

Toescu, E.C., O'Neill, S.C., Petersen, O.H., Eisner, D.A. (1992) Caffeine inhibits the agonist-evoked cytoplasmic Ca^{++} signal in mouse pancreatic acinar cells by blocking inositol trisphosphate production. *J. Biol. Chem.* **267**, 23467–23470.

Toselli, M., Taglietti, V. (1990) Pharmacological characterization of voltage-dependent calcium currents in rat hippocampal neurons. *Neurosci. Lett.* **112**, 70–75.

Toselli, M., Taglietelli, V. (1993) Baclofen inhibits high-threshold calcium currents with two distinct modes in rat hippocampal neurons. *Neurosci. Lett.* **164**, 134–136.

Toyoshima, C., Sasabe, H., Stokes, D.L.S. (1993) Three-dimensional cryo-electron microscopy of the calcium ion pump in the sarcoplasmic reticulum membrane. *Nature* **362**, 469–371.

Trejo, J., Brown, J.H. (1991) c-fos and c-jun are induced by muscarinic receptor activation of protein kinase C but are differentially regulated by intracellular calcium. *J. Biol. Chem.* **266**, 7876–7882.

Trombley, P.Q., (1992) Norepinephrine inhibits calcium currents and EPSPs via a G-protein-coupled mechanism in olfactory bulb neurons. *J. Neurosci.* **12**, 3992–3998.

Trouslard, J., Marsh, S.J., Brown, D.A. (1993) Calcium entry through nicotinic receptor channels and calcium channels in cultured rat superior cervical ganglion cells. *J. Physiol. (Lond.)* **468**, 53–71.

Trudeau, L.-E., Baux, G., Fossier, P., Tauc, L. (1993) Transmitter release and calcium currents at an *Aplysia* buccal ganglion synapse. I. Characterization. *Neuroscience* **53**, 571–580.

Tsai, T.D., Barish, M.E. (1991) Ryanodine sensitivity of caffeine-induced intracellular calcium release in cultured embryonic mouse cortical neurones. *Biophys. J.* **59**, 599a.

Turner, T.J., Adams, M.E., Dunlap, K. (1992) Calcium channels coupled to glutamate release identified by ω-Aga-IVA. *Science* **258**, 310–313.

Tymianski, M., Charlton, M.P., Carlen, P.L., Tator, C.H. (1993) Source specificity of early calcium neurotoxicity in cultured embryonic spinal cord. *J. Neurosci.* **13**, 2085–2104.

Tytgat, J., Nilius, B., Carmeliet, E. (1990) Modulation of the T-type cardiac Ca channel by changes in proton concentration. *J. Gen. Physiol.* **96**, 973–990.

Tytgat, J., Pauwels, P.J., Verecke, J., Carmeliet, E. (1991) Flunarizine inhibits a high-threshold inactivating calcium channel (N-type) in isolated hippocampal neurons. *Brain Res.* **549**, 112–117.

Uchitel, O.D., Protti, D.A., Sanchez, V. *et al.* (1992) P-type voltage-dependent calcium channel mediates presynaptic calcium influx and transmitter release in mammalian synapses. *Proc. Natl Acad. Sci. USA* **89**, 3330–3333.

Ueno, S., Harata, N., Inoue, K., Akaike, N. (1992) ATP-gated current in dissociated rat nucleus solitarii neurones. *J. Neurophysiol.* **68**, 778–785.

Usachev, Y., Verkhratsky, A. (1995) IBMX induces calcium release from intracellular stores in rat sensory neurones. *Cell Calcium* **17**, 197–206.

Usachev, Y., Shmigol, A., Pronchuk, N., Kostyuk, P., Verkhrtasky, A. (1993) Caffeine-induced calcium release from internal stores in rat sensory neurones. *Neuroscience* **57**, 845–859.

Usowicz, M.M., Porzig, H., Becker, C., Reuter, H. (1990) Differential expression by nerve growth factor of two types of Ca channels in rat pheochromocytoma cell lines. *J. Physiol. (Lond.)* **46**, 95–116.

Usowicz, M.M., Sugimori, M., Cherskey, B., Llinas, R. (1992) P-type calcium channels in the somata and dendrites of adult cerebellar Purkinje cells. *Neuron* **9**, 1185–1199.

Utzschneider, D.A., Rand, M.N., Waxman, S.G., Kocsis, J.D. (1994) Nuclear and cytoplasmic Ca^{2+} signals in development of rat dorsal root ganglion neurones studied in excised tissue. *Brain Res.* **635**, 231–237.

Vacher, P., McKenzie, J., Duffy, B. (1989) Arachidonic acid affects membrane ionic conductances of GH_3 pituitary cells. *Am. J. Physiol.* **257**, E203–E211.

Valdivia, H.H., Fuentes, O., El-Hayek, R., Morrissette, J., Coronado, R. (1991) Activation of the ryanodine receptor Ca^{2+} release channel of sarcoplasmic reticulum by a novel scorpion venom. *J. Biol. Chem.* **266**, 19135–19138.

Valdivia, H.H., Kirby, M.S., Lederer, W.J., Coronado, R. (1992) Scorpion toxins targeted against the sarcoplasmic reticulum Ca^{++}-release channel of skeletal and cardiac muscle. *Proc. Natl Acad. Sci. USA* **89**, 12185–12189.

Valentijn, J.A., Vaudry, H., Cazin, L. (1993) Multiple control of calcium channel gating by dopamine D_2 receptors in frog pituitary melanotrophs. *Ann. NY Acad. Sci.* **680**, 211–228.

Valera, S., Hussy, N., Evans, R.J. *et al.* (1994) A new class of ligand-dated ion channels defined by P_{2x} receptor for extracellular ATP. *Nature* **371**, 516–519.

Van den Pol, A.N., Finkbeiner, S.M., Cornell-Bell, A.H. (1992) Calcium excitability and oscillations in suprachiasmatic nucleus neurones and glia *in vitro. J. Neurosci.* **12**, 2648–2664.

Vercesi, A.E., Moreno, S.N., Bernardes, C.F. *et al.* (1993) Thapsigargin causes Ca^{2+} release and collapse of the membrane potential of *Trypanosoma brucei* mitochondria in situ and of isolated rat liver mitochondria. *J. Biol. Chem.* **268**, 8564–8568.

Verdoorn, T.A., Draguhn, A., Ymer, S., Seeburg, P.H., Sakmann, B. (1990) Functional properties of recombinant rat $GABA_A$ receptors depend upon subunit composition. *Neuron* **4**, 919–928.

Verhage, M., McMahon, H.T., Ghijsen, W.E.J.M. *et al.* (1991) Differential release of amino acids, neuropeptides and catecholamines from nerve terminals. *Neuron* **6**, 517–524.

Verhage, M., Ghijsen, W.E., Lopes da Silva, F.H. (1994) Presynaptic plasticity: the regulation of Ca^{++}-dependent transmitter release. *Prog. Neurobiol.* **42**, 539–574.

Verkhratsky, A.N., Trotter, J., Kettenmann, H. (1990) Cultured glial precursor cells from mouse cortex express two types of calcium currents. *Neurosci. Lett.* **112**, 194–198.

Verkhratsky, A., Shmigol., A., Kirischuk, S., Pronchuk, N., Kostyuk, P. (1994) Age-dependent changes in calcium currents and calcium homeostasis in mammalian neurons. *Ann. NY Acad. Sci.* **747**, 365–381.

Vernino, S., Amador, M., Luetje, C.W., Patrick, J., Dani, J.A. (1992) Calcium modulation and high calcium permeability of neuronal nicotinic acetylcholine receptors. *Neuron* **8**, 127–134.

Vernino, S., Rogers, M., Radcliffe, K.A., Dani, J.A. (1994) Quantitative measurement of calcium flux through muscle and neuronal nicotinic acetylcholine receptors. *J. Neurosci.* **14**, 5514–5524.

Veselovsky, N.S., Fedulova, S.A. (1983) Two types of calcium channels in the somatic membrane of rat dorsal ganglion neurons. *Doklady AN SSSR* **268**, 747–750.

Vidnyanszky, Z., Hamori, J., Neguessy, L. *et al.* (1995) Cellular and subcellular localization of the mGluR5a metabotropic glutamate receptor in rat spinal cord. *NeuroReport* **6**, 209–213.

Villa, A., Podini, P., Clegg, D.O., Pozzan, T., Meldolesi, J. (1991) Intracellular Ca^{2+} stores in chicken Purkinje neurones: differential distribution of the low-affinity high capacity Ca^{2+}-binding protein calsequestrin, of Ca^{2+}-ATPase and of the ER luminal protein Bip. *J. Cell Biol.* **113**, 779–791.

Villa, A., Sharp, A.H., Racchetti, G. *et al.* (1992) The endoplasmic reticulum of Purkinje neuron body and dendrites: molecular identity and specializations for Ca^{2+} transport. *Neuroscience* **49**, 467–477.

Villa, A., Podidni, P., Panzeri, M.C., Racchetti, G., Meldolesi, J. (1994) Cytosolic Ca^{2+} binding proteins during rat brain ageing: loss of calbindin and calretinin in the hippocampus, with no changes in the cerebellum, *Eur. J. Neurosci.* **6**, 1491–1499.

Villegas, J. (1972) Axon–Schwann cell interaction in the squid nerve fibre. *J. Physiol. (Lond.)* **225**, 275–296.

Villegas, J. (1973) Effects of tubocuraine and eserine on the axon–Schwann cell relationship in the squid nerve fibre. *J. Physiol. (Lond.)* **232**, 193–208.

Villegas, J. (1978) Cholinergic systems in axon–Schwann cell interactions. *Trends Neurosci.* **1**, 66–68.

Vitorica, J., Satrustegui, J. (1986) Involvement of mitochondria in the age-dependent decrease in calcium uptake in rat brain synaptosomes. *Brain Res.* **378**, 36–48.

Vlassara, H., Bucala, L., Striker, L. (1994) Biology of disease. Pathogenic effects of advanced glycosylation: biochemical, biologic, and clinical implications for diabetes and aging. *Lab. Invest.* **70**, 138–151.

Volpe, P., Krause, K.H., Hashimoto, S. *et al.* (1988) 'Calciosome' a cytoplasmic organelle: the inositol 1,4,5-trisphosphate-sensitive Ca^{2+} store of nonmuscle cells? *Proc. Natl Acad. Sci. USA* **85**, 1091–1095.

Volpe, P., Palade, P., Costello, B., Mitchell, R.D., Fleisher, S. (1993) Spontaneous calcium release from sarcoplasmic reticulum: effect of local anesthetics. *J. Biol. Chem.* **258**, 12434–12442.

Voronin, L.L. (1993) On the quantal analysis of hippocampal long-term potentiation and related phenomena of synaptic plasticity. *Neuroscience* **56**, 275–304.

Walker, M.W., Ewald, D.A., Perney, T.M., Miller, R.J. (1988) Neuropeptide Y modulates neurotransmitter release and Ca^{++} currents in rat sensory neurons. *J. Neurosci.* **8**, 2438–2446.

Wall, M.J., Dale, N. (1994) $GABA_B$ receptors modulate an ω-conotoxin-sensitive calcium current that is required for synaptic transmission in the *Xenopus* embryo spinal cord. *J. Neurosci.* **14**, 6248–6255.

Walseth, T.F., Aarhus, R., Zeleznikar, R.J., Jr, Lee, H.C. (1991) Determination of endogenous levels of cyclic ADP-ribose in rat tissues. *Biochim. Biophys. Acta* **1094**, 113–120.

Walton, P.D., Airey, J.A., Sutko, J.L. *et al.* (1991) Ryanodine and inositol trisphosphate receptors coexist in avian cerebellar Purkinje neurones. *J. Cell. Biol.* **113**, 1145–1157.

Walz, W., MacVicar, B. (1988) Electrophysiological properties of glial cells: comparison of brain slices with primary cultures. *Brain Res.* **443**, 321–324.

Walz, W., Ilschner, S., Ohlemeyer, C., Banati, R., Kettenmann, H. (1993) Extracellular ATP activates a cation conductance and a K^+ conductance in cultured microglial cells from mouse brain. *J. Neurosci.* **13**, 4403–4411.

Walz, W., Gimpl, G., Ohlemeyer, C., Kettenmann, H. (1994) Extracellular ATP induced currents in astrocytes: involvement of a cation channel. *J. Neurosci. Res.* **38**, 12–18.

Wand, H.-L., Reisine, T, Dichter, M. (1990) Somatostatin-14 and somatostatin-28 inhibit calcium currents in rat neocortical neurons. *Neuroscience* **38**, 335–342.

Wang, R., Karpinski, E., Wu, L.Y., Pang, P.K.T. (1990) Flunarizine selectively blocks transient calcium channel currents in N1E-115 cells. *J. Pharmacol. Exp. Ther.* **254**, 1006–1011.

Wang, R., Pang, P.K.T., Wu, L. *et al.* (1994) Enhanced calcium influx by parathyroid hormone in identified *Helisoma trivolvis* snail neurons. *Cell Calcium* **15**, 89–98.

Wang, X., Treistman, S.N., Lemos, J.R. (1992) Two types of high-threshold calcium currents inhibited by ω-conotoxin in nerve terminals of rat neurohypophysis. *J. Physiol. (Lond.)* **445**, 181–199.

Wang, X., Treistman, S.N., Lemos, J.R. (1993a) Single channel recordings of N_t-and L-type Ca^{2+} currents in rat neurohypophyseal terminals. *J. Neurophysiol.* **70**, 1617–1628.

Wang, X., Treistman, S.N., Wilson, A., Nordmann, J.J., Lemos, J.R. (1993b) Ca^{2+} channels and peptide release from neurosecretory terminals. *News Physiol. Sci.* **8**, 64–66.

Wang, X., Wang, G., Lemos, J.R., Treistman, S.N. (1994) Ethanol directly modulates gating of a dihydropyridine-sensitive Ca^{2+} channel in neurohypophyseal terminals. *J. Neurosci.* **14**, 5453–5460.

Wang, X.-L., Rinzel, J., Rogawski, M.A. (1991) A model of the T-type calcium current and the low-threshold spike in thalamic neurons. *J. Neurophysiol.* **66**, 839–850.

Webb, T.E., Simon, J., Krishek, B.J. *et al.* (1993) Cloning and functional expression of a brain G-protein coupled ATP receptor. *FEBS Lett.* **324**, 219–225.

Werlen, G., Belin, D., Conne, B. *et al.* (1993) Intracellular Ca^{2+} and the regulation of early response gene expression in HL-60 myeloid leukemia cells. *J. Biol. Chem.* **268**, 16596–16601.

Werz, M.A., Elmslie, K.S., Jones, S.W. (1993) Phosphorylation enhances inactivation of N-type calcium channel current in bullfrog sympathetic neurons. *Pflugers Arch.* **424**, 538–545.

Westbrook, G.L., Mayer, M.L. (1987) Micromolar concentrations of Zn^{2+} antagonize NMDA and GABA responses of hippocampal neurons. *Nature* **328**, 640–643.

Westenbroek, R.E., Ahlijanian, M.K., Catterall, W.A. (1990) Clustering of L-type Ca channels at the base of major dendrites in hippocampal pyramidal neurons. *Nature* **347**, 281–284.

Wheeler, D.B., Randall, A., Tsien, R.W. (1994) Roles of N-type and Q-type Ca^{2+} channels in supporting hippocampal synaptic transmission. *Science* **264**, 107–111.

White, A., Watson, S.P., Galione, A. (1993) cADP-ribose-induced calcium release from brain microsomes. *FEBS Lett.* **318**, 21–24.

White, G., Lovinger, D.M., Weight, F.F. (1989) Transient low-threshold Ca current triggers burst firing through an afterdepolarizing potential in an adult mammalian neuron. *Proc. Natl Acad. Sci. USA* **86**, 6802–6806.

Whitham, E.M., Challiss, R.A., Nahorski, S.R. (1991) M_3 muscarinic cholinoreceptors are linked to phosphoinositide metabolism in rat cerebellar granule cells. *Eur. J. Pharmacol.* **206**, 181–189.

Wicher, D., Penzlin, H. (1994) Ca^{2+} currents in cockroach neurones: properties and modulation by neurohormone D. *NeuroReport* **5**, 1023–1026.

Wier, W.G. (1990) Cytoplasmic $[Ca^{2+}]$ in mammalian ventricle: dynamic control by cellular processes. *Annu. Rev. Physiol.* **52**, 467–485.

Wiley, J.W., Gross, R.A., Lu, Y., Macdonald, R.L. (1990) Neuropeptide Y reduces calcium current and inhibits acetylcholine release in nodose neurons via a pertussis toxin-sensitive mechanism. *J. Neurophysiol.* **63**, 1499–1507.

Wiley, J.W., Gross, R.A., Macdonald, R.L. (1993) Agonists for neuropeptide Y receptor subtypes NPY-1 and NPY-2 have opposite actions on rat nodose neuron calcium currents. *J. Neurophysiol.* **70**, 324–330.

Wilk-Blaszczak M.A., Gutowski S., Sterwein P.C., Belardetti F. (1994) Bradykinin modulates potassium and calcium currents in neuroblastoma hybrid cells via different pertussis toxin-insensitive pathways. *Neuron* **12**, 109–116.

Williams, M.E., Feldman, D.H., McCue, A.F. *et al.* (1992a) Structure and functional expression of an omega-conotoxin-sensitive human N-type calcium channel. *Science* **257**, 389–395.

Williams, M.E., Feldman, M.E., McCue, A.F. *et al.* (1992b) Structure and functional expression of α_1, α_2 and β subunits of a novel human neuronal calcium channels subtype. *Neuron* **8**, 71–84.

Williams, M.E., Marubio, L.M., Deal, C.R. *et al.* (1994) Structure and functional characterization of neural α_{1E} calcium channel subtypes. *J. Biol. Chem.* **269**, 22347–22357.

Williams, P.J., MacVicar, B.A., Pittman, Q.J. (1990) Synaptic modulation by dopamine of calcium currents in rat pars intermedia. *J. Neuroscience* **10**, 757–763.

Williams, P.J., Pittman, Q.J., MacVicar, B.A. (1991) Ca- and voltage-dependent inactivation of Ca current in rat intermediate pituitary. *Brain Res.* **564**, 12–18.

Wisden, W., Seeburg, P.H. (1993) Mammalian ionotropic glutamate receptors. *Curr. Opinion Neurobiol.* **3**, 291–298.

Witcher, D.R., Kovacs, R.J., Schulman, H., Cefali, D.C., Jones, L.R. (1991) Unique phosphorylation site on the cardiac ryanodine receptor regulates calcium channel activity. *J. Biol. Chem.* **266**, 11144–11152.

Witcher, D.R., De Waard, M., Campbell, K.P. (1993) Characterization of the purified N-type Ca^{2+} channel and the cation sensitivity of ω-conotoxin GVIA binding. *Neuropharmacology* **32**, 1127–1139.

Wood, A., Wing, M.G., Benham, C.D., Compston, D.A.S. (1993) Specific induction of intracellular calcium oscillations by complement membrane attack on oligodendroglia. *J. Neurosci.* **13**, 3319–3332.

Worley, P.F., Baraban, J.M., Supattapone, S., Wilson, V.S., Snyder, S.H. (1987) Characterization of inositol trisphosphate receptor binding in brain. Regulation by pH and calcium. *J. Biol. Chem.* **262**, 12132–12136.

Wu, L., Karpinski, E., Wang, R., Pang, P.K.T. (1992) Modification by solvents of the action of nifedipine on calcium channel currents in neuroblastoma cells. *Naunyn Schmiedebergs Arch. Pharmacol.* **345**, 478–484.

Wyllie, D.J.A., Mathie, A., Symonds, C.L., Cull-Candy, S.G. (1991) Activation of glutamate receptors and glutamate uptake in identified macroglial cells in rat cerebellar cultures. *J. Physiol. (Lond.)* **432**, 235–259.

Xu, X., Best, P.M. (1992) Postnatal changes in L-type calcium current density in rat atrial myocytes. *J. Physiol. (Lond.)* **454**, 657–672.

Yakel, J.L. (1992) Inactivation of the Ba^{2+} current in dissociated *Helix* neurons: voltage dependence and the role of phosphorylation. *Pflugers Arch.* **420**, 470–478.

Yamada, W.M., Zucker, R.S. (1992) Time course of transmitter release calculated from simulations of a calcium diffusion model. *Biophys. J.* **61**, 671–682.

Yanai, K., Maeyama, K., Nakahata, N., Nakahishi, H., Watanabe, T. (1992) Calcium mobilization and its desensitization induced by endothelins and safrotoxin in human astrocytoma cells (1321N1): comparison of histamine-induced calcium mobilization. *Naunyn Schmiedebergs Arch. Pharmacol.* **346**, 51–56.

Yatani, A., Brown, A.M. (1989) Rapid β-adrenergic modulation of cardiac calcium channel currents by a fast G protein pathway. *Science* **245**, 71–74.

Yau, K.-W. (1994) Cyclic nucleotide-gated channels: an expanding new family of ion channels. *Proc. Natl Acad. Sci. USA* **91**, 3481–3483.

Yawo, H., Chuhma, N. (1993) Preferential inhibition of ω-conotoxin-sensitive presynaptic Ca^{2+} channels by adenosine autoreceptors. *Nature* **365**, 256–258.

Ye, J.H., Akaike, N. (1993) Calcium currents in pyramidal neurons acutely dissociated from the rat frontal cortex: a study by the nystatin perforated patch technique. *Brain Res.* **606**, 111–117.

Yoder, E., Lev-Ram, V., Ellisman, M.H. (1992) [Ca] transients in cultured Schwann cells evoked by activation of nicotinic AChRs. *Soc. Neurosci. Abstr.* **18**, 626.1.

Yoshii, M., Watanabe, S. (1994) Enhancement of neuronal calcium channel current by the nootropic agent, nefiracetam (DM-9384), in NG108-15 cells. *Brain Res.* **642**, 123–131.

Yuste, R., Katz, L.C. (1991) Control of postsynaptic Ca^{2+} influx in developing neurocortex by excitatory and inhibitory neurotransmitters. *Neuron* **6**, 333–344.

Zacchetti, D., Clementi, E., Fasolato, C. *et al.* (1991) Intracellular Ca^{2+} pools in PC12 cells: a unique, rapidly exchanging pool is sensitive to both inositol 1,4,5-trisphosphate and caffeine–ryanodine. *J. Biol. Chem.* **266**, 20152–20158.

Zeilhofer, H.U., Muller, T.H., Swandulla, D. (1993) Inhibition of high voltage-activated calcium currents by l-glutamate receptor-mediated calcium influx. *Neuron* **10**, 879–887.

Zhang, J.-F., Ellinor, P.T., Randall, A.D. *et al.* (1993) Functional expression of a novel neuronal voltage-dependent calcium channel, Doe-1. In: *23rd Annual Meeting of the Society for Neuroscience, Washington*, Vol. 19, part I, p.11.

Zhao, X.-I., Gutierrez, L.M., Chang, C.F., Hosey, M.M. (1994) The α_1-subunit of skeletal muscle L-type Ca channel is the key target for regulation by A-kinase and phosphatase IC. *Biochem. Biophys. Res. Commun.* **198**, 166–173.

Zhou, Z., Neher, E. (1993a) Calcium permeability of nicotinic acetylcholine receptor channels in bovine adrenal chromaffin cells. *Pflugers Arch.* **425**, 511–517.

Zhou, Z., Neher, E. (1993b) Mobile and immobile calcium buffers in bovine adrenal chromaffin cells. *J. Physiol. (Lond.)* **469**, 245–273.

Zhu, P.C., Thureson-Klein, A., Klein, R.L. (1986) Exocytosis from large dense-core vesicles outside the active synaptic zones of terminals within the trigeminal subnucleus caudalis: a possible mechanism for neuropeptide release. *Neuroscience* **19**, 43–54.

Zhu, Y., Ikeda, S.R. (1993) Adenosine modulates voltage-gated Ca^{2+} channels in adult rat sympathetic neurons. *J. Neurophysiol.* **70**, 610–620.

Zirpel, L., Lachica, E.A., Rubel, E.W. (1995) Activation of a metabotropic glutamate receptor increases intracellular calcium concentrations in neurones of the avian cochlear nucleus. *J. Neurosci.* **15**, 214–222.

Zona, C., Avoli, M. (1990) Effects induced by the antiepileptic drug valproic acid upon the ionic currents recorded in rat neocortical neurons in cell culture. *Exp. Brain Res.* **81**, 313–317.

Zong, X., Lux, H.D. (1994) Augmentation of calcium channel currents in response to G protein activation by GTPγS in chick sensory neurons. *J. Neurosci.* **14**, 4847–4853.

Zorzato, F., Fujii, J., Otsu, K. *et al.* (1990) Molecular cloning of cDNA encoding human and rabbit forms of the Ca^{2+} release channel (ryanodine receptor) of skeletal muscle sarcoplasmic reticulum. *J. Biol. Chem.* **265**, 2244–2256.

Zucker, R.S. (1989) Short-term synaptic plasticity. *Annu. Rev. Neurosci.* **12**, 13–31.

Zucker, R.S. (1993) Calcium and transmitter release. *J. Physiol. (Paris)* **87**, 25–36.

Zufall, F., Firestein, S., Shepherd, G.M. (1991) Analysis of single cyclic nucleotide-gated channels in olfactory receptor cells. *J. Neurosci.* **11**, 3573.

Zweifach, A., Lewis, R.S. (1993) Mitogen-regulated Ca^{2+} current of T lymphocytes is activated by depletion of intracellular Ca^{2+} stores. *Proc. Natl Acad. Sci. USA* **90**, 6295–6299.

Index

Index compiled by Liza Weinkove